Complementary and Alternative Medicine and Kidney Health

Mayuree Tangkiatkumjai
Srinakharinwirot University, Thailand

Annalisa Casarin
The NIHR Research Design Service East of England, UK

Li-Chia Chen
University of Manchester, UK

Dawn-Marie Walker
University of Southampton, UK

A volume in the Advances in Medical Diagnosis, Treatment, and Care (AMDTC) Book Series

IGI Global
DISSEMINATOR OF KNOWLEDGE

Published in the United States of America by
IGI Global
Medical Information Science Reference (an imprint of IGI Global)
701 E. Chocolate Avenue
Hershey PA, USA 17033
Tel: 717-533-8845
Fax: 717-533-8661
E-mail: cust@igi-global.com
Web site: http://www.igi-global.com

Library of Congress Cataloging-in-Publication Data

Names: Tangkiatkumjai, Mayuree, 1976- editor. | Walker, Dawn-Marie, editor. | Chen, Li-Chia, editor. | Casarin, Annalisa, editor.
Title: Complementary and alternative medicine and kidney health / Mayuree Tangkiatkumjai, Annalisa Casarin, Li-Chia Chen, and Dawn-Marie Walker.
Description: Hershey, PA : Medical Information Science Reference, [2018] | Includes bibliographical references.
Identifiers: LCCN 2017011897| ISBN 9781522528821 (hardcover) | ISBN 9781522528838 (eBook)
Subjects: | MESH: Complementary Therapies--standards | Clinical Decision-Making | Kidney Diseases--therapy
Classification: LCC R733 | NLM WB 890 | DDC 615.5/3--dc23 LC record available at https://lccn.loc.gov/2017011897

This book is published in the IGI Global book series Advances in Medical Diagnosis, Treatment, and Care (AMDTC) (ISSN: 2475-6628; eISSN: 2475-6636)

British Cataloguing in Publication Data
A Cataloguing in Publication record for this book is available from the British Library.

All work contributed to this book is new, previously-unpublished material.
The views expressed in this book are those of the authors, but not necessarily of the publisher.

For electronic access to this publication, please contact: eresources@igi-global.com.

Advances in Medical Diagnosis, Treatment, and Care (AMDTC) Book Series

ISSN:2475-6628
EISSN:2475-6636

MISSION

Advancements in medicine have prolonged the life expectancy of individuals all over the world. Once life-threatening conditions have become significantly easier to treat and even cure in many cases. Continued research in the medical field will further improve the quality of life, longevity, and wellbeing of individuals.

The **Advances in Medical Diagnosis, Treatment, and Care (AMDTC)** book series seeks to highlight publications on innovative treatment methodologies, diagnosis tools and techniques, and best practices for patient care. Comprised of comprehensive resources aimed to assist professionals in the medical field apply the latest innovations in the identification and management of medical conditions as well as patient care and interaction, the books within the AMDTC series are relevant to the research and practical needs of medical practitioners, researchers, students, and hospital administrators.

COVERAGE

- Internal Medicine
- Critical Care
- Alternative Medicine
- Patient-Centered Care
- Experimental Medicine
- Disease Prevention
- Cancer Treatment
- Diagnostic Medicine
- Medical Testing
- Patient Interaction

IGI Global is currently accepting manuscripts for publication within this series. To submit a proposal for a volume in this series, please contact our Acquisition Editors at Acquisitions@igi-global.com or visit: http://www.igi-global.com/publish/.

The Advances in Medical Diagnosis, Treatment, and Care (AMDTC) Book Series (ISSN 2475-6628) is published by IGI Global, 701 E. Chocolate Avenue, Hershey, PA 17033-1240, USA, www.igi-global.com. This series is composed of titles available for purchase individually; each title is edited to be contextually exclusive from any other title within the series. For pricing and ordering information please visit http://www.igi-global.com/book-series/advances-medical-diagnosis-treatment-care/129618. Postmaster: Send all address changes to above address.

Titles in this Series

For a list of additional titles in this series, please visit:
https://www.igi-global.com/book-series/advances-medical-diagnosis-treatment-care/129618

Sustainable Health and Long-Term Care Solutions for an Aging Population
Ben Fong (The Hong Kong Polytechnic University, Hong Kong) Artie Ng (The Hong Kong Polytechnic University, Hong Kong) and Peter Yuen (The Hong Kong Polytechnic University, Hong Kong)
Medical Information Science Reference • ©2018 • 441pp • H/C (ISBN: 9781522526339) • US $225.00

Emerging Applications, Perspectives, and Discoveries in Cardiovascular Research
Ashim Malhotra (Pacific University, USA) and Shivani Soni (California State University, Fullerton, USA & Chapman University, USA & Alabama State University, USA)
Medical Information Science Reference • ©2017 • 439pp • H/C (ISBN: 9781522520924) • US $225.00

Healthcare Community Synergism between Patients, Practitioners, and Researchers
Valerie C. Bryan (Florida Atlantic University, USA) and Jennifer Lynne Bird (Florida Atlantic University, USA)
Medical Information Science Reference • ©2017 • 348pp • H/C (ISBN: 9781522506409) • US $210.00

Transformative Healthcare Practice through Patient Engagement
Guendalina Graffigna (Catholic University of the Sacred Heart, Italy)
Medical Information Science Reference • ©2017 • 382pp • H/C (ISBN: 9781522506638) • US $215.00

Promoting Patient Engagement and Participation for Effective Healthcare Reform
Guendalina Graffigna (Catholic University of the Sacred Heart of Milan, Italy)
Medical Information Science Reference • ©2016 • 357pp • H/C (ISBN: 9781466699922) • US $220.00

For an enitre list of titles in this series, please visit:
https://www.igi-global.com/book-series/advances-medical-diagnosis-treatment-care/129618

IGI Global
DISSEMINATOR OF KNOWLEDGE

701 East Chocolate Avenue, Hershey, PA 17033, USA
Tel: 717-533-8845 x100 • Fax: 717-533-8661
E-Mail: cust@igi-global.com • www.igi-global.com

Editorial Advisory Board

Table of Contents

Foreword

Complementary and alternative medicine stems from ancient and have been used throughout history. Use of complementary and alternative medicines for preventive and therapeutic purposes has increased tremendously over the last two decades globally. Although modern medicine has developed tremendously, complementary and alternative medicine will always have their place as they are useful for treating conditions which no satisfactory conventional medical intervention exists, or to complement conventional medicine in promoting well-being, or helping to alleviate symptoms associated with a disease such as fatigue, or indeed side effects from pharmaceutical treatments.

Complementary and Alternative Medicine and Kidney Health comprehensively explores gaps of modern medicine, provides information how complementary and alternative medicine fills these gaps and how to consider complementary and alternative medicines for patient benefit. Without scientific and systemic evaluation of a complementary medicine's safety and efficacy, patients can be exploited by companies who sell unproven, and sometimes dangerous, remedies. There are common situations, especially in low- and middle-income countries, who may have less intense regulations, where complementary and alternative medicine are abused in this way.

There is currently a global pandemic of end stage renal disease. This catastrophic illness not only causes financial burdens to individuals and their countries, but also causes patients panic and disability. Dialysis as a treatment for end stage renal disease can be perceived as palliative treatment, and complementary and alternative medicine are often used in the hope that dialysis may be avoided or delayed.

Complementary and Alternative Medicine and Kidney Health defines the types of methods used in research in this area, the prevalence of use, and the characteristics of patients including the attitudes of users especially in relation to chronic kidney disease. The book also explores the effect of culture, including the Western and Asian perspectives, and how the behaviour and beliefs of each population differently handles complementary and alternative medicine and how the differences should be seen through the vision of the regulatory agencies. *Complementary and Alternative Medicine and Kidney Health* is a source of reference for people interested in conducting complementary and alternative medicine research, including highlight gaps in knowledge, and suggestions of how clinical research in this field should be designed.

The most important issue to consider regarding complementary and alternative medicine is the evaluation of benefits and toxicity. *Complementary and Alternative Medicine and Kidney Health* comprehensively explores the evidence of both benefits and safety, critical knowledge for health care professionals and patients, including Chinese herbal medicines, aristolochic acid, acupuncture, yoga, aromatherapy and unregistered herbal products from India and China. These unregistered products are not required to submit proof of safety or efficacy to the Food and Drug Administration of the nation before their launch in the market. Therefore of concern, are not only benefits and toxicities of products, but also the issue of drug interactions, either herb-drug or herb-herb. The strict regulation and pharmacopoeias for ready references are needed.

Complementary and Alternative Medicine and Kidney Health offers suggestions for how to conduct benefit evaluations, toxicity assessments and economic evaluations through evidence-based medicine process. These important steps offer critical scientific information for decision-making and for informing guidelines. Evidence based complementary and alternative medicine can only be possible via integrative medicine models, and prospective research, such as randomized controlled trials and adverse effect studies, cohort, pragmatic clinical trials and multiple randomized controlled trials.

Chatchai Kreepala
Srinakharinwirot University, Thailand

Mymoona Akhter
Hamdard University, India

Win Winit-Watjana
Srinakharinwirot University, Thailand

Preface

BACKGROUND

Traditional medicine is embedded in Asian regions and health care providers in this area are more likely to have experience in this field. As a pharmacist with speciality in chronic kidney disease (CKD), I always receive questions about herbal medicine from patients with CKD. Received common questions are, "Could I use herbal medicine?", "Which herbal medicine can improve my illness?", and "Is it safe to use herbal medicine?" Due to being trained in only the modern concept of health care, I struggled to answer such questions. Colleagues faced similar questions from patients and came to me as a multidisciplinary team expects a pharmacist to answer such questions as they perceive that a pharmacist well know about conventional medication, including herbal medicine. This situation led me to study and build up knowledge about herbal medicine in CKD. During conducted research in this field, I learned many aspects of complementary and alternative medicine (CAM) that I did not expect. The more I learned, the more I understood. Now I am well placed to answer questions from patients and colleagues, but also thought it would be useful to write a textbook for a novice and health care providers who are interested in this field, and who may have similar questions posed to them. This book aims to bridge the gap of concepts between conventional medicine and CAM.

CONTENTS AND ORGANISATION

CAM has become more popular in the last decade and health expenditure on CAM has been increasing worldwide. People seek an alternative treatment when they are disappointed in conventional medicine, and believe CAM to be safer than pharmaceutical interventions. Additionally, in some parts of the world, people cannot access conventional medicine; therefore CAM is a mainstream of their health care system. In other countries, traditional medicine is embedded in their culture, and therefore remains the main health care system. Reasons for using CAM in patients with kidney disease are similar to the general population's. However, patients with renal insufficiency are more vulnerable to adverse effects of CAM, particularly herbal medicine.

Health care providers, who have been trained in conventional medicine, are less likely to trust CAM and argue that the efficacy and safety of CAM as supported by scientific evidence, are lacking. However, health professionals have limited time to search and evaluate evidence in the CAM field. This results in health care providers to suggest their patient to avoid using CAM due to unknown efficacy or safety. Patients therefore may lose an opportunity to use CAM, which may improve their illness. Meanwhile, CAM practitioners are strongly confident that CAM is useful despite a lack of scientific evidence. They argue that research methodologies for conventional medicine are unsuitable for CAM. However, CAM is still required to develop its research methodologies and establish sufficient evidence in order to convince health professionals to recommend CAM. The concept of evidence based medicine is applied to form the structure and contents of this book. The authors attempted to present mutual concepts between CAM and conventional medicine and consists of ten chapters:

- Chapter 1 gives an overview of CAM including CAM definitions and types of CAM. The prevalence and demographic characteristics of CAM use in general populations and patients with kidney disease worldwide are indicated, including reasons for CAM use in both populations. Placebo effects are discussed in this chapter.
- Chapter 2 presents similarities and differences in perspectives regarding CAM between Western and Eastern populations, and compares the prevalence of CAM use, factors related to CAM use, and disclosure of CAM use in both populations. Regulation of CAM and CAM practitioners, and legislation for herbal medicinal products are provided.
- Chapter 3 reviewed the quantity and quality of clinical research in CAM worldwide and shows a trend in CAM research in terms of descriptive studies, and a gap regarding efficacy and safety research in CAM. Publication bias in CAM, particularly open-access journals, are discussed, and a guideline for choosing trusted journals is presented.

- Chapter 4 provides a basic knowledge about how to evaluate the benefits and adverse effects of CAM in kidney disease. It focuses on chronic kidney disease, dialysis therapy, kidney transplantation, and urolithiasis due to there being a high number of such patients. Assessment of clinical outcomes related to positive and negative effects of CAM in kidney diseases is presented. This chapter also suggests standard questionnaires to measure the quality of life, and individual symptoms in CAM users with kidney disease. The modified Naranjo algorithm is proposed as a way to evaluate renal adverse effects of herbal medicine.
- Chapter 5 describes a method of systematic searching and critiquing scientific evidence on CAM, and suggests assessment of web based CAM information that nowadays is a main information source. CAM databases and standard questionnaires to evaluate scientific papers are indicated. Finally, a way of decision making based on evidence is proposed.
- Chapter 6 points out that many guidelines for chronic illnesses, e.g., chronic kidney disease, asthma, cancer, etc., suggests using CAM. The author summarises which CAM has, or has not, been recommended in a guideline or illness. Suggestions for CAM in guidelines is inconsistent and is discussed. This chapter also provides details of standard tools for guideline appraisal.
- Chapter 7 provides evidence for the efficacy and nephrotoxicity of CAM, focussing on herbal medicine that is the most common CAM for treating kidney diseases. Other CAMs for relieving uraemic symptoms are mentioned. Such information is presented based on existing scientific evidence. This chapter also proposes recommendations for preventing acute kidney injury from using herbal and dietary supplements.
- Chapter 8 discusses herb-drug interactions and focuses on herbal medicine for kidney diseases that interact with conventional medicine or other herbal products. The author also explains the basic mechanisms of herb-drug interactions, i.e. pharmacokinetic and pharmacodynamic effects, and summarises common herb-drug interactions in a table.
- Chapter 9 explains a basic concept of economic evaluation and interpretations of economic results. Decision making for using CAM considers not only the efficacy and safety of CAM, but also economic evaluation. The authors summarise economic evaluation research regarding CAM, although there is a lack of such research in kidney diseases.

- Chapter 10 presents models of CAM integrated into conventional medicine in Western and Eastern regions and definitions of integrative medicine. This chapter highlights the limitations of clinical research in CAM and proposes alternative appropriate methodologies for CAM research. International and national organisations of CAM research are mentioned.

Scientific evidence on CAM is frequently published and research methodologies in are developing. Therefore readers should keep in mind that some contents in this book may be subject to change.

CONTRIBUTION

This book amalgamates recent and essential knowledge of CAM, and is presented from a scientific perspective. Although this book mainly contributes to CAM for kidney diseases, it also provides the general concept of CAM from research to practice. It prepares health care providers to be ready to work in an era of increasing CAM use, especially professionals who take care of patients with kidney disease. This book is appropriate for health care providers who are either unfamiliar with CAM, or are interested in CAM. Additionally, this book suggests future research in the CAM field and would be useful for health researchers.

Chapter 1
An Overview of Complementary and Alternative Medicine

Annalisa Casarin
The NIHR Research Design Service East of England, UK

Mayuree Tangkiatkumjai
Srinakharinwirot University, Thailand

Dawn-Marie Walker
University of Southampton, UK

ABSTRACT

A treatment that is not recognised as conventional medicine is frequently referred to as part of complementary and alternative medicine (CAM) methods. This Chapter will provide an overview of the several CAM definitions currently proposed and the types of CAM methods. The prevalence of CAM use and the characteristics and attitudes of CAM users will be also explored with a focus on patients with kidney diseases. The reasons for CAM use and the literature on the placebo effects as a debated hypothesis of CAM mechanism of action is presented.

DOI: 10.4018/978-1-5225-2882-1.ch001

INTRODUCTION

Complementary and alternative medicine (CAM) has existed in Asian cultures for centuries, recently it has become prominent in the western world. A study published in 2008 showed that 38% of adults and 12% of children used CAM in the United States in 2007 (Barnes, et al. 2008). Most recently, a survey conducted under the cross European CAMbrella project, showed that in Europe one in two surveyed people had used CAM between 2010 and 2012 (EuroCAM, 2014), and it is evident that ancient therapies have been re discovered by patients in order to find solutions to their increasing numbers of health issues. Writing an overview of CAM is difficult. While the definition of orthodox medicine is well established, CAM techniques are so widely spread across the world and embedded in different cultures that giving CAM a single definition is a challenge. Not only do different organisations define CAM in various ways, but also they include or exclude techniques within this term according to the organisation's beliefs and culture. For example, some people may identify dietary advice, exercise or prayer as CAM, but Asian people do not think that prayer is an alternative medicine as it is a part of their religion.

The interest in CAM may possibly be due to the rising number of concerns that patients have towards orthodox, western medicine. This in turn has led to a call for regulation and proof of efficacy. International establishments like the World Health Organization (WHO), recognize that it is essential to guide this process by suggesting the development of country specific policies (WHO, 2013). The goal of WHO, and CAM practitioner associations, is to analyse the value and safety of CAM interventions with scientific methods in order to best advise patients.

This chapter aims to: explain the difficulties in collating different understanding of CAM practices by Western organisations; discuss the prevalence of CAM use; explore the penchant for CAM seen in patients with renal conditions; and discuss the placebo effect, an important part of all healing processes. Suggestions of future research directions will be presented at the end of this and the following chapters.

DEFINITION OF COMPLEMENTARY AND ALTERNATIVE MEDICINE

A complementary technique is considered as one which falls beyond the scope of orthodox medicine, but which may be used alongside it (www.OxfordDictionaries.com [last accessed 17/03/17]), while an alternative method may be used instead of conventional medicine. Whether a healing method is considered as a CAM depends on the context, or culture in which is used. For example, herbal medicine is considered as traditional and integrative in China, and complementary or alternative in Europe. In regards to context, herbs can be used as a complementary therapy for infertility whilst they can be used as an alternative treatment to medications for urological conditions. In cases of incurable conditions, like end stage kidney failure where only conventional treatment will save the patient, CAM can be offered in order to relieve symptoms associated with the technique or the disease (Barnes et al., 2008). In this case the techniques may be considered complementary because they cannot be offered as alternative to dialysis. Another term frequently used and recently adopted to indicate a combination of CAM techniques and conventional medicine is integrative. In this case, Asian countries led the way in adopting the integration between systems. As Bodeker stated (2001), the Asian experience should be used by western countries when developing policies for integrating two health systems. Chapter 10 will explore the integration concept in depth.

Each CAM may also have differential definitions. Acupuncture, for example, has many different definitions according to context. The Chinese Medicine acupuncture practitioner looks at the symptoms in order to detect energy blocks, and healing ability depends upon emotions that the patient experiences during the appointment. Whilst in the western world, medical acupuncture practitioners evaluate symptoms and deliver treatments thinking of neuromodulating endogenous systems (International Council of Medical Acupuncture and Related Techniques, 2015). Therefore, the definition of a single technique may have different meanings. This makes defining CAM even more difficult.

Several Western health organisations have endeavoured to define CAM, and CAM research leaders of a number of countries, have aimed to develop a general, open, pan European definition (Table 1) that includes all systems able to maintain and improve health (Falkenberg et al., 2012). One shared understanding of CAM may be useful to overcome barriers to research and the development of international policies and regulations. But a worldwide definition of CAM looks like far from being realistic. The first obstacle is the different views between East and West. In East Asian countries, like China, Korea and Japan CAM is considered as traditional medicine. As stated in Table 1, traditional medicine is defined by the WHO (2012) as 'indigenous medicine that is used to maintain health and to diagnose, prevent, and treat mental and physical illnesses differently from conventional medicine based on beliefs, theories, and experiences'. In fact, each Asian countries has developed their own health systems according to their culture and history. Moreover, unlike CAM in Western countries, traditional medicine is an integral part of the health care and co-exist as part of a dual medical system. The same concept is applicable to Ayurveda in India and Thai medicine in Thailand (Park et al., 2012).

In the West, several countries host CAM practitioners' organisations. Following the appeal of WHO to consider increasing the use of CAM, CAM groups evaluate efficacy, and regulate CAM practitioners in order to safeguard the public. Although the definition of CAM varies slightly among associations, a common feature is that CAM is not part of the country's own health system and are not yet integrated, but instead are linked with population-specific philosophies and beliefs (WHO, 2000; Wieland et al., 2011; Falkenberg et al., 2012; NICM, 2015).

WHO is the agency of the United Nation that directs international public health issues and respond to global health threats. In 2013, WHO published an updated *Traditional Medicine Strategy 2014–2023*. In the publication, WHO tackles the rising concerns on policies and regulations of CAM practitioners (WHO, 2013).

The *Cochrane Collaboration* is a global, independent network that evaluates evidence of effects of healthcare interventions and ensures that updated and accurate information are freely available. It is renowned worldwide for its guidelines database.

The *National Center for Complementary and Integrative Health* (NCCIH) is the United States of America (USA) Government's lead agency for scientific research on health care systems, practices, and products that are not generally considered part of conventional medicine. Named NCCIH since 2014, it was

Table 1. Different organizations' definition of CAM

World Health Organization	The terms "complementary medicine" or "alternative medicine" are used interchangeably with traditional medicine in some countries. They refer to a broad set of health care practices that are not part of that country's own tradition and are not integrated into the dominant health care system. Traditional medicine is the sum total of the knowledge, skills, and practices based on the theories, beliefs, and experiences indigenous to different cultures, whether explicable or not, used in the maintenance of health as well as in the prevention, diagnosis, improvement or treatment of physical and mental illness (WHO, 2000, 2013).
Cochrane Collaboration	CAM is a broad domain of healing resources that encompasses all health systems, modalities, and practices and their accompanying theories and beliefs, other than those intrinsic to the politically dominant health system of a particular society or culture in a given historical period' (Wieland et al., 2011).
The National Center for Complementary and Integrative Health (NCCIH, formerly NCCAM) (USA)	CAM is a group of diverse medical health care systems, practices, and products that are not generally considered to be part of conventional medicine; that is, medicine as practiced by holders of medical doctor or doctor of osteopathy degrees and their allied health professionals, such as physical therapists, psychologists, and registered nurses (NCCIH, formerly called National Center for Complementary and Alternative Medicine NCCAM, 2009)
National Health Service (NHS) (UK)	Complementary and alternative medicines are treatments that fall outside of mainstream healthcare (NHS, 2016)
House of Lords (UK)	CAM is a title used to refer to a diverse group of health-related therapies and disciplines which are not considered to be a part of mainstream medical care (House of Lords, 2000).
CAMbrella (Europe)	The definition, and also the provision of different types of CAM alter from country to country. CAM, as utilized by European citizens, represents a variety of different medical systems and therapies based on the knowledge, skills and practices derived from theories, philosophies and experiences used to maintain and improve health, as well as to prevent, diagnose, relieve or treat physical and mental illnesses. CAM therapies are mainly used outside conventional health care, but in many countries some therapies are being adopted or adapted by conventional health care (Falkenberg et al., 2012).
EFCAM (Europe)	CAM is a diverse range of autonomous healthcare practices used for health maintenance, health education, health promotion, disease prevention and for the treatment of ill-health. These practices can be used independently, and, alongside conventional medical approaches to create a broad range of healthcare options for the public (EFCAM, 2016).
National Institute of Complementary Medicine (Australia)	Complementary medicine (CM) is a broad domain of healing resources that encompasses all health systems, modalities, and practices and their accompanying theories and beliefs, other than those intrinsic to the politically dominant health system of a particular society or culture in a given historical period. CM includes all such practices and ideas self-defined by their users as preventing or treating illness or promoting health and well-being. Boundaries within cm and between the CM domain and that of the dominant system are not always sharp or fixed (NICM, 2015).

Abbreviations: USA = United States of America UK = United Kingdom

previously called the National Center for Complementary and Alternative Medicine.

In the United Kingdom (UK) the *House of Lords*, part of the House of Parliament of the UK, published a report on CAM acknowledging the widespread interest in complementary therapies in the UK (House of Lords, 2000). In order to protect the public, the report invited the *National Health Service* (NHS) to create evidence on effectiveness and safety through research;

to provide information to the public and professionals through the *NHSchoices* website (National Health Service, 2016); and to regulate CAM practitioners and their training. This call for regulations and guidance, helped a number of CAM associations to flourish. Among these, the *Research Council for Complementary Medicine* produced a controlled vocabulary, *a reference tool for researchers and academics, providing a conceptual framework and an understanding of the scope of CAM terms*. The thesaurus is freely available at www.rccm.org.uk/node/229 [last accessed 19/03/17] (RCCM, 2013).

In Europe, a research network called *CAMbrella* conducted a study into the situation of CAM in Europe between 2010 and 2012. The study was funded by the European Commission. The definition of CAM, according to this project, is different among countries and in some of them CAM methods are incorporated in conventional treatment programs (Falkenberg et al., 2012). CAMbrella attempted to give CAM a pragmatic definition that could be accepted Europe-wide, as seen in Table 1. Moreover, the recommendations for regulation and research of the CAMbrella review were followed by the publication of *CAM 2020: The Contribution of Complementary and Alternative Medicine to Sustainable Healthcare in Europe*. This is a booklet published by *EuroCAM*, an association of 12 European CAM bodies (EuroCAM, 2014).

The *European Federations of CAM (EFCAM)* links different European associations on specific CAM modalities, for example reflexology and shiatsu, and national CAM organisations of multi modalities. EFCAM promotes equality of access to holistic healthcare and supports the right to practice for all trained CAM professionals (EFCAM, 2016).

In Australia, the *National Institute of Complementary Medicine (NICM)* was established after the 2003 recommendation by an Expert Committee of the Australian Health System who stated that the government has the responsibility to fund complementary medicine research given the widespread public use of CAM. The NICM definition of CAM follows the one from the Cochrane Collaboration (NICM, 2015).

TYPES OF COMPLEMENTARY AND ALTERNATIVE MEDICINE

As the definition of CAM, the lists of techniques considered complementary and alternative differ among associations. Again, the main difference is between the East and West. Unfortunately, the evidence available from

Eastern societies is not easily accessible due to language barriers. Western organisations such as NCCIH and CAMbrella, propose specific classifications. Others like Cochrane and EuroCAM, only provide a list of techniques. The comprehensive list provided by the Cochrane Collaboration is available in chapter 6.

NCCIH/NCCAM (USA) classification of CAM can be summarised as follows:

- Mind-Body Medicine, which aims to enhance the mind's ability to affect symptoms.
- Natural Product or Biologically Based Therapies, which promotes health using substances found in nature as herbs, vitamins, minerals and probiotics.
- Manipulative and Body-Based Practices, based on manipulation and/or movements.
- Energy Medicine, which involves the use of electromagnetic fields.
- Whole, Alternative Medical Systems, which are complete systems of theory and practice outside the conventional allopathic (mainstream) model.

This classification has no clearly defined boundaries. Yoga, chiropractic and osteopathic manipulation, meditation, and massage therapy (the most popular practices used by US adults [NCCAM, 2012]), can be part of mind and body practices as well as the manipulative/movements class. Considering acupuncture, this technique can be part of mind and body practices, but also the alternative medical systems class together with methods like homeopathic medicine, naturopathic medicine, anthroposophic medicine, neural therapy, Ayurveda, and Tibetan medicine. In general, when mainstream therapies are combined with methods supported by high quality scientific evidence of safety and effectiveness, the method is called integrative (NCCIH, 2015).

EuroCAM (Europe) lists CAM as the following methods: acupuncture, ayurveda, anthroposophic medicine, chiropractic, herbal medicine, homeopathic medicine, kinesiology, naturopathic medicine, osteopathy, reflexology, shiatsu, traditional Chinese medicine, Tibetan medicine, and yoga (EuroCAM, 2014).

CAMbrella (Europe) proposes the following: CAM-disciplines/methods, may be provided by medical doctors, practitioners but also used as self-treatments. This includes traditional European naturopathy; special European medicinal systems (e.g. homeopathy, anthroposophy); adapted methods/

medicinal systems from non-European traditional systems; and other unconventional medicinal methods used in Europe (Uehleke, et al., 2012).

EFCAM (Europe) acknowledges that CAM modalities have a distinct philosophical, diagnostic and methodological basis. The characteristics EFCAM considers as belonging to CAM are: holistic; natural; curative; preventive; health supporting methods which are open to innovation; traditional and established. They need to be safe for both patients and users and enhance self-healing capacities; whilst promoting self-responsibility for health. They will be able to be used either in combinations or individually; therefore increasing the range of options available for patient care. So far the federation has provided a description of acupuncture, homeopathy, reflexology, shiatsu, and traditional Chinese medicine among the CAM modalities they recognise as such (EFCAM, 2016).

The *NICM* (Australia) embraces the NICCH tendency of classifying CAM methods in 5 domains: mind and body medicine; biologically based products; manipulative and body based practices; or energy medicine (NICM, 2015).

In East Asian countries the main therapeutic methods of traditional medicine consist of acupuncture, moxibustion, cupping, herbal medicines, and manual therapies (Park et al., 2012). In these cultures they are not considered alternatives but part of the range of healthcare options. In the West, the list of methods that are considered CAM is an extensive one and depends on the CAM definition adopted by the regulatory organizations. Some specify practices, others cluster methods together according to recurrent themes. This heterogeneity in understanding among stakeholders may be why WHO called for the development of regulations and policies applicable worldwide and for collaborative research.

PREVALENCE AND REASONS FOR CAM USE

CAM use has been rising amongst the general population worldwide. This spread is dependent on the patients' culture, society, and economy. The number of surveys on this issue has been increasing over the last decade, leading to an improved knowledge of the prevalence of CAM use (e.g. Harris, et al., 2012). Between 1998 and 2011, the 12 months prevalence for CAM practitioners' visits varied from 1.8 to 9.8, and use from 48.7% to 76% in 15 countries (Harris, et al., 2012). A study about child use of CAM in Europe showed a mean prevalence of 52% after adjustment for the size of the population of each country (Zuzak et al., 2013). The specifics of the prevalence of CAM use in each region, particularly the comparison of CAM use between Western and Eastern countries, will be discussed in Chapter 2. Governments in many countries acknowledge the high prevalence of CAM use and call for a comparison of cost-effectiveness between CAM and conventional medicine before adding CAM to standard guidelines for maintaining well-being or for treating illnesses (Bridges, et al., 2010; Canadian Agency for Drugs and Technologies in Health, 2006; National Institute for Health and Care Excellence, 2012). Chapter 9 will give an overview of the economic evaluation of CAM.

CAM use is associated with two possible meanings. Some studies identify health treatment as the purpose for CAM use, whilst others focus on attitudes that influence using CAM, such as safety or affordability of CAM. This section focuses on the second meaning as it indicates which factors impact on decision making for using CAM. Several authors systematically reviewed 83 quantitative and qualitative studies of the reasons for use and non-use of CAM in both general and patient populations worldwide. They found that the top three reasons for CAM use in either populations were a perception of CAM benefits, dissatisfaction with conventional medicine, and the perceived safety of CAM (Tangkiatkumjai, et al., 2017). Other reasons for CAM use are willingness to try, belief in a holistic approach, easy access to CAM, and affordability of CAM (Tangkiatkumjai, et al., 2017). It has been reported that the mass media, e.g. newspapers, television, internet, etc., also influences people to use CAM (Alkhateeb, et al., 2006; Levine, et al., 2009; Ock, et al., 2009). In addition, CAM is used as a last resort in patients who are hopeless with their therapy, such as some of those with cancer or life threatening co-morbidities (Verhoef, et al., 2005).

It is worrying that in a high percentage of all clinicians are not aware of their patients' propensity of using CAM (Zuzak et al., 2013). Knowing the reasons for using CAM would guide practitioners to learn about the existence of CAM and to ask their patients about them. If practitioners would not like their patients to use CAM, they should discuss this as well as the patient's complaints about the side effects of conventional medicine. When their patients are using CAM, practitioners should be able to suggest whether the CAM has any scientific evidence about the efficacy or safety. Chapter 5 will provide information on how to search CAM databases and critique studies in CAM.

CHRONIC KIDNEY DISEASE PATIENTS AND CAM USE

Chronic kidney disease (CKD) is an illness that either gradually decreases kidney function or damages the kidney structure for more than 3 months. Common causes of CKD are diabetes and hypertension. Chapter 4 will explain more detail about what CKD is, severity of CKD, and how to evaluate benefits and adverse effects of CAM in kidney disease. A gold standard conventional treatment for CKD focuses on slowing the progression of CKD, whilst patients with end-stage renal disease (ESRD) require treatment for CKD complications, i.e. fatigue, pruritus, edema, anaemia, hyperkalemia, hyperphosphatemia, metabolic acidosis, and hypertension. Controlled blood pressure and blood sugar are the key to slowing the progression of CKD, including the restriction of protein intake. The main conventional medications for slowing the progression of CKD are angiotensin-converting enzyme inhibitors (ACEIs), and angiotensin II receptor antagonists (ARBs) (KDIGO, 2012). Dialysis is a gold standard therapy for ESRD and removes a toxin called uraemia from the body. Kidney transplant is also another standard treatment for ESRD; however, kidney transplant recipients need to take immunosuppressants for the rest of their life.

Since conventional medicine cannot cure CKD nor its symptoms, patients with CKD, particularly in Asian countries, are more likely to seek alternative medicine in order to delay receiving dialysis, relieve their symptoms, such as fatigue and pruritus, and decrease the side effects of their conventional medication. Herbal medicine that may slow the progression of CKD or relieve ESRD symptoms and acupuncture for pruritus are commonly used in patients with kidney disease. Chapter 7 will elaborate on studies of benefits from CAM in patients with kidney disease. Similarly, general populations are more likely to use herbal medicines or dietary supplements than other types of CAM, such as acupuncture, homeopathy, chiropractic, or massage (House of Lords, 2000; Barnes, et al., 2004; Ock, et al., 2009; Singh, et al., 2004; Eardley, et al., 2012).

CAM use in patients with kidney diseases is almost twice the prevalence of that found in the general population (Harris et al., 2012). The prevalence of CAM use in patients with CKD as detected in six countries ranges from 17.6% to 64.0% (Grabe & Garrison, 2004; Osman, et al., 2015; Shah, et al., 2013; Spanner & Duncan, 2005; Tangkiatkumjai, et al., 2013; Wazaify, et al., 2013). This prevalence is not different from other patient populations, such as cancer patients (7-64%) (Ernst, & Cassileth, 1998). To be noted is that the lowest prevalence of CAM use in patients with CKD (17.6%) is still almost twice the prevalence of CAM use in general populations (9.8%) (Harris et al., 2012). Likewise, patients with other chronic diseases, such as diabeties, are more likely to use CAM than general populations (Egede, et al., 2002). Amongst patients receiving dialysis and kidney transplant recipients, the prevalence of CAM use internationally is between 12% and 64% (Birdee, et al., 2013; Hess, et al., 2009; Kara, 2009; Nowack et al., 2009; Osman, et al., 2015; Zyoud, et al., 2016). These published surveys on prevalence showed that kidney transplant recipients are less likely to use CAM than patients with CKD or those receiving dialysis because transplant patients may be concerned about the interaction between their immunosuppressants and CAM. Another reason is that they may be less poorly and be less likely to need treatments.

Considering only studies in kidney patient populations, the evidence reveals that characteristics of patients with kidney disease who use CAM are inconsistent worldwide. Three surveys of herbal use in patients with CKD or receiving dialysis in Turkey, Thailand, and the US compared demographic characteristics between the users and non-users and found that both groups had no difference in age, sex, education, or income (Kara, 2009; Spanner & Duncan, 2005; Tangkiatkumjai, et al., 2013). However, this finding differs from demographics of CAM use in general populations where people who are older, female or better educated are more likely to use CAM, especially in Western countries (Thomson, et al., 2012; Marques-Vidal, et al., 2009; Guo, et al., 2009). Meanwhile, demographic characteristics are similar between the users and non-users of CAM in Asian populations perhaps because they perceive CAM and conventional medicine similarly (Lee and Kim, 2009; Araz, et al, 2009).

Demographics of kidney transplant recipients and dialysis patients in some countries may differ from patients with CKD as above. Kidney transplant recipients using CAM in European countries are more likely to be female (Hess, et al., 2009; Nowack, et al., 2009), whilst those in Egypt tend to be male (Osman, et al., 2015). Patients receiving dialysis and kidney transplant recipients who use CAM in the Middle Eastern region tend to have higher incomes (Osman, et al., 2015; Zyoud, et al., 2016). In an Indian survey of 52 dialysis patients using CAM, its use was highest in those aged between 50 and 64 (67%), and 63% were upper middle class (Arjuna Rao, et al., 2016).

Based on existing evidence on types of CAM used in patients with kidney disease, herbal medicine is the commonest CAM modality among US and Palestinian patients with CKD, dialysis patients and kidney transplant recipients, followed by mind-body practices, massage and acupuncture

(Birdee, et al., 2013; Zyoud et al., 2016). However, patients with CKD in India tend to use yoga, homeopathy and Ayurveda (Shah, et al., 2013). In a survey of 52 Indian renal patients on maintenance haemodialysis, Arjuna Rao et al (2016) found that Ayurveda was the most frequently used CAM, alone and in combination with other methods, followed by acupuncture and herbal therapy. In Switzerland, kidney transplant recipients are more likely to use homeopathy than herbal medicine (Hess, et al., 2009). A survey of CAM use amongst kidney transplant recipients in Egypt also reported that these patients are more likely to use non-herbal medicine than patients with CKD and dialysis patients (Osman, et al., 2015). In conclusion, there is a variety of CAM techniques used by patients with kidney diseases. It can be hypothesized that both the patient's culture, together with the availability of CAM and access to CAM practitioners influences the decision on using CAM.

Only three surveys in Canada, India, and Thailand reported reasons for CAM use in patients with CKD. They showed that the major reasons were the perceived benefits and safety of CAM, together with a dissatisfaction of conventional medicine, including having side effects, dissatisfaction with a doctor or the high costs of conventional medicine (Shah, et al., 2013; Spanner & Duncan, 2005; Tangkiatkumjai, et al., 2014). The main reasons for CAM use in patients with CKD are similar to the reasons given by other populations: patients with kidney disease use CAM for maintaining well-being, and treating their illness. Despite the fact that studies about the reasons for CAM use in dialysis patients and kidney transplant recipients are not found, it is possible to extrapolate that they do so for the same reasons as patients with CKD. However, further studies are required to explore the reasons why dialysis patients and kidney transplant recipients use CAM.

The high prevalence of CAM use in patients with kidney disease should alert health care providers to regularly ask their patients about CAM, and provide information about the efficacy and safety of CAM. This is because herbal products can either accumulate or cause interactions with other medications (Arjuna Rao, et al., 2016). Chapter 8 discusses the issue of herb-drug interactions.

The underpinning mechanism of action of CAM is difficult to determine since the techniques are so different. One of the commonly acclaimed mechanisms is the controversial contribution of the placebo effect. This concept applies to both western and eastern medicine and the literature has being abundant on its role within the healing process.

PLACEBO EFFECT

A placebo is an inert medical intervention which often takes the form of sugar pills, inert creams, or even sham surgery. It is designed to make the participant feel like they are taking the active ingredient. This can result in an effect on their condition, i.e. the placebo effect. The placebo effect can result in clinically significant improvements in many disorders such as depression, or pain. However, placebos may relieve but do not cure. Placebos do not alter the pathophysiology of a disease, but rather eases the comorbid, subjective symptoms (Kaptchuk & Miller, 2015). However, co-morbid symptoms such as mood disorders, are common factors in chronic medical conditions such as diabetes and cancer (Melek & Norris, 2008). This is evident even in children. A study of paediatric epilepsy found that comorbid psychiatric disorders such as depression, or anxiety at an age of approximately 4 years, was associated with a significantly poorer quality of life 9 years later (Baca, et al., 2011). Therefore, although the placebo may not affect the objective measures of a disease, it may increase a patient's wellbeing and ultimately, the way they respond to that disease so it may be less disabling. Patients may also experience adverse effects from placebo, i.e., nocebo. This is due to participants having expectations of side effects, not only benefits. It is estimated that between 4% and 26% of patients randomly assigned to placebo, discontinue the trial due to perceived adverse effects (Kaptchuk & Miller, 2015).

Although historically the placebo effect was thought to be due to an expectation response, i.e. the participant thought they were taking the real intervention so received benefit from it, it has been shown that even open label placebo, where participants are told they are taking a placebo, still result in a significant placebo effect. Ted Kaptchuk is one of the leading placebo researchers. He and his team conducted a trial in which he recruited 80 participants with irritable bowel syndrome. They were randomised to receive no care, or open label placebos. They found that the open label placebo group produced significant improvements in both the short term (11 days) and the longer term (21 days after intervention) (Kaptchuk et al., 2010).

The placebo effect is part of any treatment's result. For example, in trials of antidepressants where only subjective measures of the severity can be used, the placebo accounts for between 65%-85% of the drug's effect (Kirsch, 2000). Indeed, in cough medicines, 85% of the reduction in coughs is attributable to placebo (Eccles, 2002). A significant proportion of new treatments and interventions routinely fail to demonstrate a benefit greater than that of placebos in clinical trials. It is argued that the therapeutic effect of an intervention includes the specific effect related to the treatment itself, but also the contextual effect, i.e., how the intervention is delivered (Kaptchuk et al., 2008). These contextual effects are often clinically significant. For example, the majority of the treatment effect for pain in osteoarthritis are due to these (Zhang, 2013). A systematic review have studied these effects, and the patient-practitioner interaction appears to be the most powerful (Di Blasi, et al., 2001). This includes both verbal and nonverbal communication.

Because of this, any new intervention needs to prove significant clinical efficacy over and above the placebo effect. Therefore, a placebo is usually the control in randomised controlled trials of new interventions, where the participant is randomly allocated to receive either the new intervention or the placebo to which they are blinded (they don't know which group they are in). This allows researchers to ascertain whether their intervention benefits patients over and above the placebo effect. Because of this, great effort is taken in conducting trials of CAM to see whether they are more effective than placebo, and time and time again failing to do so. This is partly due to the fact that it is almost impossible to conduct a gold standard randomised trial in CAM as blinding participants is difficult. For example, to blind a participant in acupuncture and they are not needled they would be able to tell. Although attempts have been made to validate a sham procedure such as The Park Sham Device, it is debatable whether it truly blinds participants (Park, et al., 2002; Tan, et al., 2009).

There is a further argument; however, that actually the placebo effect is an integral part of the effect from CAM. The placebo effect is essentially a body's mechanism for healing and works in a holistic way, which is fundamentally the way CAM works also. CAM's effect is complex. Their way of achieving efficacy is nonspecific. "These CAM methods spur the organism to do something by itself to find its original balance" (Walach, 2001, p. 214). So rather than the placebo being 'noise' to overcome, the placebo is enhanced via factors such as context including having a discussion about the patient's wellbeing, and also therapeutic touch being part of any CAM consultation. Improvements in patients' symptoms due to placebo are attributable to their 'participation in the therapeutic encounter, with its rituals, symbols, and interactions. (Kaptchuk & Miller, 2015).

These contextual factors may be another reason why CAM is set up to fail when being studied as part of a trial. To blind a researcher in a trial it may be one person taking the medical history, and another delivering the intervention, thus altering the context and diminishing the nonspecific factors being derived from this (Walach, 2001). Indeed, as mentioned earlier, a significant amount of conventional medication's effect is due to non-specific, or placebo effects (Eccles, 2002; Kirsch, 2000). Walach terms this the 'placebo trap' where only specific effects over and above the placebo or nonspecific effects are worth achieving. He argues that this is not appropriate for complex interventions such as CAM as they do not have an effect on one specific outcome in a mechanistic method such as pharmaceutical interventions do. But rather they stimulate organisms toward self-healing actions (Walach, 2001).

CAM critics often mention the placebo effect as the reason why it should not be considered scientifically accepted. But the reported evidence of the existence of this effect in conventional medicine as well, and the positive impact it may have on patients' healing, should not deter practitioners to suggest CAM when appropriate and patients are willing to adopt it. The contextual effect is part of the holistic nature of CAM treatments and should be considered an asset instead of a detrimental factor. New research methodologies should then be suggested in order to embed these influences and validate techniques studying them in real life conditions.

FUTURE RESEARCH DIRECTIONS

CAM is a flourishing source of research since validation of practices in various different health conditions is far from achieved. Since the main obstacle to CAM being integrated into conventional systems is the paucity of good quality, scientific evidence, several aspects still need to be explored in order to create evidence based recommendations. The upcoming chapters will further explore some of these topics. As on overview, some of the frequently mentioned areas for potential research are listed here:

- Periodic surveys of population-level CAM use in western and eastern countries are needed to inform healthcare bodies on the prevalence and attitudes of CAM users (CAMbrella, 2012; Fischer et al., 2014).
- Cost-effectiveness and comparative evaluations between CAM and conventional medicine should be conducted in specific settings before adding CAM to standard guidelines (CAMbrella, 2012; Fischer et al., 2014).

- The impact of teaching of CAM principles in western medical education may benefit the relationship between practitioners and patients should be explored further (Bodeker, 2001).
- Policy development and regulations of CAM practitioners are needed in order to appropriately train professionals and guarantee safety of practice (CAMbrella, 2012).
- Investment to develop effective services and ensure affordability to all levels of society are desirable, otherwise poor standards and low quality practices may persist (Bodeker, 2001).
- Evidence on which illnesses are best treated through which approach, safety of herbal medicines, and conservation of herbal species needs to be generated (Bodeker, 2001).
- Rural communities should be investigated as they are the most likely to use CAM. Research on their use, practice, decision making processes and patient – practitioner interaction should be promoted (Wardle et al., 2012).
- Comparison of policies and practices among countries should be conducted in order to adopt worldwide the best possible solution taking into account specific contexts (Bodeker, 2001).
- CAM's methodological challenges such as the use of placebos should be studied and alternatives to common study designs developed (CAMbrella, 2012).
- Strategies in order to centralise and regulate centrally the education and provision of CAMs should be promoted (CAMbrella, 2012; Fischer et al., 2014).
- Within cancer research, the development of new cancer therapies derived from botanicals, supplements, and other natural products should be supported (Deng et al., 2009).

CONCLUSION

CAM is a term that refers to many prevention and treatment techniques. Its definition depends on different cultures, professionals' experience and patients' beliefs. This chapter explored several definitions and the classification of CAM techniques as provided by Western organisations. Eastern countries' perspectives differ since CAM methods are often embedded in the health systems as part of an integrative medicine approach. The prevalence of CAM use is increasing worldwide and reasons for CAM use in the general population and renal patients are linked to a dissatisfaction with conventional medicine. The placebo and contextual effects are part of both mainstream and complementary techniques and needs to be further explored with innovative research designs. Since the evidence on the efficacy of CAM is overall limited, the opportunities for research are abundant and research funding bodies should promote studies in this field.

REFERENCES

Alkhateeb, F. M., Doucette, W. R., & Ganther-Urmie, J. M. (2006). Influences on consumer spending for herbal products. *Research in Social & Administrative Pharmacy*, *2*(2), 254–265. doi:10.1016/j.sapharm.2006.03.001 PMID:17138511

Araz, A., Harlak, H., & Mese, G. (2009). Factors related to regular use of complementary/alternative medicine in Turkey. *Complementary Therapies in Medicine*, *17*(5-6), 309–315. doi:10.1016/j.ctim.2009.09.002 PMID:19942111

Arjuna Rao, A. S., Phaneendra, D., Pavani, C. D., Soundararajan, P., Rani, N. V., Thennarasu, P., & Kannan, G. (2016). Usage of complementary and alternative medicine among patients with chronic kidney disease on maintenance hemodialysis. *J Pharm Bioallied Sci*, *8*(1), 52–57. doi:10.4103/0975-7406.171692 PMID:26957870

Baca, C. B., Vickrey, B. G., Caplan, R., Vassar, S. D., & Berg, A. T. (2011). Psychiatric and Medical Comorbidity and Quality of Life Outcomes in Childhood-Onset Epilepsy. *Pediatrics, 128*(6), e1532-e1543.

Barnes, P. M., Bloom, B., & Nahin, R. L. (2008). Complementary and alternative medicine use among adults and children: United States, 2007. *National Health Statistics Reports*, (12): 1–23. PMID:19361005

Barnes, P. M., Powell-Griner, E., McFann, K., & Nahin, R. L. (2004). Complementary and alternative medicine use among adults: United States 2002. *Advance Data*, *343*, 1–19. PMID:15188733

Birdee, G. S., Phillips, R. S., & Brown, R. S. (2013). Use of complementary and alternative medicine among patients with end-stage renal disease. *Evidence-Based Complementary and Alternative Medicine*, *2013*, 654109. doi:10.1155/2013/654109 PMID:23710227

Bridges, J. F., Cohen, J. P., Grist, P. G., & Mühlbacher, A. C. (2010). International experience with comparative effectiveness research: Case studies from England/Wales and Germany. *Advances in Health Economics and Health Services Research*, *22*, 29–50. doi:10.1108/S0731-2199(2010)0000022005 PMID:20575227

Canadian Agency for Drugs and Technologies in Health. (2006). *Guidelines for the economic evaluation of health technologies*. Author.

Deng, G. E., Frenkel, M., Cohen, L., Cassileth, B. R., Abrams, D. I., Capodice, J. L., …, , & Sagar, S. (2009). Evidence-based clinical practice guidelines for integrative oncology: Complementary therapies and botanicals. *Journal of the Society for Integrative Oncology*, *7*(3), 85–120. PMID:19706235

Di Blasi, Z., Harkness, E., Ernst, E., Georgiou, A., & Kleijnen, J. (2001). Influence of context effects on health outcomes: A systematic review. *Lancet*, *357*(9258), 757–762. doi:10.1016/S0140-6736(00)04169-6 PMID:11253970

Eardley, S., Bishop, F. L., Prescott, P., Cardini, F., Brinkhaus, B., Santos-Rey, K., & Lewith, G. et al. (2002). A systematic literature review of complementary and alternative medicine prevalence in EU. *Forschende Komplementarmedizin*, *19*(s2), 18–28. doi:10.1159/000342708 PMID:23883941

Eccles, R. (2002). The powerful placebo in cough studies. *Pulmonary Pharmacology & Therapeutics*, *15*(3), 303–308. doi:10.1006/pupt.2002.0364 PMID:12099783

Egede, L. E., Ye, X., Zheng, D., & Silverstein, M. D. (2002). The prevalence and pattern of complementary and alternative medicine use in individuals with diabetes. *Diabetes Care*, *25*(2), 324–329. doi:10.2337/diacare.25.2.324 PMID:11815504

Ernst, E., & Cassileth, B. R. (1998). The prevalence of complementary/alternative medicine in cancer: A systematic review. *Cancer*, *83*(4), 777–782. doi:10.1002/(SICI)1097-0142(19980815)83:4<777::AID-CNCR22>3.0.CO;2-O PMID:9708945

Falkenberg, T., Lewith, G., Roberti di Sarsina, P., von Ammon, K., Santos-Rey, K., Hök, J., & Uehleke, B. et al. (2012). Towards a pan-European definition of complementary and alternative medicinea realistic ambition? *Forschende Komplementarmedizin*, *19*(s2), 6–8. doi:10.1159/000343812 PMID:23883939

Fischer, F. H., Lewith, G., Witt, C. M., Linde, K., von Ammon, K., Cardini, F., & Brinkhaus, B. et al. (2014). High prevalence but limited evidence in complementary and alternative medicine: Guidelines for future research. *BMC Complementary and Alternative Medicine*, *14*, 46.

Grabe, D. W., & Garrison, G. D. (2004). Comparison of natural product use between primary care and nephrology patients. *The Annals of Pharmacotherapy*, *38*(7-8), 1169–1172.

Guo, X., Willows, N., Kuhle, S., Jhangri, G., & Veugelers, P. J. (2009). Use of vitamin and mineral supplements among Canadian adults. *Canadian Journal of Public Health, 100*(4), 357–360. PMID:19994737

Harris, P. E., Cooper, K. L., Relton, C., & Thomas, K. J. (2012). Prevalence of complementary and alternative medicine (CAM) use by the general population: A systematic review and update. *International Journal of Clinical Practice*, *66*(10), 924–939. doi:10.1111/j.1742-1241.2012.02945.x PMID:22994327

Hess, S., De Geest, S., Halter, K., Dickenmann, M., & Denhaerynck, K. (2009). Prevalence and correlates of selected alternative and complementary medicine in adult renal transplant patients. *Clinical Transplantation*, *23*(1), 56–62. doi:10.1111/j.1399-0012.2008.00901.x PMID:18786136

House of Lords. (2000). *Complementary and alternative medicine: Science and technology, sixth report*. Author.

Kaptchuk, T. J., Friedlander, E., Kelley, J. M., Sanchez, M. N., Kokkotou, E., Singer, J. P., & Lembo, A. J. et al. (2010). Placebos without Deception: A Randomized Controlled Trial in Irritable Bowel Syndrome. *PLoS ONE*, *5*(12), e15591. doi:10.1371/journal.pone.0015591 PMID:21203519

Kaptchuk, T. J., Kelley, J. M., Conboy, L. A., Davis, R. B., Kerr, C. E., Jacobson, E. E., & Lembo, A. J. et al. (2008). Components of placebo effect: Randomised controlled trial in patients with irritable bowel syndrome. *BMJ (Clinical Research Ed.)*, *336*(7651), 999–1003. doi:10.1136/bmj.39524.439618.25 PMID:18390493

Kaptchuk, T. J., & Miller, F. (2015). Placebo Effects in Medicine. *The New England Journal of Medicine*, *373*(1), 8–9. doi:10.1056/NEJMp1504023 PMID:26132938

Kara, B. (2009). Herbal product use in a sample of Turkish patients undergoing haemodialysis. *Journal of Clinical Nursing*, *18*(15), 2197–2205. doi:10.1111/j.1365-2702.2008.02730.x PMID:19207805

Kidney Disease: Improving Global Outcome (KDIGO). (2012). KDIGO clinical practice guideline for the management of blood pressure in chronic kidney disease. *Kidney International. Supplement*, *2*(5), 340–397.

Kirsch, I. (2000). Are drug and placebo effects in depression additive? *Biological Psychiatry*, *47*(8), 733–735. doi:10.1016/S0006-3223(00)00832-5 PMID:10773181

Lee, J. S., & Kim, J. (2009). Factors affecting the use of dietary supplements by Korean adults: Data from the Korean National Health and Nutrition Examination Survey III. *Journal of the American Dietetic Association*, *109*(9), 1599–1605. doi:10.1016/j.jada.2009.06.374 PMID:19699841

Levine, M. A. H., Xu, S., Gaebel, K., Brazier, N., Bédard, M., Brazil, K., & MacLeod, S. M. et al. (2009). Self-reported use of natural health products: A cross-sectional telephone survey in older Ontarians. *The American Journal of Geriatric Pharmacotherapy*, *7*(6), 383–392. doi:10.1016/j.amjopharm.2009.12.003 PMID:20129259

Marques-Vidal, P., Pecoud, A., Hayoz, D., Paccaud, F., Mooser, V., Waeber, G., & Vollenweider, P. (2009). Prevalence and characteristics of vitamin or dietary supplement users in Lausanne, Switzerland: The CoLaus study. *European Journal of Clinical Nutrition*, *63*(2), 273–281. doi:10.1038/sj.ejcn.1602932 PMID:17940542

Melek, S., & Norris, D. (2008). *Chronic conditions and comorbid psychological disorders*. Milliman.

National Institute for Health and Care Excellence. (2012). *Process and methods guides: The guidelines manual*. Retrieved from www.nice.org.uk/Media/Default/About/what-we-do/our-programmes/developing-NICE-guidelines-the-manual.pdf

Nowack, R., Ballé, C., Birnkammer, F., Koch, W., Sessler, R., & Birck, R. (2009). Complementary and alternative medications consumed by renal patients in Southern Germany. *Journal of Renal Nutrition*, *19*(3), 211–219. doi:10.1053/j.jrn.2008.08.008 PMID:19251442

Ock, S. M., Choi, J. Y., Cha, Y. S., Lee, J., Chun, M. S., Huh, C. H., & Lee, S. J. et al. (2009). The use of complementary and alternative medicine in a general population in South Korea: Results from a national survey in 2006. *Journal of Korean Medical Science*, *24*(1), 1–6. doi:10.3346/jkms.2009.24.1.1 PMID:19270805

Osman, N. A., Hassanein, S. M., Leil, M. M., & NasrAllah, M. M. (2015). Complementary and alternative medicine use among patients with chronic kidney disease and kidney transplant recipients. *Journal of Renal Nutrition*, *25*(6), 466–471. doi:10.1053/j.jrn.2015.04.009 PMID:26093884

Park, J., White, A., Stevinson, C., Ernst, E., & James, M. (2002). Validating a new non-penetrating sham acupuncture devise: Two randomized controlled trials. *Acupuncture in Medicine*, *20*(4), 168–174. doi:10.1136/aim.20.4.168 PMID:12512790

Shah, S., Singh, N. P., & Qureshi, W. (2013). Prevalence of complementary and alternative medicine in patients with chronic kidney disease in India. *American Journal of Kidney Diseases*, *61*(4), B88. doi:10.1053/j.ajkd.2013.02.295

Singh, V., Raidoo, D. M., & Harries, C. S. (2004). The prevalence, patterns of usage and peoples attitude towards complementary and alternative medicine (CAM) among the Indian community in Chatsworth, South Africa. *BMC Complementary and Alternative Medicine*, *4*(1), 3. doi:10.1186/1472-6882-4-3 PMID:15018622

Spanner, E. D., & Duncan, A. M. (2005). Prevalence of dietary supplement use in adults with chronic renal insufficiency. *Journal of Renal Nutrition*, *15*(2), 204–210. doi:10.1053/j.jrn.2005.01.005 PMID:15827893

Tan, C. W., Christie, L., St-Georges, V., & Telford, N. (2009). Discrimination of real and sham acupuncture needles using the park sham device: A preliminary study. *Archives of Physical Medicine and Rehabilitation*, *90*(12), 2141–2145. doi:10.1016/j.apmr.2009.08.142 PMID:19969182

Tangkiatkumjai, M., Boardman, H., Praditpornsilpa, K., & Walker, D.-M. (2013). Prevalence of herbal and dietary supplement usage in Thai outpatients with chronic kidney disease: A cross-sectional survey. *BMC Complementary and Alternative Medicine*, *13*(1), 153. doi:10.1186/1472-6882-13-153 PMID:23815983

Tangkiatkumjai, M., Boardman, H., Praditpornsilpa, K., & Walker, D.-M. (2014). Reasons why Thai patients with chronic kidney disease use or do not use herbal and dietary supplements. *BMC Complementary and Alternative Medicine*, *14*(1), 473. doi:10.1186/1472-6882-14-473 PMID:25481733

Tangkiatkumjai, M., Boardman, H., & Walker, D.-M. (2017). *Comparing reasons for users and non-users of complementary and alternative medicine among various populations worldwide: a narrative review*. Unpublished.

Thomson, P., Jones, J., Evans, J. M., & Leslie, S. J. (2012). Factors influencing the use of complementary and alternative medicine and whether patients inform their primary care physician. *Complementary Therapies in Medicine*, *20*(1-2), 45–53. doi:10.1016/j.ctim.2011.10.001 PMID:22305248

Uehleke, B., Falkenberg, T., von Ammon, K., Lewith, G., Lazarus, A., & Roberti di Sarsina, P. (2012). *A pan-European research network for Complementary and Alternative Medicine*. CAMbrella.

Verhoef, M. J., Balneaves, L. G., Boon, H. S., & Vroegindewey, A. (2005). Reasons for and characteristics associated with complementary and alternative medicine use among adult cancer patients: A systematic review. *Integrative Cancer Therapies*, *4*(4), 274–286. doi:10.1177/1534735405282361 PMID:16282504

Walach, H. (2001). The efficacy paradox in randomised controlled trials of CAM and elsewhere: Beware of the placebo trap. *Journal of Alternative and Complementary Medicine (New York, N.Y.)*, *7*(3), 213–218. doi:10.1089/107555301300328070 PMID:11439833

Wazaify, M., Alawwa, I., Yasein, N., Al-Saleh, A., & Afifi, F. U. (2013). Complementary and alternative medicine (CAM) use among Jordanian patients with chronic diseases. *Complementary Therapies in Clinical Practice*, *19*(3), 153–157. doi:10.1016/j.ctcp.2013.03.001 PMID:23890462

Zyoud, S. H., Al-Jabi, S. W., Sweileh, W. M., Tabeeb, G. H., Ayaseh, N. A., Sawafta, M. N., & Awang, R. et al. (2016). Use of complementary and alternative medicines in haemodialysis patients: A cross-sectional study from Palestine. *BMC Complementary and Alternative Medicine*, *16*(1), 204. doi:10.1186/s12906-016-1196-8 PMID:27400742

KEY TERMS AND DEFINITIONS

Alternative Medicine: A healing method used instead of orthodox treatment.

Complementary Medicine: A technique that is used along with conventional medicine.

Evidence: Information indicating a fact is true and valid.

Integrative Medicine: The combination of complementary or alternative technique with conventional medicine.

Nocebo: Negative response to a treatment due to psychological factors.

Placebo Effect: The positive effect that a treatment or intervention has on a patient that has no treatment properties, but works based on the patient's belief.

Regulation: A directive made by an authority or organization with authority in a field.

Traditional Medicine: Healthcare practices based on theories, beliefs and principles owned by a specific culture.

Chapter 2
CAM Use From Western and Asian Perspectives:
Overview of Different Cultural Beliefs of CAM Medicine and Prevalence of Use

Dawn-Marie Walker
University of Southampton, UK

Mayuree Tangkiatkumjai
Srinakharinwirot University, Thailand

ABSTRACT

This chapter will discuss the impact on the provision and integration of complementary and alternative medicine (CAM) into the patient's medical pathway and in turn, the prevalence of usage, not only for treatment but also prevention. Similarities and differences of these issues between Western and Asian perspectives will be presented. The authors will provide an overview of regulatory organisations which influence this provision, as well as advertising within the cultures which will have impact on belief of efficacy, which in turn will increase the placebo effect (thereby increasing efficacy). Due to a lack of evidence for CAM advertising in Asian cultures, further research is needed.

DOI: 10.4018/978-1-5225-2882-1.ch002

GENERAL PERSPECTIVES ON CAM

With a long history of complementary and alternative medicine (CAM) use in certain cultures, CAM appears far more integrated in some nations rather than others. This integration seems to be due to the concurrent use of CAM with the development of orthodox medicine. Also CAM emerged prior to the need for evidence based medicine, which demands a significant p-value in a randomised controlled trial. CAM had built a good anecdotal evidence base by the time orthodox medicine emerged, which then enabled its use to be maintained over recent years within certain cultures, such as Asian ones. For example, the Thai population began to use herbal medicine for the treatment of various symptoms and diseases and for promoting well-being before 1238 A.D (He, 2015). Indeed, Thai traditional medicine has been the main intervention for health care until the early 20th. Century (Chokevivat, & Chuthaputti, A. 2005). Prior to this, traditional Chinese medicine (TCM) was born in the Chinese culture with its roots within a philosophy such as Buddhism, more than 2,500 years ago (He, 2015). During the Ming and Qing dynasties (1368AD-1911AD) thanks to the advancement of paper making and printing, TCM spread to other countries of the Western continent (He, 2015). However, as the word spread from Asia about TCM, so the news reached Asia about orthodox medicine, leading to a change in cultural beliefs. In 1928, the Central Committee on Hygiene of China, put forward a motion to 'abolish Chinese medicine in order to remove the obstacles to the cause of orthodox medicine and hygiene.' (Wang, 2013). In 1949, the People's Republic of China, outlawed the use of Chinese medicine in hospitals, and during the Cultural Revolution in 1966-1976 many practitioners were either jailed or killed (Wang, 2013). Therefore, in 1976, a document was submitted to the Chinese government, saying that there were almost no traditional doctors left (Wang, 2013). This led to the establishment in 1979 of the National Association of Chinese Medicine, and many traditional texts were edited and republished (Wang, 2013). Now CAM use, especially TCM, is accepted more by governments in Asian rather than Western areas (Bautista, et al., 2011). For example, there is still a department within the Ministry of Public Health in China, specifically dealing with TCM (Hesketh & Zhu, 1997). Its aim is to support the use and integration of TCM within cultures and to create a framework in which CAM can be delivered. Today, China is regarded as one of the most integrated health systems in the world where TCM is embedded within medical training (Chung et al., 2011). Furthermore, a study found that 82% of orthodox medical doctors in China had referred patients to TCM practitioners (Harmsworth & Lewith, 2001), compared to 41% in the UK (Lewith, et al., 2001).

PREVALENCE OF CAM USE

The prevalence of the use of CAM varies between countries due to economic, cultural and social factors. For example, in countries where CAM has cultural and historical influences, such as Singapore and Korea, although orthodox health care systems are quite well established, 76% and 86% of their population still use TCM (World Health Organisation, 2012). CAMs are widely used and valued around the globe. These medicines, which are often proven to be safe, ensures that all people have access to care, when many have no access to orthodox medicine. For example, the ratio of traditional healers to population in Africa is 1:500 whilst to medical doctors it is 1:40,000 (Abdullahi, 2011). Indeed for many millions of people, herbal medicines and traditional treatments are the main, and sometimes only source of healthcare (World Health Organisation, 2014). Furthermore, it is argued that CAM may reduce healthcare costs and contribute to the economic development of a number of countries, thanks to not only the agriculture incentive to grow herbs, but also to the internet which has made buying herbs and other CAM products easier globally (World Health Organisation, 2014).

The use of CAM is highest in East Asian countries such as Japan with 76% of patients using CAM (Yamashita, et al., 2002), Malaysia with 69.4% (Siti, et al., 2009), and South Korea with 74.8% using CAM (Ock, et al., 2009). A study in India found that 89% of the doctors which responded to their survey had used CAM (Telles, et al., 2011). A report on the prevalence of use in 2007 in the US, found that 38.8% (83 million) adults and 11.8% (8.5 million) children used CAM (Barnes, et al., 2008), with the estimated total out of pocket expense on CAM for adults in 2007 being approximately $33.9 billion per year (Nahin, et al., 2009) with the most common condition treated being described as musculoskeletal (Barnes, et al., 2008). Whilst in Australia, the number of people reporting to have consulted a CAM therapist in the two weeks prior to being questioned rose from 500,000 in 1995, to 750,000 in 2005 (Australian Bureau of Statistics, 2008). Indeed, Australia has some of the highest CAM usage in the developed world (Andrews, et al., 2012), with visits to CAM practitioners accounting for about ½ of all health consultations (Xue, et al., 2007). In some geographical areas there are more CAM practitioners than medical ones (Wardle, et al., 2011), especially in rural areas (Wardle, et al., 2012). In the UK, the prevalence of use in the population ranges from 41% - 50% (Posadzki, et al., 2013), where a survey found that herbal medicine was the most popular CAM used.

Worldwide, acupuncture seems to be one of the most used and recognised CAMs. According to the World Health Organisation (2014), Acupuncture was recognised in 80% of its 129 member states, although there are many other traditional medicines from Asia used in Western countries, such as Traditional Chinese Medicine, or Ayurvedic medicine from India. The increasing prevalence of CAM use in Western cultures, is not only due to the growing awareness of CAM, but also to the spread of complex multi-factorial chronic diseases and comorbidities. For example, in England, the number of people with comorbidities is set to rise from 1.9 million in 2008, to 2.9 million by 2018 (Department of Health, 2012). This rise in comorbidities is, in turn, related to the rise of people living with chronic conditions. The global burden of chronic diseases was 46% in 2001 (World Health Organization, 2002) which is expected to rise to 57% by 2020 (World Health Organization, 2002). In the US, the presence of a chronic disease is the main cause of disability and is the main reason why people seek health care, taking up 70% of all healthcare spending (Holman & Lorig, 2000). CAM appears to be an excellent option for this relentless rise of chronic disease globally (World Health Organization, 2014), and it is seen by people as effective for the treatment of chronic conditions, though not superior to orthodox medicine (Vincent & Furnham, 1994). Also, being that co-morbidities arise alongside chronic conditions, this supports the need of an holistic approach to care, which is at the heart of any CAM therapy.

PERCEIVED CAM EFFECTIVENESS AND SAFETY

Major factors influencing the use of CAM in both Western and Asian countries are social, cultural, medical reasons, and costs of health care (Table 1). A study which compared the attitudes of patients attending a CAM clinic, to those visiting a General Practitioner's surgery, found that the CAM patients believed in the impact of psychological factors on a physical illness (which denotes the belief in, and need for, holistic approaches), and were more fearful of the harmful effects of orthodox medicine (Vincent & Furnham, 1997). They see CAM as 'natural', and 'better than taking drugs' as there are less side effects (Williamson, et al., 2008). This belief in holism, has been borne out in further research (Barrett et al., 2004; Bishop, et al., 2007). People may also use CAM when in good health to keep that status. For example, an Australian survey study found that 61% of the CAM users who responded described their health as very good/excellent, compared to 50% of the general Australian population (Williamson, et al., 2008). The CAM users may feel in good shape because they use CAM to prevent diseases.

Another Australian cross-sectional study found that consumers of CAM thought differently about CAMs when asked to compare them to orthodox medicine. They saw them as 'natural' and a holistic way of achieving and maintaining good health. They also saw them as 'safer' (Williamson, et al., 2008). People who use CAM are more likely to have healthy behaviours such as eating the recommended amount of fruit and vegetables, and exercising (Australian Bureau of Statistics, 2008). Whereas a person who has a very positive attitude to science, will believe in orthodox medicine more (Vincent & Furnham, 1997). Regarding information seeking on CAMs, the process seemed to be biased in that 56% of respondents seek information regarding benefits, but only 24% seek information on adverse effects (Vincent & Furnham, 1997). This is possibly linked to their perception that CAM is 'safer'. They mainly obtain information about CAM from people they know (55%) and the internet (51%).

However, although the benefits of CAM are recognized, CAM is mostly thought of as complementary rather than alternative in Western cultures. For example, just under one third of respondents to a survey in Australia who had visited a CAM therapist, had visited an orthodox doctor within the 2 weeks prior, rising to 63% within the 3 months prior (Australian Bureau of Statistics, 2008). CAM is commonly used in developed societies as an adjunct therapy to orthodox medicine for chronic diseases such as cancers (Harris, et al., 2003; Molassiotis, et al., 2005), where it has been found that 91% of patients who have received chemo or radiotherapy had received some sort of CAM (Yates, et al., 2005). In Western cultures, people often turn to CAM when orthodox medicine has failed (Sharples, et al., 2003; Williamson, et al., 2008), such as to self-manage chronic conditions such as back pain (National Institute for Health and Clinical Excellence (NICE), 2009). NICE, in the UK, write guidelines which medical doctors turn to for advice in delivering care. The NICE guideline for low back pain treatment, suggests treating adults with opioids (NICE, 2009), despite a meta-analyses of opioids compared to placebo showing no significant effect for treating chronic back pain (Martell, et al., 2007). Therefore, although people may utilize orthodox medicine initially, they may turn to CAM due to unsatisfactory results, or medication side effects. Opioids can cause nausea and may cause addiction if taken over an extended period of time for example.

The use of CAM in Western cultures is linked to affordability of CAM, therefore usage is often linked to whether the therapy is covered by insurance or provided free of charge by the national healthcare provider. In Australia for example, 66% of people who had visited a chiropractor, had this therapy covered by their health insurance (Australian Bureau of Statistics, 2008). In the UK, CAM is not routinely provided by the National Health Service (NHS) (their health care provider), thus only 1/3 of GPs had referred a patient for a CAM in 2000 (Thomas, et al., 2001). Instead CAM had been provided by either one of the primary health care team, or a therapist who is employed by the GP practice (Thomas, et al., 2001). Indeed, in the UK, although 1 in 10 of the adult population have used CAM, 90% of this was delivered outside of the NHS (Thomas, et al., 2001). Cost issues such as these has led to most CAM users in Western societies being higher educated and belonging to a middle to high income bracket (Barnes, et al., 2008; Williamson, et al., 2008).

In many Asian cultures, CAM is not perceived as a complementary medicine, and instead is the main form of health care (Peltzer, et al., 2016). Asian people perceive CAM as the only type of medicine and use it for treating both acute and chronic illnesses (Pandey, et al., 2013; Sydara, et al., 2005; Tangkiatkumjai, et al., 2014). In Asia herbal medicine is the most frequently used CAM followed by acupuncture, and massage. Some types of CAM are embedded in Asian countries because they are affordable, such as TCM in China and Vietnam, Ayurvedic medicine in India, and herbal medicine in Thailand, Laos and Cambodia (Table 1). There are different characteristics of CAM users in Asian populations, compared with Western populations; Asian users are ordinary people, not wealthy or educated (Tangkiatkumjai, et al., 2014). However, some CAMs which are imported from other countries, such as dietary supplements, are expensive (Tangkiatkumjai, et al., 2014). Thus, affordability is not always the reason why Asians use CAM. Most Asian people frequently use traditional medicine for their self-care management. Due to the close knit family culture in Asian countries, it is common that parents give traditional medicine to their children; relatives recommend that their family members use CAM; or friends suggest CAM to a member of their social network. Therefore, the social network strongly influences decision regarding CAM use in Asian cultures when compared with Western cultures

Table 1. Common factors that influence CAM use between Western and Asian populations

Factors	Western	Asian
Perspective on CAM	Holistic approach	Familiarity and trust
Culture	Scientific base	Traditional base
Common access to health system	Orthodox medicine	Traditional medicine
Affordability of orthodox medicine	Fully	Limited
Affordability of CAM	Expensive	Cheap
Medical reasons for CAM use	- Failure or dissatisfaction with orthodox medicine	Efficacy and safety of CAM
	- Efficacy and safety of CAM	
	- CAMs complement orthodox medicine	

(Tangkiatkumjai, et al., 2016). Other factors linked to CAM use in Asian cultures are similar to those in Western cultures; CAM is used for both the promotion of well-being and treatment of illnesses, and is perceived as being safer than orthodox medicine. In many Asian countries orthodox medicine is widely available, so their citizens are likely to use CAM as a complement to orthodox medicine when affected by chronic diseases.

DISCLOSURE OF CAM USE

In an Australian cross sectional study, only 50% of respondents who used CAM told their doctors, or discussed this with them (Williamson, et al., 2008). This disclosure is even lower in the USA where about 38% of those using CAM tell their doctor (Eisenberg, et al., 1998). However, although one may assume that disclosure would be higher in a culture where CAM is embedded, this is not necessarily the case. A study in 2001 found no significant difference in the rate of disclosure between elderly Japanese and elderly US patients (Flaherty, et al., 2001), whilst 84% of respondents in CAM users in Singapore didn't tell their doctor (Lee, et al., 2004). In contrast, Western patients with chronic kidney disease or end-stage renal disease are more likely to inform their doctor about CAM use (Bonevski, et al., 2008; Nowack, et al., 2009; Tangkiatkumjai, et al., 2016), compared with renal patients in Asian and Middle Eastern countries (Kara, 2009; Osman, et al., 2015; Tangkiatkumjai, et al., 2013).

REGULATION OF CAM

Due to this increased awareness and use of CAM in Western cultures, there has been a concurrent need for legislation for the safe use of CAM. The most notable legislation has grown around the use of herbal medicines. As herbal medicines are ingested, arguably herb use poses a higher risk to public health, for example if they were poisonous. Some CAM practitioners will argue that the efficacy of their intervention is, in part, due to having the possibility of altering their treatments according to the symptomatology and unique requirements of the patient. However, if the CAM is to be ingested, such as in the case of herbal medicine, quick fix adjustments are not possible in Western cultures as there are very strict regulations over the freedom to prescribe and take these herbs. They need to be tested and a safety profile of them developed. Without this, one wouldn't be able to prescribe them, and also wouldn't be able to buy them in Western countries. Meanwhile, herbal medicine assumes the form of freely available plants in Asian countries. People sometimes collect it from tropical forests or their gardens, to self-manage their health. Crude herbal medicine is classified as dietary and a specific legislation is not required. Herbal medicines which are transformed from the original plants however, need to be registered similar to Western countries, although Asian laws are less strict than European (EU) legislation. The World Health Organisation (WHO) is still working on a global harmonised regulation of herbal medicine under the International Regulatory Cooperation for Herbal Medicines (IRCH). Currently, there are regional regulatory networks, in Europe and Asia.

Regulation of CAM Practitioners

There are various regulatory bodies governing CAM practice. For example, there are 28 different systems of regulation of CAM in the EU alone, however most of these are self monitoring and voluntary. Regulation of CAM practice in Europe varies from country to country, for example in the UK only two CAM professions are subject to statutory regulation, i.e. osteophathy and chiropractic. Indeed a report in 2012 stated 'The only common factor we have found across all 39 nations is the amazing ability they have demonstrated of structuring legislations and regulation differently in every single country, no matter how small the size of the population (Fonnebo, 2012, page 9). Due to this lack of regulation, anyone can practice CAM (excluding the above mentioned regulated ones). However, in the absence of formal regulation, various professional bodies have developed their own regulatory system, including registers of practitioners who abide by their code of ethics and who have the correct experience and/or qualifications, for example, The Dutch Council of Classical Homeopathy has set educational requirements in line with the European Council for Classical Homeopathy. There has been work however to standardise regulation across Europe which is inclusive of all treatment modalities. It is argued that this will need to be voluntary rather than EU wide, as the EU have consistently reiterated that they will leave this matter to the individual country (Fonnebo, 2012). In south Asian countries however, they are much more harmonious with over 70% of the countries having policy and regulation and therefore are world leaders in regards to policy development and research (WHO, 2005). In accordance with this, often their requirements for practitioner qualifications/experience are stringent. For example, in Japan most practitioners must complete at least 3 years of training (King's Fund, 2008). Furthermore, in some countries, including Japan and Germany, training in CAM is a formal part of the curriculum for medical practitioners (King's Fund, 2008). Many countries who have a practitioner register or license, also have requirements for continuing professional development (King's Fund, 2008).

EU LEGISLATION FOR HERBAL MEDICINAL PRODUCTS

EU legislation was introduced in 2004 and is similar to legislation on pharmaceutical products for human use. The legislation aimed to safeguard public health, and facilitate the free movement of herbal products across the EU. They simplified this process by stating that if an herbal medicine has been used over the previous 30 years, and 15 of those in an EU community, they would not need to obtain and provide data from trials regarding safety or efficacy. They would however need to obtain EU approval. This approval includes a review of safety carried out by a doctor, pharmacist, or herbal practitioner, a summary of the product's characteristics, assurance of appropriate manufacturing standards, and the submission of patient appropriate information about the herb, together with a fee of over £2,000. There are over 100 herbal medicinal products approved. The list of herbs which are already approved is available at: www.gov.uk/government/publications/herbal-medicines-granted-a-traditional-herbal-registration-thr/herbal-medicines-granted-a-traditional-herbal-registration [last accessed 24/03/17] which includes herbs such as Arnica, black cohosh, and St. John's Wort. There is also a list of banned or restricted herbs: www.gov.uk/government/publications/list-of-banned-or-restricted-herbal-ingredients-for-medicinal-use/banned-and-restricted-herbal-ingredients [last accessed 24/03/17]. Evidence of whether the herb is effective or not, is not required. If an herbal medicine product has obtained the approval, it will be registered under the Traditional Herbal Registration scheme. All products which are registered should have a logo incorporating the initials THR. This logo denotes that the product has met the quality standards related to safety and manufacturing. However, this is only a requirement in the EU.

The only herbal medicines exempt from this authorization are those unlicensed remedies that are made up for a patient following a consultation with an herbalist. However, these herbalists need to be registered, such as with The National Institute of Medical Herbalists in the UK.

ASEAN LEGISLATION FOR HERBAL MEDICINAL PRODUCTS

In 2015, the Association of Southeast Asian Nations (ASEAN) Economic Community was established and launched the ASEAN Harmonisation of Traditional Medicines and Health Supplements (TMHS) initiative. The TMHS is developing the ASEAN guidelines on limits of contaminants for herbal and dietary supplements (HDS), stability and shelf-life of HDS, safety and efficacy of HDS, also good manufacturing practice and labelling requirements for HDS (Health Sciences Authority, 2015). It will be implemented in 2021.

With respect to the efficacy of traditional medicine and health supplements, claims of traditional medicines are classified into 3 types: traditional health use, traditional treatment, and scientifically established treatment. The first two types require well-documented traditional use to prove their efficacy. Traditional use for health maintenance is defined as the use of traditional medicine for at least 40 years by a general population. Approving the efficacy via the third type needs human studies which may be supplemented by non-clinical studies. Meanwhile, claims of health supplements are classified into i) general or nutritional, ii) functional, and iii) disease risk reduction. Functional claims require published and unpublished studies and should be supported by empirical or historical data. Disease risk reduction claims need human studies which may be supplemented with non-clinical studies. The safety of most products is argued by anecdotes and documents regarding historical use. However, a new ingredient or new combination of the products requires additional scientific evidence, including toxicity data from animal and/or human studies, to prove their safety (WHO, 2014).

ADVERTISING CAM

Not only do beliefs, cultures, and traditions influence CAM use, but also CAM advertising via television, radio, newspaper, and the internet. The mass media have mainly advertised positive effects of CAM and poorly report CAM risks (Weeks & Strudsholm, 2008). They commonly cite evidence from anecdotes. CAM advertising via newspapers, the internet or television in Australia was analysed for accuracy and sufficiency of information. This showed a lack of data about the efficacy, safety and costs of CAM (Bonevski, et al., 2008). However, Bonevski et al. did not critique the accuracy of CAM information. Therefore, it raises concerns about the data quality and health care providers should warn their patients of this.

Both Western and Asian health providers have growing concerns about misleading or deceptive claims for CAM and report many complaints about these issues (Smith, et al., 2014; Wardle, et al., 2014). For example, there was a report that a patient with chronic kidney disease died during detoxification programme in Australia. Media influence may also cause indirect harm, such as delaying diagnosis and financial exploitation. CAM regulations worldwide are still tackling this problem. Further research is required due to a lack of studies assessing the quality of CAM advertising in Asian countries.

CONCLUSION

The prevalence of CAM has been increasing worldwide. Affluent and well educated Westerners are more likely to use CAM, whilst there are no differences in characteristics between CAM users and non-users in Asian populations. This is due to CAM having been embedded in Asian cultures for a long time and is no longer considered an alternative medicine. Social, cultural, and medical reasons, advertising, and costs of health care mainly influence people's choice on their use of CAM. The tone of the mass media is commonly positive and there is a lack of reporting on the risks of using CAM. Misleading and deceptive advertising about CAM is a major concern, which regulatory bodies worldwide are attempting to deal with.

REFERENCES

Abdullahi, A. A. (2011). Trends and Challenges of Traditional Medicine in Africa. *African Journal of Traditional, Complementary, and Alternative Medicines*, *8*(5Suppl), 115–123. PMID:22754064

Andrews, G., Adams, J., Segrott, J., & Lui, C. (2012). The Profile of Complementary and Alternative Medicine Users and Reasons for Complementary and Alternative Medicine Use. In J. Adams, G. Andrews, J. Barnes, P. Magin, & A. Broom (Eds.), *Traditional, Complementary and Integrative Medicine: An International Reader*. London: Palgrave Macmillan. doi:10.1007/978-1-137-26559-3_2

Australian Bureau of Statistics. (2008). *Australian Social Trends, 2008: Complementary therapies*. Retrieved from www.abs.gov.au/AUSSTATS/abs@.nsf/Lookup/4102.0Chapter5202008

Barnes, P. M., Bloom, B., & Nahin, R. L. (2008). *Complementary and alternative medicine use among adults and children: United States, 2007*. Hyattsville, MD: National Center for Health Statistics.

Barrett, B., Marchand, L., Scheder, J., Plane, M. B., Maberry, R., Appelbaum, D., & Rabago, D. et al. (2004). Themes of Holism, Empowerment, Access, and Legitimacy Define Complementary, Alternative, and Integrative Medicine in Relation to Conventional Biomedicine. *Journal of Alternative and Complementary Medicine (New York, N.Y.)*, *9*(6), 937–947. doi:10.1089/107555303771952271 PMID:14736364

Bautista, C., Joubert, R., & Moehler, T. (2011). *CAM use in Asia-Pacific*. Retrieved from www.appliedclinicaltrialsonline.com/cam-use-asia-pacific

Bishop, F. L., Yardley, L., & Lewith, G. T. (2007). A systematic review of beliefs involved in the use of complementary and alternative medicine. *Journal of Health Psychology*, *12*(6), 851–867. doi:10.1177/1359105307082447 PMID:17956965

Bonevski, B., Wilson, A., & Henry, D. A. (2008). An analysis of News media coverage of complementary and alternative medicine. *PLoS ONE*, *3*(6), e2406. doi:10.1371/journal.pone.0002406 PMID:18545688

Chokevivat, V., & Chuthaputti. (2005). *The Role of Thai Traditional Medicine in Health Promotion.* Dept. for the Development of Thai Traditional and Alternative Medicine, Ministry of Public Health, 6GCHP Bangkok.

Chung, V. C., Hillier, S., Lau, C. H., Wong, S. Y., Yeoh, E. K., & Griffiths, S. M. (2011). Referral to and attitude towards traditional Chinese medicine amongst western medical doctors in postcolonial Hong Kong. *Social Science & Medicine*, *72*(2), 247–255. doi:10.1016/j.socscimed.2010.10.021 PMID:21145150

Department of Health. (2012). *Long Term Conditions Compendium of Information* (3rd. ed.). Retrieved from www.gov.uk/government/uploads/system/uploads/attachment_data/file/216528/dh_134486.pdf

Eisenberg, D. M., Davis, R. B., Ettner, S. L., Appel, S., Wilkey, S., Van Rompay, M., & Kessler, R. C. (1998). Trends in Alternative Medicine Use in the United States, 1990-1999: 7 Results of a Follow-up National Survey. *Journal of the American Medical Association*, *280*(18), 1569–1575. doi:10.1001/jama.280.18.1569 PMID:9820257

Flaherty, J. H., Takahashi, R., Teoh, J., Kim, J. I., Habib, S., Ito, M., & Matsushita, S. (2001). Use of Alternative Therapies in Older Outpatients in the United States and Japan: Prevalence, Reporting Patterns, and Perceived Effectiveness. *J Geron: Medical Sciences*, *56A*(10), M650–M655. doi:10.1093/gerona/56.10.M650 PMID:11584039

Fonnebo, V. (2012). *Legal status and regulation of CAM in Europe*. Retrieved from www.cam-europe.eu/dms/files/CAMbrella_Reports/CAMbrella-WP2-part_1final.pdf

Harmsworth, K., & Lewith, G. (2001). Attitudes to traditional Chinese medicine amongst western trained doctors in the Peoples Republic of China. *Social Science & Medicine*, *52*(1), 149–153. doi:10.1016/S0277-9536(00)00124-6 PMID:11144912

Harris, P., Finlay, I. G., Cook, A., Thomas, K. J., & Hood, K. (2003). Complementary and alternative medicine use by patients with cancer in Wales: A cross sectional survey. *Complementary Therapies in Medicine*, *11*(4), 249–253. doi:10.1016/S0965-2299(03)00126-2 PMID:15022659

He, K. (2015). Traditional Chinese and Thai medicine in a comparative perspective. *Complementary Therapies in Medicine*, *23*(6), 821–826. doi:10.1016/j.ctim.2015.10.003 PMID:26645523

Health Sciences Authority. (2015). *ASEAN Harmonization of Traditional Medicines and Health Supplements*. Retrieved from www.hsa.gov.sg/content/hsa/en/Health_Products_Regulation/Complementary_Health_Products/Overview/ASEAN_Harmonization_of_Traditional_Medicines_and_Health_Supplements.html

Hesketh, T., & Zhu, W. X. (1997). Traditional Chinese Medicine: One Country Two Systems. *BMJ (Clinical Research Ed.)*, *315*(7100), 115–117. doi:10.1136/bmj.315.7100.115 PMID:9240055

Holman, H., & Lorig, K. (2000). Patients as partners in managing chronic disease. *BMJ (Clinical Research Ed.)*, *320*(7234), 526–527. doi:10.1136/bmj.320.7234.526 PMID:10688539

Kara, B. (2009). Herbal product use in a sample of Turkish patients undergoing haemodialysis. *Journal of Clinical Nursing*, *18*(15), 2197–2205. doi:10.1111/j.1365-2702.2008.02730.x PMID:19207805

King's Fund. (2008). *Regulating Complementary Medical Practitioners*. Retrieved from www.kingsfund.org.uk/sites/files/kf/Research%20summary1.pdf

Lee, G. B. W., Charn, T. C., Chew, Z. H., & Ng, T. P. (2004). Complementary and alternative medicine use in patients with chronic diseases in primary care is associated with perceived quality of care and cultural beliefs. *Family Practice*, *21*(6), 654–660. doi:10.1093/fampra/cmh613 PMID:15531625

Lewith, G. T., Hyland, M., & Gray, S. F. (2001). Attitudes to and use of complementary medicine among physicians in the United Kingdom. *Complementary Therapies in Medicine*, *9*(3), 167–172. doi:10.1054/ctim.2001.0475 PMID:11926430

Martell, B. A., OConnor, P. G., Kerns, R. D., Becker, W. C., Morales, K. H., Kosten, T. R., & Fiellin, D. A. (2007). Systematic Review: Opioid Treatment for Chronic Back Pain: Prevalence, Efficacy, and Association with Addiction. *Annals of Internal Medicine*, *146*(2), 116–127. doi:10.7326/0003-4819-146-2-200701160-00006 PMID:17227935

Molassiotis, A., Fernadez-Ortega, P., Pud, D., Ozden, G., Scott, J. A., & Panteli, V. et al.. (2005). Use of complementary and alternative medicine in cancer patients: A European survey. *Annals of Oncology*, *16*(4), 655–663. doi:10.1093/annonc/mdi110 PMID:15699021

Nahin, R. L., Barnes, P. M., Stussman, B. J., & Bloom, B. (2009). Costs of complementary and alternative medicine (CAM) and frequency of visits to CAM practitioners: United States, 2007. *National Health Statistics Reports*, (18): 1–14. PMID:19771719

National Institute for Health and Clinical Excellence (NICE). (2009). *Early management of persistent non-specific low back pain: NICE clinical guideline 88.* Retrieved from www.nice.org.uk/guidance/cg88?unlid=78007570201689060

Nowack, R., Ballé, C., Birnkammer, F., Koch, W., Sessler, R., & Birck, R. (2009). Complementary and alternative medications consumed by renal patients in Southern Germany. *Journal of Renal Nutrition*, *19*(3), 211–219. doi:10.1053/j.jrn.2008.08.008 PMID:19251442

Ock, S. M., Choi, J. Y., Cha, Y. S., Lee, J., Chun, M. S., Huh, C. J., & Lee, S. J. et al. (2009). The Use of Complementary and Alternative Medicine in a General Population in South Korea: Results from a National Survey in 2006. *Journal of Korean Medical Science*, *24*(1), 1–6. doi:10.3346/jkms.2009.24.1.1 PMID:19270805

Osman, N. A., Hassanein, S. M., Leil, M. M., & NasrAllah, M. M. (2015). Complementary and alternative medicine use among patients with chronic kidney disease and kidney transplant recipients. *Journal of Renal Nutrition*, *25*(6), 466–471. doi:10.1053/j.jrn.2015.04.009 PMID:26093884

Pandey, M. M., Rastogi, S., & Rawat, A. K. S. (2013). Indian traditional Ayurvedic system of medicine and nutritional supplementation. *Evidence-Based Complementary and Alternative Medicine*, *2013*, 376327. doi:10.1155/2013/376327 PMID:23864888

Peltzer, K., Pengpid, S., Puckpinyo, A., Yi, S., & Anh, L. V. (2016). The utilization of traditional, complementary and alternative medicine for non-communicable diseases and mental disorders in health care patients in Cambodia, Thailand, and Vietnam. *BMC Complementary and Alternative Medicine*, *16*(1), 92. doi:10.1186/s12906-016-1078-0 PMID:26952043

Posadzki, P., Watson, L. K., & Ernst, E. (2013). Prevalence of use of complementary and alternative medicine (CAM) by patients/consumers in the UK: Systematic review of surveys. *Clinical Medicine (London, England), 13*(2), 126–131. doi:10.7861/clinmedicine.13-2-126 PMID:23681857

Sharples, F. M. C., Van Haselen, R., & Fisher, P. (2003). NHS patients perspective on complementary medicine: A survey. *Complementary Therapies in Medicine, 11*(4), 243–248. doi:10.1016/S0965-2299(03)00107-9 PMID:15022657

Siti, Z. M., Tahir, A., Farah, A., Fazlin, S. M., Sondi, S., Azman, A. H., & Zaleha, W. C. W. et al. (2009). Use of traditional and complementary medicine in Malaysia: A baseline study. *Complementary Therapies in Medicine, 17*(5-6), 292–299. doi:10.1016/j.ctim.2009.04.002 PMID:19942109

Smith, A., Jogalekar, S., & Gibson, A. (2014). Regulation of natural health products in Canada. *Journal of Ethnopharmacology, 158*, 507–510. doi:10.1016/j.jep.2014.06.037 PMID:24969823

Sydara, K., Gneunphonsavath, S., Wahlström, R., Freudenthal, S., Houamboun, K., Tomson, G., & Falkenberg, T. (2005). Use of traditional medicine in Lao PDR. *Complementary Therapies in Medicine, 13*(3), 199–205. doi:10.1016/j.ctim.2005.05.004 PMID:16150374

Tangkiatkumjai, M., Boardman, H., Praditpornsilpa, K., & Walker, D.-M. (2013). Prevalence of herbal and dietary supplement usage in Thai outpatients with chronic kidney disease: A cross-sectional survey. *BMC Complementary and Alternative Medicine, 13*(1), 153. doi:10.1186/1472-6882-13-153 PMID:23815983

Tangkiatkumjai, M., Boardman, H., & Walker, D.-M. (2014). Herbal and dietary supplement use in Bangkok: A survey. *J Complement Integr Med, 11*(3), 203–211. PMID:24914729

Tangkiatkumjai, M., Boardman, H., & Walker, D-M. (2016). *Comparison of reasons for users and non-uses of complementary and alternative medicine among various populations worldwide: A narrative review*. Manuscript submitted for publication (CTIM-D-14-00500R1).

Telles, S., Gaur, V., Sharma, S., & Balkrishna, A. (2011). Attitude of Conventional and CAM Physicians Toward CAM in India. *Journal of Alternative and Complementary Medicine (New York, N.Y.), 17*(11), 1069–1073. doi:10.1089/acm.2010.0407 PMID:22070443

Thomas, K., Nicholl, J., & Coleman, P. (2001). Use and expenditure on complementary medicine in England: A population based survey. *Complementary Therapies in Medicine*, *9*(1), 2–11. doi:10.1054/ctim.2000.0407 PMID:11264963

Thomas, K. J., Nicholl, J., & Fall, M. (2001). Access to complementary medicine via general practice. *The British Journal of General Practice*, *51*(462), 25–30. PMID:11271869

Vincent, C. A., & Furnham, A. (1994). The perceived efficacy of orthodox and complementary medicine: Preliminary findings and the development of a questionnaire. *Complementary Therapies in Medicine*, *2*, 128–134. doi:10.1016/0965-2299(94)90110-4

Vincent, C. A., & Furnham, A. (1997). The perceived efficacy of complementary and orthodox medicine: A replication. *Complementary Therapies in Medicine*, *5*(2), 85–89. doi:10.1016/S0965-2299(97)80004-0

Wang, J. H. (2013). *Historical Timeline of Chinese Medicine*. Retrieved from www.traditionalstudies.org/historical-timeline-of-chinese-medicine/

Wardle, J., Adams, J., Soares Magalhães, R. J., & Sibbritt, D. (2011). Distribution of complementary and alternative medicine (CAM) providers in rural New South Wales, Australia: A step towards explaining high CAM use in rural health?. *The Australian Journal of Rural Health*, *19*(4), 197–204. doi:10.1111/j.1440-1584.2011.01200.x PMID:21771161

Wardle, J., Lui, C. W., & Adams, J. (2012). Complementary and alternative medicine in rural communities: Current research and future directions. *The Journal of Rural Health*, *28*(1), 101–112. doi:10.1111/j.1748-0361.2010.00348.x PMID:22236320

Wardle, J., Weir, M., Marshall, B., & Archer, E. (2014). Regulatory and legislative protections for consumers in complementary medicine: Lessons from Australian policy and legal developments. *European Journal of Internal Medicine*, *6*(4), 423–433.

Weeks, L. C., & Strudsholm, T. (2008). A scoping review of research on complementary and alternative medicine (CAM) and the mass media: Looking back, moving forward. *BMC Complementary and Alternative Medicine*, *8*(1), 43. doi:10.1186/1472-6882-8-43 PMID:18638413

Williamson, M., Tudball, J., Toms, M., Garden, F., & Grunseit, A. (2008). *Information Use and Needs of Complementary Medicines Users*. Retrieved from www.nps.org.au/__data/assets/pdf_file/0010/66619/Complementary_Medicines_Report_-_Consumers.pdf

World Health Organisation. (2002). *The World Health Report 2002: Reducing risks, promoting healthy life*. Retrieved from www.who.int/whr/2002/en/

World Health Organisation. (2005). *National policy on traditional medicine and regulation of herbal medicines: Report of a WHO global survey*. Retrieved from http://apps.who.int/medicinedocs/en/d/Js7916e/

World Health Organisation. (2012). *The global burden of chronic*. Retrieved from www.who.int/nutrition/topics/2_background/en/

World Health Organisation. (2014). *WHO Traditional Medicine Strategy 2014-2023*. WHO.

Xue, C., Zhang, A., Lin, V., Da Costa, C., & Story, D. (2007). Complementary and alternative medicine use in Australia: A national population-based survey. *Journal of Alternative and Complementary Medicine (New York, N.Y.)*, *13*(6), 643–650. doi:10.1089/acm.2006.6355 PMID:17718647

Yamashita, H., Tsukayama, H., & Sugishita, C. (2002). Popularity of complementary and alternative medicine in Japan: A telephone survey. *Complementary Therapies in Medicine*, *10*(2), 84–93. doi:10.1054/ctim.2002.0519 PMID:12481956

Yates, J. S., Mustian, K. M., Morrow, G. R., Gillies, L. J., Padmanaban, D., Atkins, J. N., & Colman, L. K. et al. (2005). Prevalence of complementary and alternative medicine use in cancer patients during treatment. *Supportive Care in Cancer*, *13*(10), 806–811. doi:10.1007/s00520-004-0770-7 PMID:15711946

KEY TERMS AND DEFINITIONS

Disclosure: An act of giving individual information, such as history of medication.

Legislation: A law on the quality of health products.

Orthodox Medicine: Treatment is conventional medicine, particularly Western medicine.

Perspective: Thinking is influenced by individual experience.

Prevalence: A number of people under a specific time, place, and condition.

Regulation: An official rule aims to control the quality of CAM services.

Traditional Medicine: Treatment is used for a long time.

Chapter 3
An Overview of Publications of Complementary and Alternative Medicine Research

Mayuree Tangkiatkumjai
Srinakharinwirot University, Thailand

ABSTRACT

This chapter presents an overview of the quantity and quality of clinical research in CAM and publication bias. Descriptive studies and their systematic reviews on CAM, e.g., prevalence and reasons for CAM use, have been widely conducted worldwide. The findings of the efficacy of herbal medicine, traditional Chinese medicine and acupuncture for treating various illnesses, have been highly published. Publications of CAM safety are limited. A number of clinical studies of CAM in treating kidney diseases were lower than other illnesses. Studies of Ayurveda and other CAMs are still lacking. The quality of CAM publications is described based on systematic reviews of assessing CAM publications. Publication bias is explained in terms of selective publications and location bias, language bias and conflict of interest. The mainstream journals are more likely to publish positive findings. Predatory open access and recommendations for assessing predatory journals are addressed in this chapter.

DOI: 10.4018/978-1-5225-2882-1.ch003

INTRODUCTION

The amount of complementary and alternative medicine (CAM) research has been rapidly increasing over recent years (Figure 1). CAM publications slowly increased in number prior to 2000, dramatically rising in number after 2000. Several aspects of CAM research have been explored, e.g. prevalence of use, attitudes of CAM users and practitioners, the efficacy, safety, and cost-effectiveness of CAM, methodologies used in CAM research, and CAM regulation. In addition, the number of systematic reviews and meta-analyses of CAM research has been growing since 2010. High quality CAM research has been accepted for publishing in mainstream biomedical journals, e.g. *Annals of Internal Medicine*, *British Medical Journal*, *The Lancet*, *The Journal of the American Medical Association*, and *The New England Journal of Medicine* (Fontanarosa, 2001). This chapter gives an overview of CAM publications worldwide, any publication bias, their quality, and presents the common types and research topics of CAM published. This chapter will also identify any gaps in CAM research.

OVERVIEW OF GLOBAL PUBLICATIONS IN CAM

Five major publishers based in Europe and the US, i.e. Elsevier, Springer, Wiley, Tayor & Francis, and Sage, dominate CAM publishing. The prominent journals based on their impact factors in this area are the *Journal*

Figure 1. Trends in publications on CAM in the medical literature
(Treister-Goltzman et al., 2015)

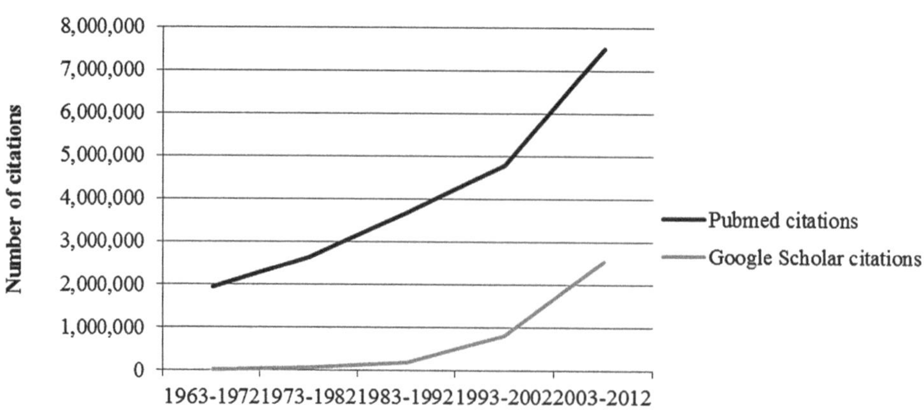

of Ethnopharmacology, Phytomedicine, The American Journal of Chinese Medicine, Chinese Medicine, and *Complementary Therapies in Medicine* (Fan, 2015). Other reliable journals in this field are *The Journal of Alternative and Complementary Medicine, Evidence Based Complementary and Alternative Medicine, BMC Complementary and Alternative Medicine, Journal of Manipulative and Physiological Therapeutics, Alternative Medicine Review, Integrative Cancer Therapies, Alternative Therapies in Health and Medicine, Forsch Komplementmed, Homeopathy,* and *Chinese Journal of Integrative Medicine* (Fu et al., 2011).

The Cochrane CAM group have been collecting details of published randomised controlled trials in CAM since 1996 in order to support the development of systematic reviews of CAM. The Cochrane Central Register of Controlled Trials (CENTRAL) indicates that the most frequent studies of CAM were non-vitamin, non-mineral dietary supplements, such as glucosamine or fish oil; Chinese herbal medicine, diet-based therapies; vitamin and mineral interventions; and acupuncture. This may be due to the Cochrane CAM group being based at the University of Maryland, and collaborates with the National Center for Complementary and Integrative Health in the US where researchers are more likely to focus on dietary supplements. Frequently reported medical purposes for using CAM by the Cochrane CAM group were heart and circulation, pain, mental health, and endocrine and metabolic conditions. In addition, the group published several systematic reviews regarding treating kidney diseases (see Chapter 7). Regarding the quality of CENTRAL, this database covers controlled trials in CAM from the Medical Literature Analysis and Retrieval System Online (MEDLINE), Excerpta Medica Database (EMBASE) and non-MEDLINE resources; 28% of CAM RCTs in CENTRAL were not included in either MEDLINE or EMBASE (Wieland et al., 2013). Therefore, CENTRAL is more likely to cover a higher number of controlled trials in CAM than MEDLINE or EMBASE.

Research on herbal medicine has the highest number of studies worldwide, compared to other CAMs. Popović et al. (2016) reviewed publications in herbal medicine between 2001 and 2013 over which they found a 6.3x increase in the number of articles. The top three regions producing publications in herbal medicine are Africa (34%), Asia (31%), and Europe (17%). Although the top three regions producing CAM publications in general are the US, East Asia, and Europe (Fu, et al., 2011). *In vitro* (4,589 articles), and animal studies (3,275 articles) were the most prevalent study types, whilst in humans there were 1,285 articles (Popović et al., 2016). This small number of publications in humans may be due to the fact that this review focused on pharmacological effects of herbal medicine in conditions such as cardiovascular diseases, gastrointestinal diseases, cancer, neurological disorders, respiratory diseases, infectious diseases and urinary disorders.

Regarding traditional Chinese medicine (TCM), Chan et al. (2015) reviewed articles about from 20 selected journals. They found the main themes of TCM research were quality of ingredients, toxicity/safety (including regulation), and efficacy. The methods used were *in vitro, in vivo,* clinical trials, and *in silico*, i.e. results generated using a computer (Ekins et al., 2007). The clinical trials were mainly regarding the efficacy and safety of acupuncture (Chan et al., 2015). Acupuncture is quite well researched via various methods, such as RCTs. The research has mainly tested the efficacy of acupuncture on pain, cardio-cerebrovascular diseases, and the neuropsychological system (Chan et al., 2015). However approximately 30% of systematic reviews and 21% of RCTs regarding TCM are published in China (Cai et al., 2012). Therefore, a high percentage of acupuncture research is published in the Chinese language that is difficult for many people to access.

The publications of other CAMs, such as Ayurveda are fewer, compared to publications on herbal medicine, acupuncture or TCM. The most common use of Ayurveda was for treating diabetes, asthma and hypertension (Sridharan, et al., 2016). Yoga has been increasing in publications since 2011 and frequent uses of yoga were cited for treating pain, stress, anxiety, depression, and cancer (Field, 2016). It should be noted that India and the US most often publish RCTs on yoga. Publications of manipulative therapy are numerous, and a systematic review found 72 systematic reviews, 96 RCTs, and 10 non-RCTs (Clar, et al., 2014). This review reports both efficacy and adverse effects for manipulative therapy for both musculoskeletal and non-musculoskeletal conditions, e.g. asthma, cancer, gastrointestinal illnesses, etc.

SCOPE AND QUALITY OF EXISTING CAM RESEARCH

This section outlines the prevalence of CAM use, attitudes of CAM users, and publication bias based on information from systematic reviews.

Descriptive Studies

The prevalence of CAM use has been widely published with prevalence rates given for both general populations, and patients with specific illnesses such as cancer, diabetes, cardiovascular diseases, kidney diseases, and mental illnesses. Specific populations, e.g. older adults, children, pregnant women, pharmacists, doctors, college students, etc. are also well studied. The author of this chapter systematically searched the PubMed, EMBASE, and ScienceDirect databases up to 2010 and found 48 studies on the prevalence of CAM use in general and patient populations worldwide, including five surveys of CAM use in patients with kidney diseases (Tangkiatkumjai, 2014). Surveys are the main methodology used, however there are inconsistencies with the definition of CAM use and period of CAM use, e.g. 6 months, 12 months, or lifetime. Most surveys used the CAM definition of the World Health Organisation (WHO), the US Food and Drug Administration, or the National Center for Complementary and Integrative Health, together with a 12-month period of use. Since 2010, five systematic reviews of the prevalence of CAM use have been published (Cooper et al., 2013; Harris et al., 2012, 2014; Posadzki et al., 2013a; Posadzki et al., 2013b).

Attitudes of CAM users and practitioners has been largely explored. The author of this chapter systematically searched Pubmed, EMBASE and ScienceDirect databases from 2003 to 2013 and used key search terms of CAM and attitude. The databases returned 743 articles, 776 articles, and 986 articles, respectively. Only one mixed methods study reported attitudes towards the use of herbal and dietary supplements in patients with chronic kidney disease (Tangkiatkumjai et al., 2014). Most studies were conducted using qualitative or quantitative methods, and systematic reviews, and mixed methods research on this topic are still lacking.

Since the prevalence of CAM use worldwide, and attitudes of CAM users appears to be well-established; many prominent journals are unlikely to publish prevalence papers, and instead choose to publish papers regarding the efficacy and safety of CAM.

Efficacy of CAM

This section focuses on systematic reviews regarding CAM efficacy which although is the most reliable evidence, should be interpreted with caution such as when included RCTs are biased the findings of the review would be questionable. The quality of reporting and conducting RCTs in CAM are discussed in Chapter 10.

One hundred and thirty-one non-Cochrane systematic reviews of CAM were retrieved from the Medline database (2010 – 2011) and were assessed their quality (Turner et al., 2013). The US, UK, and China were the main contributors to these systematic reviews. The top three areas reported by them were the musculoskeletal system and connective tissue, mental and behavioural disorders, and the circulatory system. The authors compared the quality between CAM-related non-Cochrane systematic reviews, and conventional non-Cochrane reviews. The CAM reviews less frequently reported publication bias (5%) than the conventional reviews (46%), and underreported the source of funding. Only 2% of the reviews adhered to the reporting guideline Preferred Reporting Items for Systematic Reviews and Meta-Analyses (PRISMA, www.prisma-statement.org) [last accessed 17/03/17]. Therefore, non-Cochrane systematic reviews of CAM urgently need to be improved and should be interpreted with caution.

The Cochrane CAM group is a reliable organisation which has published a high number of systematic reviews. However, the quality of Cochrane systematic reviews and meta-analyses was raised as a concern by Fønnebø (2011). The major risks of bias are that the interventions in publications may not reflect the best practice of CAM practitioners, or test an irrelevant CAM technique. The outcome measured may also not be appropriate (Fønnebø, 2011). For instance, included studies may measure only one component of the overall outcome. A systematic review of CAM is likely to be broad in order to obtain a high number of qualified studies. As a result, the included studies may have a great variety of interventions and outcomes which can lead to a lack of conclusive findings. However, this may be due to the limited number of high quality RCTs in CAM.

The quality of systematic reviews and meta-analyses of RCTs on acupuncture published by the Cochrane CAM group was assessed and found that most of them included studies only in the English language which led to inconclusive findings (69% included only English language papers vs. 31% in both English and Chinese languages) even though significantly more studies of acupuncture were published ($p < 0.01$) in the Chinese language (53%) than in English (Lui et al., 2010). This review suggests that systematic reviews on acupuncture should include publications in both English and Chinese languages. The top three countries publishing acupuncture research between 2000 and 2014 were the US, China, and South Korea (Moré et al., 2016). However, researchers should be aware of publication bias as almost all of the RCTs on acupuncture published in Chinese journals report positive effects (Wang et al., 2014). Researchers also should assess risk of bias using the STandards for Reporting Interventions in Clinical Trials of Acupuncture (STRICTA) (see Chapter 5).

Systematic reviews of Chinese herbal medicine (CHM) have been published in Medline, EMBASE, Cochrane Database of Systematic Reviews, and Database of Abstracts of Reviews of Effect (DARE). Two hundred and one meta-analyses were published between 1993 and 2013, and report CHM for treating various illnesses, i.e. cardiovascular diseases, cancer, gastrointestinal illnesses, mental disorders, infectious diseases, and genitourinary illnesses (Chung et al., 2015). Nearly 60% of the reviews included meta-analyses and at least one third assessed the risk of bias of the primary studies using a Cochrane risk of bias tool or Jadad score. The weaknesses of these reviews and meta-analyses were the high heterogeneity of dosage forms and routes of CAM administration (34% did not report the route), whilst half of them did not report their funding source. These findings would suggest that improvement in the quality of reviews and meta-analyses of CHM is required.

A systematic review of manipulative therapy reported that a high number of poor quality of RCTs showed positive effects for musculoskeletal conditions, cervicogenic headaches, and cervicogenic dizziness. Meanwhile, negative effects were found for asthma, cancer, infant colic, and dysmenorrhea (Clar, et al., 2014). This review found that the majority of the RCTs had poor methodologies, such as small sample sizes, unclear randomisation and allocation concealment, and unblinding. Researchers should address these issues in future. Furthermore systematic reviews for kidney disease are lacking.

Safety of CAM

A meta-review regarding the safety of CAM retrieved 88 reviews from the National Health System (NHS) evidence base, DARE, the Allied and Complementary Medicine Database (AMED), British Nursing Index, EMBASE, Ovid, Medline, and PsycINFO from 2009 to 2010 (Pilkington et al., 2012). Sixty nine percent of the publications reported adverse effects of herbal medicine and dietary supplements whilst safety reports of other CAMs were limited (9% acupuncture, 1% moxibustion, 13% body-based therapies, and 2% homoeopathy). The main information sources were clinical trials (12 systematic reviews) and case reports (6 systematic reviews). Case reports addressed rare or serious adverse effects of herbal medicine or spinal manipulation. Other information sources were from experts on spinal manipulation, herbs, massage, acupuncture, or homoeopathy (28 systematic reviews), manufacturers (21 systematic reviews), adverse drug reactions reporting schemes (15 systematic reviews), or professional organisations that reviewed the safety of acupuncture, herbs, dietary supplements and massage (12 systematic reviews). One meta-analysis and one systematic review indicated adverse effects of manipulative therapy (Carnes et al., 2010; Clar, et al., 2014). Mild to moderate adverse effects, e.g. increased pain, headaches, dizziness, nausea and vomiting, etc., commonly occurred within 24 hours after manipulative therapy and resolved within 72 hours (Clar, et al., 2014). Whilst Carnes et al. (2010) reported between 22% and 41% mild to moderate transient adverse effects, with 0.13% being major adverse effects, such as stroke. It would therefore appear that although the efficacy of manipulative therapy is unclear, the risk of adverse effects is high.

PUBLICATION BIAS

Publication bias is the tendency of investigators, reviewers, and editors to differentially submit or accept manuscripts for publication based on the direction or strength of the findings (Cook et al., 1993). Publication bias consists of; (1) selective publications, e.g. frequently published positive findings, and location bias; (2) language bias; and (3) conflicts of interest among people involved in making a decision on publications. Several systematic reviews analysed publication bias in CAM research. Sood et al. (2007) evaluated CAM publications in the four highest impact factor general medical journals, i.e. *The Lancet*, *British Medical Journal*, *New England Journal of Medicine* and *Journal of American Medical Association* from 1965 to 2004. These journals were more likely to publish positive findings, and European journals tended to publish positive results more than US ones. This may be due to the fact that CAM is more embedded in Europe, compared to the US. Likewise, during 2005, CAM journals in PubMed which reported positive findings increased 6.3-fold compared to negative (Coelho et al., 2007). CAM journals tend to publish fewer negative papers than biomedical journals (Caufield et al., 2005). This publication bias could skew or mislead trends in the efficacy of CAMs as systematic reviews that cannot include non-significant findings due to their lack of publication may overestimate treatment effects. Although this issue can be remedied through including grey literature, only 15% of systematic reviews of CAM included data from unpublished studies (Turner, et al., 2013).

Homoeopathy has a higher number of negative findings published (Caufield et al 2005), so it would seem that biomedical journals do not believe in the efficacy of homoeopathy and therefore are more likely to publish studies reporting negative findings (Caufield et al 2005). Meanwhile, CAM journals seem to support the efficacy of homoeopathy and publish positive findings of homoeopathy more than negative findings (Caufield et al 2005). To reduce selective publications, the registration of all studies at inception is required and journals should balance positive and negative findings.

Regarding language bias, a systematic review of CAM systematic reviews reported that 49% of CAM systematic reviews included both English and non-English articles (Turner, et al., 2013). Systematic reviews should include all languages as they are significantly different to reviews that include only English articles (Pham et al., 2005). Moreover, systematic reviews of Traditional Chinese medicine must include articles published in Chinese in order to decrease language bias (Wu et al., 2013).

Finally, conflicts of interest could influence publication bias. For example, an article supported by CAM companies may tend to report more positive findings. Conflicts of interest should include both financial and non-financial support. For instance, CAM practitioners tend to believe in the positive effects of CAM, and Ernst (2007) suggested that "selective evidence can be worse than no evidence at all" (pg 60).

PREDATORY OPEN ACCESS

The number of open-access journals have been dramatically increasing. These journals provide free access to a full-text and aim to decrease the dominance of mainstream journals. However, a high number of predatory open access journals undermines the benefit of open access journal (Figure 2). Seventy thousand biomedical articles were identified as predatory publications with India and North America being the main contributors (Shen et al., 2015).

Predatory journals or publishers are publications that charge scientists fees to publish research, but do not offer proper services, e.g. peer review, or make misleading claims on impact factors or indexing. However determination of predatory is often based on the journal or publishers' websites and less likely to be from direct contact with editors or publishers (Butler, 2013). Some critics say that labelling a journal as predatory may ruin start-up open access journals in developing countries, such as India and China. Therefore, researchers should consider this issue when publishing their work.

Figure 2. Rapid growth of predatory open access journals from 2010 to 2014 (Shen, et al., 2015)

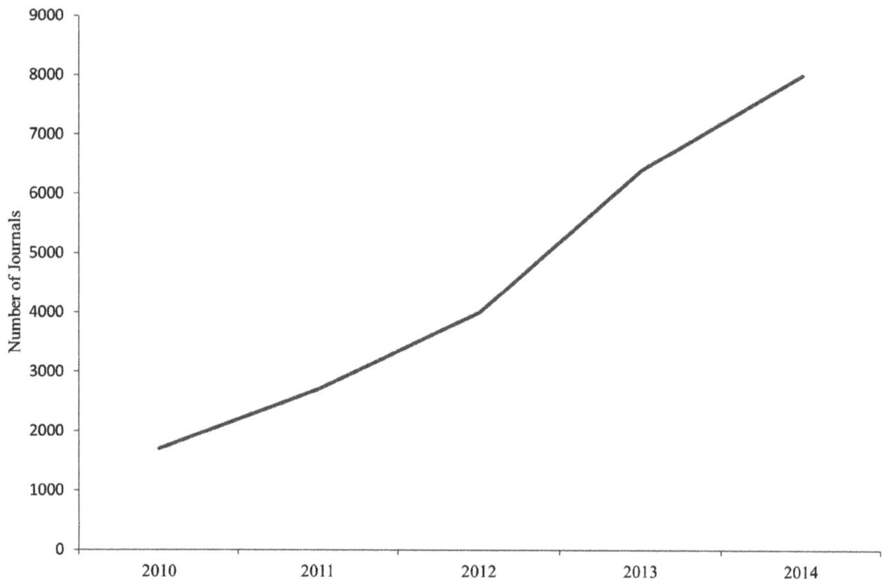

Journals or publishers that comply with the International Committee of Medical Journal Editors (ICMJE) Recommendations for the Conduct, Reporting, Editing and Publication of Scholarly Work in Medical Journals are classified into a non-predatory list (Table 1). The complete list is available at www.icmje.org/journals-following-the-icmje-recommendations [last accessed 17/03/17]. They use an honour system to comply with the criteria. As a result, journals on this list are not 100% guaranteed not to be predatory. For example, *International Journal of Research in Ayurveda and Pharmacy,* and *Journal of Ayurveda and Integrated Medical Sciences* have been listed on both predatory and non-predatory lists. Therefore, readers should analyse the quality of journals (Table 2).

CONCLUSION

The number of systematic reviews and meta-analyses in CAM research on the prevalence of CAM use, the efficacy of herbal medicine, traditional Chinese medicine, acupuncture, or manipulative therapy, have been dramatically increasing, as has research evaluating the quality of CAM publications. The

Table 1. Predatory CAM journals in 2016

Predatory	Non-Predatory
African Journal of Traditional	Acupuncture in Medicine
Complementary and Alternative Medicines	Advanced Herbal Medicine
Asian Pacific Journal of Natural Products	Advancement in Medicinal Plant Research
International Ayurvedic Medical Journal	Alternative Therapies in Health And Medicine
International Journal of Ayurveda and Pharma Research	Australian Journal of Herbal Medicine
International Journal of Ayurveda and Pharmaceutical Chemistry	Ayurpub.Com (International Ayurveda Publication)
International Journal of Herbal Medicine	British Homoeopathic Journal
Journal of Ayurveda and Holistic Medicine	Chiropractic Journal of Australia
Journal of HerbMed Pharmacology	European Journal of Medicinal Plants
Journal of Intercultural Ethnopharmacology	International Archives of Integrated Medicine
Journal of Natural Products	International Journal of Ayurveda & Alternative Medicine
Plants Journal / Journal of Medicinal Plants Studies	International Journal of Medicinal Plants and Alternative Medicine
Journal of Research in Traditional Medicine	Journal of Chiropractic Medicine
	Journal of Integrative Medicine
	Journal of Integrative Medicine & Therapy
	Journal of Research in Traditional Medicine
	Medical Acupuncture
	World Journal of Acupuncture-Moxibustion

Table 2. Recommendations for assessing journals or publishers (Butler, 2013)

1. Check that the publisher provides full, verifiable contact information, including address, on the journal site. Be cautious of those that provide only web contact details.
2. Check that a journal's editorial board lists recognised experts with full affiliations. Contact some of them and ask about their experience with the journal or publisher.
3. Check that the journal prominently displays its policy for author fees.
4. Be wary of e-mail invitations to submit to journals or to become editorial board members.
5. Read some of the journal's published articles and assess their quality. Contact past authors to ask about their experience.
6. Check that a journal's peer-review process is clearly described and try to confirm that a claimed impact factor is correct.
7. Find out whether the journal is a member of an industry association that vets its members, such as the Directory of Open Access Journals (www.doaj.org) or the Open Access Scholarly Publishers Association (www.oaspa.org) [both last accessed 17/03/17].
8. Use common sense, as you would when shopping online; if something looks odd, proceed with caution.

quality of clinical research in CAM has been gradually improving also. The publication bias in CAM is mainly due to mainstream journals tending to publish positive findings. Systematic reviews of CAM should include both English and non-English articles as a high number of CAM studies are published in Non-English journals such as in Chinese publications. Authors and readers should be aware of predatory journals.

REFERENCES

Butler, D. (2013). The dark side of publishing. *Nature*, *495*(7442), 433–435. doi:10.1038/495433a PMID:23538810

Cai, Y., Shen, J., Zhong, D., Li, Y., & Wu, T. (2012). Status quo, issues, and challenges for acupuncture research evidence: An overview of clinical and fundamental studies. *J Evid Based Med*, *5*(1), 12–24. doi:10.1111/j.1756-5391.2012.01163.x PMID:23528116

Carnes, D., Mars, T. S., Mullinger, B., Froud, R., & Underwood, M. (2010). Adverse events and manual therapy: A systematic review. *Manual Therapy*, *15*(4), 355–363. doi:10.1016/j.math.2009.12.006 PMID:20097115

Caufield, T., & DeBow, S. (2005). A systematic review of how homeopathy is represented in conventional and CAM peer reviewed journals. *BMC Complementary and Alternative Medicine*, *5*(1), 12. doi:10.1186/1472-6882-5-12 PMID:15955254

Chan, K., Hu, X. Y., Razmovski-Naumovski, V., & Robinson, N. (2015). Challenges and opportunities of integrating traditional Chinese medicine into mainstream medicine: A review of the current situation. *European Journal of Internal Medicine*, *7*(1), 67–75.

Chung, V. C. H., Ho, R. S. T., Wu, X., Fung, D. H. Y., Lai, X., Wu, J. C. W., & Wong, S. Y. S. (2015). Are meta-analyses of Chinese herbal medicine trials trustworthy and clinically applicable? a cross-sectional study. *Journal of Ethnopharmacology*, *162*, 47–54. doi:10.1016/j.jep.2014.12.028 PMID:25554640

Clar, C., Tsertsvadze, A., Court, R., Hundt, G. L., Clarke, A., & Sutcliffe, P. (2014). Clinical effectiveness of manual therapy for the management of musculoskeletal and non-musculoskeletal conditions: Systematic review and update of UK evidence report. *Chiropr Man Therap*, *22*(1), 12. doi:10.1186/2045-709X-22-12 PMID:24679336

Coelho, H. F., Pittler, M. H., & Ernst, E. (2007). An investigation of the contents of complementary and alternative medicine journals. *Alternative Therapies in Health and Medicine*, *13*(4), 40–44. PMID:17658121

Cook, D. J., Guyatt, G. H., Ryan, G., Clifton, J., Buckingham, L., Willan, A., . . . Oxman, A. D. (1993). Should unpublished data be included in meta-analyses? current convictions and controversies. *JAMA, 269*(21), 2749-2753.

Cooper, K. L., Harris, P. E., Relton, C., & Thomas, K. J. (2013). Prevalence of visits to five types of complementary and alternative medicine practitioners by the general population: Systematic review. *Complementary Therapies in Clinical Practice*, *19*(4), 214–220. doi:10.1016/j.ctcp.2013.06.006 PMID:24199976

Ekins, S., Mestres, J., & Testa, B. (2007). *In silico* pharmacology for drug discovery: Methods for virtual ligand screening and profiling. *British Journal of Pharmacology*, *152*(1), 9–20. doi:10.1038/sj.bjp.0707305 PMID:17549047

Ernst, E. (2007). Publication bias in complementary/alternative medicine. *Journal of Clinical Epidemiology*, *60*(11), 1093–1094. doi:10.1016/j.jclinepi.2007.07.002 PMID:17938049

Ernst, E. (2012). Conflicts of interest. *Focus Altern Complement Ther*, *17*(3), 141. doi:10.1111/j.2042-7166.2012.01161.x

Fan, K. W. (2015). Bias and other limitations affect measures of journals in integrative and complementary medicine. *Journal of the Medical Library Association: JMLA*, *103*(3), 148–151. doi:10.3163/1536-5050.103.3.009 PMID:26213508

Field, T. (2016). Yoga research review. *Complementary Therapies in Clinical Practice*, *24*, 145–161. doi:10.1016/j.ctcp.2016.06.005 PMID:27502816

Fønnebø, V. (2011). Cochrane CAM reviews commentary: Is there more to quality than the research method itself? *Explore (New York, N.Y.)*, *7*(1), 53–54. doi:10.1016/j.explore.2010.10.010 PMID:21194673

Fontanarosa, P. B. (2001). Publication of complementary and alternative medicine research in mainstream biomedical journals. *Journal of Alternative and Complementary Medicine (New York, N.Y.)*, *7*(Suppl 1), S139–S143. doi:10.1089/107555301753393913 PMID:11822629

Fu, J. Y., Zhang, X., Zhao, Y. H., Huang, M. H., & Chen, D. Z. (2011). Bibliometric analysis of complementary and alternative medicine research over three decades. *Scientometrics*, *88*(2), 617–626. doi:10.1007/s11192-011-0391-0

Harris, P. E., Cooper, K. L., Relton, C., & Thomas, K. J. (2012). Prevalence of complementary and alternative medicine (CAM) use by the general population: A systematic review and update. *International Journal of Clinical Practice*, *66*(10), 924–939. doi:10.1111/j.1742-1241.2012.02945.x PMID:22994327

Harris, P. E., Cooper, K. L., Relton, C., & Thomas, K. J. (2014). Prevalence of visits to massage therapists by the general population: A systematic review. *Complementary Therapies in Clinical Practice*, *20*(1), 16–20. doi:10.1016/j.ctcp.2013.11.001 PMID:24439639

Lui, S., Smith, E. J., & Terplan, M. (2010). Heterogeneity in search strategies among Cochrane acupuncture reviews: Is there room for improvement? *Acupuncture in Medicine*, *28*(3), 149–153. doi:10.1136/aim.2010.002444 PMID:20615852

Moré, A. O., Tesser, C. D., da Silva, J. B., & Min, L. S. (2016). Status and impact of acupuncture research: A bibliometric analysis of global and Brazilian scientific output from 2000 to 2014. *Journal of Alternative and Complementary Medicine (New York, N.Y.)*, *22*(6), 429–436. doi:10.1089/acm.2015.0281 PMID:27136034

Pham, B., Klassen, T. P., Lawson, M. L., & Moher, D. (2005). Language of publication restriction in systematic reviews gave different results depending on whether the intervention was conventional or complementary. *Journal of Clinical Epidemiology*, *58*(8), 769–776. doi:10.1016/j.jclinepi.2004.08.021 PMID:16086467

Pilkington, K., & Boshnakova, A. (2012). Complementary medicine and safety: A systematic investigation of design and reporting of systematic reviews. *Complementary Therapies in Medicine*, *20*(1-2), 73–82. doi:10.1016/j.ctim.2011.10.002 PMID:22305252

Popović, Z., Matić, R., Bojović, S., Stefanović, M., & Vidaković, V. (2016). Ethnobotany and herbal medicine in modern complementary and alternative medicine: An overview of publications in the field of I&C medicine 20012013. *Journal of Ethnopharmacology*, *181*, 182–192. doi:10.1016/j.jep.2016.01.034 PMID:26807912

Posadzki, P., Watson, L., Alotaibi, A., & Ernst, E. (2013a). Prevalence of complementary and alternative medicine (CAM)-use in UK paediatric patients: A systematic review of surveys. *Complementary Therapies in Medicine*, *21*(3), 224–231. doi:10.1016/j.ctim.2012.11.006 PMID:23642955

Posadzki, P., Watson, L. K., Alotaibi, A., & Ernst, E. (2013b). Prevalence of use of complementary and alternative medicine (CAM) by patients/consumers in the UK: Systematic review of surveys. *Clin Med (Lond)*, *13*(2), 126–131. doi:10.7861/clinmedicine.13-2-126 PMID:23681857

Shen, C., & Björk, B. C. (2015). Predatory open access: A longitudinal study of article volumes and market characteristics. *BMC Medicine*, *13*(1), 230. doi:10.1186/s12916-015-0469-2 PMID:26423063

Sood, A., Knudsen, K., Sood, R., Wahner-Roedler, D. L., Barnes, S. A., Bardia, A., & Bauer, B. A. (2007). Publication bias for CAM trials in the highest impact factor medicine journals is partly due to geographical bias. *Journal of Clinical Epidemiology*, *60*(11), 1123–1126. doi:10.1016/j.jclinepi.2007.01.009 PMID:17938053

Sridharan, K., & Sivaramakrishnan, G. (2016). Clinical trials in Ayurveda: Analysis of clinical trial registry of India. *J Ayurveda Integr Med*, *7*(3), 141–143. doi:10.1016/j.jaim.2016.08.009 PMID:27658912

Tangkiatkumjai, M. (2014). *Herbal and dietary supplement use in Thai patients with chronic kidney disease (CKD) and their association with progression of CKD*. Nottingham, UK: University of Nottingham.

Tangkiatkumjai, M., Boardman, H., Praditpornsilpa, K., & Walker, D. M. (2014). Reasons why Thai patients with chronic kidney disease use or do not use herbal and dietary supplements. *BMC Complementary and Alternative Medicine*, *14*(1), 473. doi:10.1186/1472-6882-14-473 PMID:25481733

Treister-Goltzman, Y., & Peleg, R. (2015). Trends in publications on complementary and alternative medicine in the medical literature. *J Complement Integr Med*, *12*(2), 111–115. doi:10.1515/jcim-2014-0055 PMID:25565548

Turner, L., Galipeau, J., Garritty, C., Manheimer, E., Wieland, L. S., Yazdi, F., & Moher, D. (2013). An evaluation of epidemiological and reporting characteristics of complementary and alternative medicine (CAM) systematic reviews (SRs). *PLoS ONE*, *8*(1), e53536. doi:10.1371/journal.pone.0053536 PMID:23341949

Wang, Y., Wang, L., Chai, Q., & Liu, J. (2014). Positive results in randomized controlled trials on acupuncture published in Chinese journals: A systematic literature review. *Journal of Alternative and Complementary Medicine (New York, N.Y.)*, *20*(5), A129. doi:10.1089/acm.2014.5346.abstract

Wieland, L. S., Manheimer, E., Sampson, M., Barnabas, J. P., Bouter, L. M., Cho, K., & Berman, B. M. et al. (2013). Bibliometric and content analysis of the Cochrane Complementary Medicine Field specialized register of controlled trials. *Syst Rev*, *2*(1), 51. doi:10.1186/2046-4053-2-51 PMID:23826877

Wu, X. Y., Tang, J. L., Mao, C., Yuan, J. Q., Qin, Y., & Chung, V. C. H. (2013). Systematic reviews and meta-analyses of traditional Chinese Medicine must search Chinese Databases to reduce language bias. *Evidence-Based Complementary and Alternative Medicine*, *2013*, 812179. doi:10.1155/2013/812179 PMID:24223063

KEY TERMS AND DEFINITIONS

Bias: An opinion influences unfair decision.

Bibliometrics: A study involves an analysis of publications.

Open Access: An article provides a free access to a full-text for anyone.

Publication: An academic article is published by a publisher.

Predatory Journal: A journal that charges money for publication, but does not provide academic service, such as proper peer review.

Selective Publication: A type of publication bias that tends to accept an interesting study, such as a study reporting positive findings.

Systematic Review: A study that systematically search and analyse scientific evidence.

Chapter 4
General Approach to Evaluating Beneficial and Adverse Effects of CAM Use in Kidney Diseases

Mayuree Tangkiatkumjai
Srinakharinwirot University, Thailand

Chatchai Kreepala
Srinakharinwirot University, Thailand

ABSTRACT

This chapter will address the issue of how to evaluate benefits and nephrotoxicity of complementary and alternative medicine (CAM) in chronic kidney disease, dialysis therapy, kidney transplantation, and urolithiasis. Serum creatinine, proteinuria and estimated glomerular filtration rate are standard parameters to assess kidney function. Serum creatinine is used in evaluating acute kidney injury, which is the most common nephropathy from using herbal medicine. Assessment of electrolyte imbalance and urolithiasis is included in this chapter. The modified Naranjo algorithm has been proposed as a way to evaluate renal adverse effects of herbal medicine due to a lack of disease-specific causality assessments in herbal use. Measurement of humanistic outcomes is mentioned in this chapter. The SF-36 is commonly used in evaluating quality of life in CAM users and patients with kidney diseases. The MYMOP2 is to assess individual's symptoms in CAM use and might be used in this population.

DOI: 10.4018/978-1-5225-2882-1.ch004

INTRODUCTION

Efficacy and safety of CAM on the kidneys are required to be investigated by clinical trials. This chapter will explain the principle of evaluating the benefits and adverse effects of CAM use in patients with kidney diseases, relating to conditions that include chronic kidney disease (CKD), dialysis therapy, kidney transplantation, and urolithiasis. Benefits from CAM will be measured via clinical outcomes, such as slowing the progression of CKD, preventing allograft rejection, improving CKD complications, and providing kidney stone relief. The progression of CKD is measured using an estimated glomerular filtration rate (eGFR). Benefits from CAM are not only seen in clinical outcomes, but also humanistic ones. Humanistic outcomes are defined as an individual's perspective on symptom relief, health-related quality of life, and health satisfaction (Schena, 2000). These outcomes have been measured in conventional medicine since the 20th century. Current evidence reports that conventional medicine is likely to improve the quality of life in patients with CKD (Travers et al., 2013). Patient-Reported Outcomes Measures (PROMs) are the current tool to measure humanistic outcomes (Refolo et al., 2012).

This chapter will explain how to assess potential renal adverse events associated with herbal and dietary supplements (HDS), whilst nephropathy of CAM will be addressed in Chapter 7. Common nephropathy related to herbal medicine and dietary supplements are acute kidney injuries (AKI), electrolyte imbalances, and urolithiasis. AKI is an abrupt reduction in kidney function measured by a rapid decline in glomerular filtration rate occurring over a period of minutes or days that results in the dysregulation of extracellular volume, waste products and electrolytes. The clinical spectrum of AKI can be attributed to any process that interferes with the renal structure or its function such as hypovolaemia, toxic drug induced renal tubular injury, acute glomerular renal diseases, acute interstitial nephritis or obstructive nephropathy (causing urinary blockage). Measurement of nephropathy will be explained in this chapter.

AKI has a significant impact on developing CKD and end-stage kidney disease. There are different definitions of AKI based on Risk, Injury, Failure, Loss of kidney function, and End stage kidney disease (RIFLE) classification (Bellomo et al., 2004), and the Acute Kidney Injury Network (AKIN) classification (Lopes et al., 2013). Each classification has its own advantages and disadvantages. The AKIN classification will be explained in this chapter as it is widely accepted and used. There are no specific tools to assess a likelihood of renal adverse effects related to herbal medicines. The World Health Organisation's Uppsala Monitoring Center causality assessment and the Naranjo algorithm have been globally used for assessing adverse drug reactions (Edwards et al., 2000). However, the Naranjo algorithm may not be appropriate to assess adverse effects of herbal medicines as one category in this algorithm requires evidence to confirm their negative effect. This is often lacking in herbal medicines and dietary supplements (Naranjo et al., 1981). The modified Naranjo algorithm and the World Health Organisation's Uppsala Monitoring Center causality assessment have been proposed to evaluate causal relationships of adverse events involving herbal and dietary supplements (Ide et al., 2015).

BENEFITS OF CAM

Beneficial effects of CAM in kidney diseases are assessed by the use of both clinical and humanistic outcomes. This section will focus on methods of evaluating the benefits of CAM in clinical studies, so this information could guide practitioners and researchers how to conduct studies in this field.

Clinical Outcomes

Chronic kidney disease is defined as a kidney disease with either persisting abnormalities of renal function (longer than 3 months) or structure. Thus, a patient with CKD may present with albuminuria, abnormal urinary sediments, electrolyte abnormalities, a history of kidney transplantation, or abnormal structure on imaging for at least 3 months (Kidney Disease: Improving Global Outcome (KDIGO) CKD Work Group, 2012b). There are four common outcomes that are expected from using CAM. First of all, an ultimate goal of therapy for CKD is a slower progression of CKD measured by eGFR. Estimated glomerular filtration rate (eGFR) is a standard surrogate end point in clinical trials to evaluate kidney function in patients with chronic kidney disease and kidney transplant recipients. Several studies about herbal medicine related to the progression of CKD also measure end-stage renal disease (ESRD) as a clinical end point (Lin et al., 2015; Tsai et al., 2009). End-stage renal disease is defined as having dialysis or kidney transplantation. Proteinuria is an independent factor relative to the progression of CKD, so this parameter is a further outcome to be considered. Next, to judge the efficacy of CAM in supporting kidney transplantation, one needs to assess acute renal allograft rejection and chronic renal allograft injury. Finally, the outcome of CAM for kidney stones is dissolution of the stones.

A pragmatic method to evaluate eGFR is by measurement of serum creatinine, and then calculating eGFR using validated equations, such as the Modification of Diet in Renal Disease (MDRD) or the Chronic Kidney Disease Epidemiology Collaboration (CKD-EPI) equations (Cirillo, 2010) (Table 1). Each equation has its pros and cons. The MDRD equation is more accurate in patients with less than 60 ml/min/1.73m^2 of eGFR, whilst the CKD-EPI equation is appropriate for those with eGFR of more than 60 ml/min/1.73m^2 (Earley et al., 2012). However, the MDRD equation needs to be modified for the Asian and African populations in order to improve its accuracy. This is because this equation was developed on the North American population, who have a different body mass compared with other populations and body mass influences eGFR. The CKD-EPI equation on the other hand, can be used without adjustment in Asian populations (Teo et al., 2011). Therefore, the CKD-EPI equation has been endorsed by Kidney Disease: Improving Global Outcome (KDIGO) for global use, as the glomerular filtration rate estimated by this equation predicts mortality better than the MDRD equation (Lamb et al., 2015).

There are two methods to evaluate the progression of CKD: the rate of decline in eGFR calculated by the slope of a best fit linear regression line over a period of time, and the percent change of eGFR at 12 months. Regarding the rate of a decline in eGFR, the progression of CKD is defined as a range from -3 to -5 ml/min/1.73m^2/year of eGFR. Whilst a fast progression of CKD is defined as a decline in eGFR of at least 5 ml/min/1.73m^2/year (KDIGO,

Table 1. The MDRD and CKD-EPI equations

eGFR Equation	Formulas
Reexpressed MDRD equation (ml/min/1.73 m^2)	(175 X Scr$^{-1.154}$ X Age$^{-0.203}$) Female (X 0.742)
CKD-EPI equation (ml/min/1.73 m^2)	Male: with Scr $\leq$ 0.9 mg/dL 141^{163} X (Scr/0.9)$^{-0.411}$ X (0.993)^{Age} Male: with Scr > 0.9 mg/dL 141^{163} X (Scr/0.9)$^{-1.209}$ X (0.993)^{Age} Female: with Scr $\leq$ 0.7 mg/dL 144^{166} X (Scr/0.7)$^{-0.329}$ X (0.993)^{Age} Female: with Scr > 0.7 mg/dL 144^{166} X (Scr/0.7)$^{-1.209}$ X (0.993)^{Age}

2012b; The National Collaborating Centre for Chronic Conditions, 2008). However, the rate of the progression of CKD varies based on the type of kidney disease. A faster progression of CKD has been shown in patients with diabetic kidney disease and focal segmental glomerulosclerosis (FSGS) (Badal et al., 2015; Cravedi et al., 2012; D'Agati, 2008). Therefore, a cutoff point of the progression of CKD in these populations should be defined based on their decline in eGFR over a period of time. On the contrary, patients with hypertensive kidney disease or tubulointerstitial kidney diseases have a slower progression.

If any CAM slows the progression of CKD over one-year, as measured by a decline in eGFR of less than 3 ml/min/1.73m^2/year, this CAM would be regarded as effective. This parameter also could assess worsening kidney function from using CAM. If any CAM decreases the rate of eGFR of at least 5 ml/min/1.73m^2/year, it would harm the kidneys. Therefore, patients with kidney diseases should avoid using that CAM. A limitation of this method is that there are no definite cutoff points for either slow or fast progression of CKD in patients with different causes of CKD.

The second method is to calculate the percent change in eGFR over 12 months as follows:

$$\text{Percent change in eGFR at 12 months} = [(eGFR_{12mo} - eGFR_{baseline}) / eGFR_{baseline}] \times 100\%$$

In 2014, the National Kidney Foundation proposed this method for calculating a surrogate marker for detecting earlier kidney failure, compared to measuring serum creatinine levels (Levey et al., 2014). This marker is suitable for a study conducted over a short period of time, or has a population with different causes of kidney diseases, or if it is assessing different interventions for slowing the progression of CKD. The cutoff points of 30% and 40% are recommended due to their association with the progression of CKD (Heerspink et al., 2014).

Proteinuria is a further outcome to be considered. It is mainly caused by diabetic kidney disease or glomerular diseases. Diminished proteinuria can slow the progression of CKD. Recently, standard guidelines for CKD management recommend three standard methods to measure proteinuria; the urine dipstick test, the urine protein-to-creatinine ratio (PCR), and the urine albumin-to-creatinine ratio (ACR) (National Kidney Foundation, 2002; The National Collaborating Centre for Chronic Conditions, 2008; The Nephrology Society of Thailand, 2009). Table 2 shows cutoff points of proteinuria and

Table 2. The cutoff points of quantitative assessment of proteinuria

Urine Protein Measurement	Cutoff Point of Proteinuria or Albuminuria
Urine protein-to-creatinine ratio, PCR	≥ 500 mg/g
Urine albumin-to-creatinine ratio, ACR	≥ 300 mg/g
Urine dipstick test	≥ 1+
24-hour urinary protein excretion rate, PER	≥ 500 mg/ 24 hour
24-hour urinary albumin excretion rate, AER	≥ 300 mg/ 24 hour

albuminuria. Proteinuria is defined as at least 2+ urine dipstick protein measurements for diabetic patients or at least 1+ of urine dipstick protein measurement for non-diabetic patients (National Kidney Foundation, 2002; The Nephrology Society of Thailand, 2009). Many studies measure 24-hour urinary protein excretion rate (PER) to identify proteinuria and 24-hour urinary albumin excretion rate (AER) to identify albuminuria. These methods are the gold standards for the quantitative assessment of proteinuria (National Kidney Foundation, 2002). However, 24-hour urine collection may cause errors if patients miss or improperly collect some samples. Thus leading to underestimated amounts of protein. Albuminuria is defined as an AER of equal to or more than 300 mg/ 24 hour (KDIGO, 2012b). If any CAM can diminish proteinuria in patients with diabetes or glomerular diseases, it could slow the progression of diseases.

In 2012, KDIGO proposed a new classification of CKD based on eGFR (stage 1-5 or G1-G5, see Table 3) and albuminuria (A1-A3) related to risk of cardiovascular mortality (Figure 1) (KDIGO, 2012a). A1,A2 and A3 is ACR < 30, 30-300, and > 300 mg/g, respectively.

This figure shows a relationship between albuminuria and glomerular filtration rates (GFR). A higher amount of albuminuria with lower GFR

Table 3. The classification of chronic kidney disease based on GFR

Stage	Prognosis of CKD	GFR (ml/min/1.73m^2)
1 (G1)	Normal or high	≥ 90
2 (G2)	Mild decrease	60-89
3a (G3a)	Mild to moderate decrease	45-59
3b (G3b)	Moderate to severe decrease	30-44
4 (G4)	Severe decrease	15-29
5 (G5)	Kidney failure	< 15

Figure 1. Cardiovascular mortality risk: a relationship between GFR and albuminuria

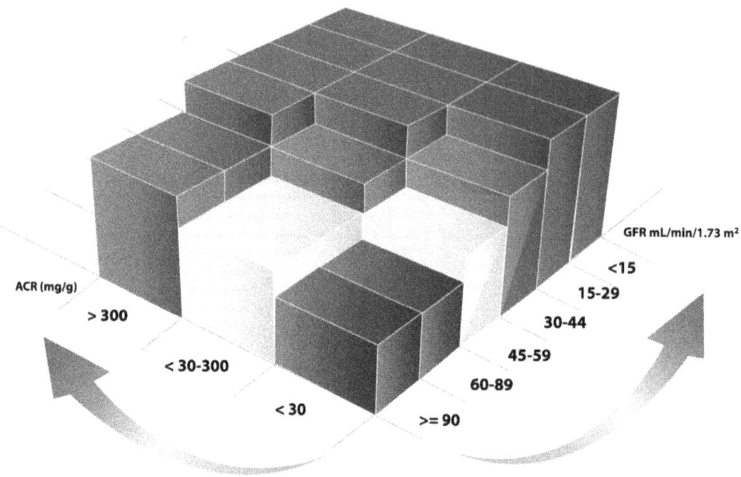

(thus, more advanced stage of CKD), the greater the risk of cardiovascular mortality. Abbreviations: ACR = Urine Albumin-to-Creatinine Ratio, GFR = Glomerular Filtration Rate. Color; Green: low risk; Yellow: moderately increased risk; Orange: high risk; Red: very high risk.

Some Chinese herbal medicines have been used as an adjunctive therapy to conventional medicine for kidney transplantation. Their target is to prevent acute renal allograft rejection and chronic renal allograft injury. An increase in serum creatinine and proteinuria are clinical manifestations of acute rejection and chronic allograft injury when other causes of graft dysfunction have been excluded. For kidney transplant recipients, the KDIGO Clinical Practice Guideline (2009) recommended biopsy to diagnose acute rejection and chronic allograft injury (Miller et al., 2007). The Banff classification is a standard international classification for the assessment of renal allograft biopsies and has been used in identifying these problems since the 1990s. The Banff 07 classification is the latest version (Bhowmik et al., 2010). Evaluating the efficacy of CAM for kidney transplantation should follow the Banff standard guidelines.

Dissolution of urolithiasis is another expected outcome from using several herbal medicines. As known, urinalysis is a basic test to monitor the outcome of treatment of urolithiasis. Microscopic urinalysis can detect crystals in urine and measure the size of the stones. Calcium oxalate crystals are the most common stones in kidneys. The efficacy of an herbal medicine for this disease can be judged by measuring the size of the stones. If the medicine is effective it would reduce the size of the stones or give stone relief.

Humanistic Outcomes

Chronic kidney disease and dialysis therapy affect patients' quality of life (QoL). Such conditions cause symptoms related to poor QoL such as fatigue, stress, anxiety, depression, insomnia, lack of mobility, and sexual dysfunction. Additionally, patients with urolithiasis suffer from pain, which is another condition related to decreased QoL (Penniston et al., 2013). These symptoms influence, most often negatively, physical, psychological and social functioning, which are related to the patients' QoL. Patients receiving dialysis therapy are not required to evaluate their kidney function as their kidneys have reached end-stage renal disease. The outcomes of their treatment are ones that alleviate the symptoms of CKD complications and improve QoL. Although some CAM may not directly cause physiological changes, they may alleviate such symptoms or improve the QoL. For example, herbal medicine, acupuncture, massage, and mind-body therapies have yielded positive evidence in the treatment of kidney diseases and associated complications. It is important to keep in mind that not only CAM influences QoL, other factors, such as standard conventional therapies, social relationships and financial concerns, are also associated with this outcome.

The World Health Organization (WHO) offers a broad definition of QoL which includes physical, mental and social well-being of an individual (The WHOQoL Group, 1995). Health-related quality of life (HRQoL) is the most common humanistic outcome to quality of life. Unruh and Hess (2007) proposed a more specific HRQoL for patients with CKD that consists of the following four domains:

1. Physical function, e.g., physical activity, fatigue, etc.
2. Psychological status, e.g., stress, anxiety, depression, cognitive function, etc.
3. Social status, e.g., family relationships, relationship stability, etc.
4. Global QoL, e.g., perceived health, daily functioning, happiness, etc.

Therefore, measurement of HRQoL in patients with kidney diseases should include these domains. In addition, Verhoef et al. (2006) proposed six domains to assess health-related outcomes from using CAM: physical, psychological, social, spiritual and holistic outcomes, quality of life, and individualised outcomes. The In-CAM database has gathered questionnaires to measure outcomes (IN-CAM, 2014). These tools have been designed for patient-centred, subjective outcome measurement. Choosing an appropriate questionnaire to measure an outcome of CAM should regard whether the questionnaire is well tested, acceptable and relevant to patients, and sensitive to change.

There are two main types of QoL questionnaires: generic or disease-specific. The generic questionnaires measure HRQoL, developed from the WHO definition in a wide range of patient populations such as patients with kidney diseases, asthma or cardiovascular diseases. The disease-specific questionnaires evaluate HRQoL in a specific disease condition, such as CKD. An ideal HRQoL questionnaire should be simple, short and easy to comprehend, as it is difficult for many patients to complete a long questionnaire.

Commonly Used HRQoL Questionnaires in Patients With Kidney Diseases

1. **Generic Questionnaires:** Table 4 shows the most common generic questionnaires, the domains they measure, the populations with kidney diseases assessed, and the availability of the questionnaires in other languages. The domains they measure are associated with the concept of QoL measurement as described above.
   a. **The Short Form 36 Health Survey (SF-36):** Is the most common generic questionnaire to measure HRQoL and has been translated and validated in more than 35 countries. This questionnaire is frequently used for patients with CKD receiving dialysis or urolithiasis (Bensalah et al., 2008; Butt et al., 2008; Merkus et al., 1997). It is also commonly used in evaluating the QoL in CAM users (Verhoef et al., 2006).
   b. **The EuroQoL Five-Dimensional Questionnaire (EQ-5D):** Is easily completed by respondents, can be used for evaluating economic outcomes, and is available in 170 different languages (Yang et al., 2015). This questionnaire is widely used in dialysis or kidney transplant patients (Sakthong et al., 2012; Wyld et al., 2012).

c. **The World Health Organization Quality of Life Brief (WHOQoL-BREF):** Is a 26-item short version of the WHOQoL and is available in 19 different languages. It has been used in patients receiving haemodialysis or kidney transplants (Sathvik et al., 2008).

d. **The Nottingham Health Profile (NHP):** Coons et al. (2000) evaluated this questionnaire and found that the NHP is simple and evaluates QoL in general, rather than from a health professionals' perspective. Part one of the NHP consists of six health domains (38 items): physical mobility, pain, sleep, energy, social isolation, and emotion. Part two is comprised of seven domains of daily life: paid employment, home duties, social life, personal relationships, sex life, hobbies and interests, and holidays. This questionnaire has been translated into 24 languages. The NHP has been used in assessing the QoL in Filipinos receiving haemodialysis and Turkish kidney transplant patients (Chuku et al., 2010; Ogutmen et al., 2006).

e. **The Sickness Impact Profile (SIP):** Is used for evaluating sickness in relation to behaviour dysfunction. This tool is to assess and discriminate the likelihood of physical functioning between patients receiving dialysis or kidney transplantations (Hart et al., 1987). The SIP consists of 136 items and therefore creates a respondent burden, whilst the SIP 68 is a short version. The SIP 136 takes 30 minutes to complete and the SIP 68 takes 15-20 minutes (Busija et al., 2011).

f. **The Dartmouth Cooperative Functional Assessment (COOP) Charts:** Are appropriate for practitioners to assess patients' QoL on a daily basis. This instrument is simple and suitable for people who have difficulty reading (Kempen et al., 1997). This tool can be used with dialysis and transplant patients.

All of these questionnaires are likely to be completed within 15 minutes, except the SIP.

2. **Disease-Specific Questionnaires:** There are several standardised questionnaires to evaluate HRQoL in patients with kidney diseases (Table 5). The questionnaires are appropriate for end-stage renal disease (ESRD), kidney transplantation, or urolithiasis.

   a. **Questionnaires for ESRD:** The four questionnaires to assess the HRQoL in patients receiving dialysis are (1) the Kidney Disease Quality of Life 36 questionnaire (KDQOL-36); (2) the Kidney

Table 4. Most common generic questionnaires about quality of life

Questionnaire Abbreviation, Number of Items (References)	Measurement of QoL Domains	Kidney Patient Populations	Languages
SF-36, 36 items (Ware et al., 1992)	Physical functioning, role physical, bodily pain, general health perceptions, vitality, social functioning, role emotional, and mental health	CKD, dialysis, kidney transplantation, urolithiasis	English, Arabic, Chinese, Danish, Dutch, Finnish, French, German, Hebrew, Italian, Japanese, Norwegian, Russian, Spanish, Swedish, Turkish, Vietnamese, Welsh, etc.
EQ-5D, 5 items (Rabin et al., 2001)	Mobility, self-care, usual activities, pain/discomfort, and anxiety/depression	Dialysis, kidney transplantation	English, Danish, Dutch, Finnish French, German, Japanese, Spanish, Thai, etc.
WHOQoL-BREF, 26 items (Skevington et al., 2004)	Physical health, psychological status, social relationships and environment	Haemodialysis, kidney transplantation	English, Chinese, Dutch, French, German, Hebrew, Japanese, Persian, Russian, Thai, etc.
NHP, 45 items (Wiklund, 1990)	6 domains of health and 7 domains of daily living	Haemodialysis, kidney transplantation	English, Danish, Dutch, French, German, Greek, Russian, Spanish, Swedish, Turkish
SIP, 136 items (Bergner et al., 1981)	Sleep and rest, emotional behaviour, body care and movement, home management, mobility, social interaction, ambulation, alertness behaviour, communication, work, eating, and recreation & pastimes	Dialysis, kidney transplantation	English, Arabic, Chinese, Danish, Dutch, Finnish, French, German, Italian, Norwegian, Portuguese, Romanian, Russian, Spanish, Swedish, Tamil, Thai
The Dartmouth COOP Charts, 7 items (Kempen et al., 1997)	Physical fitness, feelings, daily activities, social activities, change in health status, current overall health perceptions, and bodily pain	Dialysis	English, Dutch, Finnish, French, German, Hebrew, Japanese, Moroccan, Spanish, Turkish

Disease Quality of Life Short Form (KDQOL-SF); (3) the CHOICE Health Experience Questionnaire (CHEQ), and (4) the Kidney Disease Questionnaire (KDQ).

The KDQOL-36 and *the KDQOL-SF* questionnaires have been designed for ESRD. The KDQOL-36 has been translated into 24 different languages. These tools are commonly used in patients with CKD or who are receiving dialysis. The KDQOL-36 has been developed from the SF-36, but has added disease-specific items relating to the impact of disease-specific dietary restrictions and their attitudes towards the illness. The KDQOL-36 may create respondent burden due to it taking 30 minutes to complete, whilst the KDQOL-SF takes approximately 16 minutes to complete (Rettig et al., 1997). The KDQOL-SF questionnaire covers the domains of physical and mental health, and the six kidney disease issues of cognitive function, symptoms, and the effect of the kidney disease, sexual function, sleep, and patient satisfaction (Moreiras-Plaza et al., 2011). The KDQOL-SF has also been tested for validity and reliability, and used with kidney transplant recipients (Barotfi et al., 2006).

The CHOICE Health Experience Questionnaire (CHEQ) has been designed for ESRD and complements the SF-36. It has an additional eight generic domains and five ESRD-specific domains over and above the SF-36. The eight additional domains are: cognitive and sexual functioning, sleep, work, recreation, travel, finances, and general quality of life. The five ESRD-specific domains are: diet, freedom, body image, dialysis access (catheters and/or vascular), and symptoms (Wu et al., 2001).

The Kidney Disease Questionnaire (KDQ) has been constructed for patients receiving haemodialysis (Laupacis et al., 1992). Unlike other specific questionnaires, the KDQ only takes 10-15 minutes to complete (Edgell et al., 1996). However, this questionnaire does not evaluate a respondent's overall health status.

b. The two HRQoL questionnaires for kidney transplant recipients are the Kidney Transplant Questionnaire (KTQ) (Chisholm-Burns et al., 2011), and the End-Stage Renal Disease Symptom Checklist-Transplantation Module (ESRD-SCL) that is focused on transplantation-specific symptoms, psychological distress, and the side effects of immunosuppressive therapy (Franke et al., 1999).
c. The Wisconsin Stone QoL instrument (WSQ) was developed for patients with urolithiasis in 2013 (Penniston et al., 2013). However, this questionnaire is still in the process of being tested for its test-retest reliability, concurrent validity, and construct validity (Raja et al., 2014).

Three *classic administration modes for such questionnaires* are self-administered, face-to-face or over the telephone. Each method has its own advantages and disadvantages. Some advantages of self-administered surveys are that they are less expensive, more convenient, and provides more privacy than the interviews. Their disadvantages are poor response rates, and poor completion rates. Interviews provide a higher response rate than postal questionnaires and are suitable for non-readers. However, this method of data gathering is expensive in both time and money. There is also the possibility that an interviewer may bias the findings, i.e. the Hawthorne Effect. However, Unruh, et al. (2003) suggests that an interview-administered questionnaire is

Table 5. Most common disease-specific questionnaires for measuring quality of life in patients with kidney diseases

Questionnaire Abbreviation, Number of Items (References)	Dimensions	Patient Population	Languages
KDQOL-36, 36 items (Hays et al., 1994)	Physical and mental health, burden of kidney disease, symptoms, effects of kidney disease	Dialysis	English, Arabic, Chinese, French, German, Spanish, etc.
KDQOL-SF, 79 items (Hays et al., 1997)	Symptoms, burden of kidney disease, effects of kidney disease, work status, cognitive function, quality of social interaction, sexual function, sleep, social support, dialysis staff encouragement, patient satisfaction	Dialysis	English, Arabic, Hungarian, Polish, Turkish, Moroccan, Spanish
CHEQ, 83 items (Wu et al., 2001)	8 generic domains in the SF-36 combined with 8 additional generic domains and 5 ESRD-specific domains	Dialysis	English, Thai
KDQ, 26 items (Laupacis et al., 1992)	Physical symptoms, fatigue, depression, relationships, frustration	Haemodialysis	English
KTQ, 25 items (Laupacis et al., 1993)	Physical symptoms, fatigue, uncertainty/fear, appearance, and emotional status	Kidney transplantation	English, Persian, Spanish
ESRD-SCL, 43 items (Franke et al., 1999)	Limitations in the physical and cognitive capacity, cardiac and renal dysfunction, side effects of corticosteroids, increased hair growth, transplant-associated psychological disorders	Kidney transplantation	English, German, Norwegian, Spanish, Turkish
WSQ 28 item (Penniston et al., 2013)	Energy and fatigue, sleep, work and family, nutrition and pharmacological therapies, physical symptoms, concerns related to intimacy and travel, general emotional well-being	Urolithiasis	English

suitable for dialysis patients. Their study shows that patients who completed a HRQoL by themselves, had inaccurate HRQoL as dialysis patients frequently have vision problems and limited arm ranges during dialysis. Regarding *the time-period to measure the HRQoL*, this outcome can be assessed at one point, before and after interventions, or over a period of time, such as 1-2 years.

Advantages of the generic questionnaires, particularly the SF-36, are that they are able to assess the HRQoL in patients with various diseases, including kidney diseases. The findings from such tools can be compared with general populations or other patient groups. These questionnaires also take a shorter time to complete compared with the specific questionnaires, except the KDQ. However, they are sometimes unable to discriminate the HRQoL between patients who are receiving an intervention, and a placebo group; especially if the intervention improves some specific symptoms in patients with ESRD or kidney transplant recipients (Edgell et al., 1996). The disease-specific questionnaires are more responsive to detecting the treatment effects in the HRQoL related to a specific disease state. The authors of this chapter suggest that clinicians and researchers could use both generic and specific questionnaires to complement each other; the generic questionnaires can assess the HRQoL related to daily life, which is lacking in specific questionnaires. Therefore, researchers should choose the questionnaire and the method of administration that is most appropriate for their measurement objectives and their population. All of the questionnaires need permission from copyright holders before using them. Some may charge a license fee depending on whether it's for commercial or non-commercial usage, such as the SF-36, the NHP, the SIP136, the Dartmouth COOP Charts, or the KDQOL-36.

Several HRQoL tools provide a score of QoL, e.g. SF-36, KDQOL-36, etc., and it is a challenge to interpret the HRQoL scores to determine meaningful clinical practice and how to link HRQoL scores to a clinically relevant effect size. Recently, two methods have been proposed to identify a cutoff point of clinical significance in chronic diseases: anchor-based methods, and distribution-based methods (Revicki et al., 2008). *Anchor-based methods* estimate the minimal clinically important difference (MCID). The variety of MCID depends on the type of disease, the HRQoL questionnaire used, and the populations. The literature suggests that MCID for each disease is estimated by findings from clinical trials or systematic reviews. This existing evidence provides a target significant difference in HRQoL scores between treatment and control groups in patients with same disease. This difference should be associated with clinical significance. More details of the methods of estimating MCID are explained in a review of recommended methods for determining responsiveness (Revicki et al., 2008), and a paper (Hedayat et al., 2015). Unfortunately there is a lack of existing evidence to estimate MCID in patients with kidney diseases. Revicki, et al. (2008) suggests the use of a second method to determine clinically relevant effect sizes in HRQoL, i.e., *distribution-based.* This is the determination of clinically relevant effect sizes based on a distribution database of HRQoL scores in each disease. For instance, half a standard deviation of the mean HRQoL score in the population can be a cutoff point of clinical significance (Revicki et al., 2008). One major limitation of this method is that the determination of this cutoff point is mainly based on statistics and, as a result, may not relate to clinically relevant effect sizes. In addition, many factors may influence the HRQoL rather than the intervention, e.g. economic status, access to the basic needs of life, the national health system, availability of social support, etc. Lack of access to a health system is likely to cause a worsening in an individual's HRQoL, whilst having good social support seems to improve this outcome (Kang et al., 2015; Zyoud et al., 2016). Therefore, the interpretation of the HRQoL should include not only estimating a cutoff point of clinically relevant effect sizes in each kidney disease, but also other potential confounding factors related to the HRQoL scores.

Measure of Patients' Symptoms and Patient Satisfaction

Many generic and disease-specific questionnaires evaluate patients' symptoms or physical functioning; for example, SF-36, KDQoL, CHEQ, KDQ, and KTQ. These outcomes are subjective, so the data may be less accurate than objective, clinical outcomes. Validated instruments provide a more accurate measurement. The questionnaires often use a 4 or 5 point Likert scale, whilst others use Yes/No responses, visual analogue scales or 10-point scales to assess outcomes.

3. **Questionnaires to Evaluate Patients' Symptoms in Kidney Diseases:** Assessing symptoms in critically ill patients with ESRD can be adopted from symptom-specific questionnaires for patients with cancer, such as the Memorial Symptom Assessment Scale (short form), and the McGill Quality of Life questionnaire, due to such diseases having similar heath status, e.g. life-threatening (Murtagh et al., 2007). This section will focus on seven symptom-specific questionnaires validated for use in patients with CKD, receiving dialysis, or kidney transplants. Most of the questionnaires have been designed to assess the severity of symptoms in dialysis patients. Seven relevant symptom-specific questionnaires are: (1) the Palliative Care Outcome Scale-Symptoms modified for renal patients (POS-S renal), (2) the Human Activity Profile (HAP), (3) the Modified Edmonton Symptom Assessment System (ESAS), (4) the Dialysis Symptom Index (DSI), (5) the 100 Category Check List, (6) the Short-Version Check List, and (7) the Physical Symptom Distress Scale (PSDS) (Table 6). The ideal questionnaire to estimate patients' symptoms should target symptoms that have happened within the last 7 days in order to reduce recall bias, as well as being able to measure multiple symptoms (Flythe et al., 2015).

a. **The Palliative Care Outcome Scale-Symptoms modified for renal patients (POS-S Renal):** Evaluates 17 symptoms in patients with advanced CKD or end-stage renal disease (Murphy et al., 2009). Recently, the Integrated POS-Renal (IPOS-Renal) has been developed through the integration of the IPOS and POS-S Renal instruments in order to provide a short questionnaire to assess symptoms in ESRD patients (11 questions). This questionnaire is designed for clinicians but still needs to be fully validated (Palliative care Outcome Scale, 2012).

b. **The Human Activity Profile (HAP):** Has been validated in haemodialysis patients to measure physical activity and functioning (Johansen et al., 2001). This questionnaire is also used for patients with CKD and with kidney transplant recipients (Johansen et al., 2001; Robinson-Cohen et al., 2013). A total of 94 specific activities in the HAP relate to the energy expenditure required to perform a task such as getting in and out of chairs or bed, taking a bath, walking 30 yards, or climbing 6 steps. There are three options for response: (1) still doing this activity, (2) have stopped doing this activity, and (3) never did this activity.

c. **The Modified Edmonton Symptom Assessment System (ESAS):** Has been validated in both haemodialysis, and peritoneal dialysis patients. This tool assesses 10 symptoms using a visual analogue scale (0-10): pain, tiredness, well-being, drowsiness, shortness of breath, anxiety, depression, appetite, nausea, and itch (Davison et al., 2006). It is simple and suitable for clinical use.

d. **The Dialysis Symptom Index (DSI):** Has been tested for validity and reliability in patients undergoing haemodialysis, and measures a total of 30 symptoms (Weisbord et al., 2004). Examples of symptoms in the questionnaire are constipation, appetite, muscle cramps, swelling in legs, breathlessness, numbness, tiredness, pain, itch, worry, insomnia, mood, and libido.

e. **The 100 Category Check List:** Has been tested for validity and reliability in Japan (Tsutsui et al., 2014). Due to a high number of items (100), the Short Version Check List consisting of 31 categories has been developed for clinical use (Tsutsui et al., 2014). Regarding items in the short version, components are body function, and structure, activities and participation, and environmental. However, these questionnaires need to be translated and validated for other languages in other populations.

f. **The Physical Symptom Distress Scale (PSDS):** Has been developed to evaluate patients' symptoms of distress in haemodialysis (Chiou, 1998). This 16-item questionnaire is comprised of two domains: (1) fluid and electrolyte imbalance (e.g. numbness, impaired visual ability, swelling in feet, itching, fatigue, etc.), and (2) disturbance in neuromuscular function (e.g. dizziness, headache, muscle cramps, difficulty sleeping, shortness of breath, etc.).

Moreover, questionnaires have been designed to measure a specific symptom, e.g., anaemia or side effects of immunosuppressants, in patients with dialysis or kidney transplants, which are not included in the prior questionnaires. *The National Kidney Dialysis and Kidney Transplantation Study Symptom Checklist (NKDKTS)* has been validated to assess symptoms of anaemia in dialysis patients (Spiegel et al., 2009). Meanwhile, *the Transplant Symptom Occurrence and Distress Scale* evaluates symptoms of the side effects of immunosuppressants in kidney transplant recipients (Dobbels et al., 2008). However, these tools do not seem to be suitable for evaluating the severity of multiple symptoms.

Table 6. Symptoms-specific questionnaires for CKD, ESRD, and kidney transplantation

Questionnaire Abbreviation, Number of Items (References)	Dimension	Patient Population	Recall	Language
POS-S renal, 17 items (Murphy et al., 2009)	Physical symptoms, including itchy and restless legs	Advanced CKD, ESRD	3 days	English, Portuguese
HAP, 94 items (Johansen et al., 2001)	Energy expenditure required to perform the task	Haemodialysis, CKD, kidney transplantation	7 days	English, German
ESAS, 10 items (Davison et al., 2006)	Physical and psychological symptom distress	Dialysis	Present	English
DSI, 30 items (Weisbord et al., 2004)	Physical and emotional symptoms	Haemodialysis	7 days	English
100 Category Check List, 100 items (Tsutsui et al., 2014)	Body functions and structures, activities and participation, environmental factors	Haemodialysis	Unknown	Japanese
Short-Version Check List, 31 items (Tsutsui et al., 2014)	Body functions and structures, activities and participation, environmental factors	Haemodialysis	Unknown	Japanese
PSDS 16 item (Chiou, 1998)	Fluid and electrolyte imbalance and disturbance in neuromuscular function	Haemodialysis	7 days	English, Chinese

Measurement of Symptom Outcomes From Using CAM

The questionnaires measuring the improvement of symptoms in patients with kidney diseases may be applied to evaluating CAM. However, a limitation of these questionnaires is a lack of validity in CAM research, so the questionnaires should be used with caution.

Choosing a questionnaire to assess symptoms in CAM users depends on the target symptoms related to the CAM, and the population. When practitioners and researchers aim to measure a specific symptom, such as depression, they should use an available valid symptom-focused questionnaire. The Beck Depression Inventory and the Brief Pain Inventory are frequently used in evaluating depression and pain in dialysis patients (Murtagh et al., 2007). There is a validated generic questionnaire to assess the degree of any symptoms related to CAM use, i.e. the *'Measure Yourself Medical Outcome Profile' (MYMOP)*. It is used in measuring any symptom change, particularly in acute symptoms, over the period of time, and allows an individual to choose the most problematic symptom (Paterson, 1996). This questionnaire can measure an effect of a wide variety of CAMs as it is not designed to measure a specific symptom. It is simple and appropriate for CAM practitioners to use during a consultation. This tool covers the measurement of symptoms, activities, and wellbeing. The MYMOP 2 has been developed, based on limitations of the original MYMOP and added medication history for a chosen symptom (Paterson et al., 2000). The effects of several CAMs have been assessed by the MYMOP, such as acupuncture, massage therapy, and chiropractic (Hull et al., 2006; Polus et al., 2011; Wakefield, 2014). This questionnaire has also been translated from English into Chinese and validated in the Chinese population (Chung et al., 2010). Therefore, the MYMOP is recommended to assess alleviated symptoms from using CAM, although it needs to be tested for validity and reliability when used in patients with kidney diseases. A limitation of this tool is that it collects subjective data, so practitioners should interpret the findings with caution.

Questionnaires to Evaluate Patient Satisfaction

There is a lack of validated questionnaires to assess patient satisfaction in CKD patients and kidney transplant recipients. Few questionnaires assessing satisfaction in dialysis patients have been developed (Gu et al., 2015; Kirchgessner et al., 2006; RAND Health, 2015; Rubin et al., 1997;

Wasserfallen et al., 2006). They measure patient satisfaction from dialysis therapy and care, e.g. doctor and nurse services, physical environment at a dialysis clinic, etc. Health care providers use the questionnaires to improve their services. These tools therefore, need to be modified in order to assess specific CAMs, and need to be validated. However, some researchers may use their own questionnaires to evaluate patient satisfaction in CAM research (Barbadoro et al., 2011). Using standardised questionnaires to assess symptoms and patient satisfaction in CAM research provides more valid information rather than just reports of practitioner or patients' experience.

ADVERSE EFFECTS OF CAM

Potential renal side effects of herbal medicines and dietary supplements (HDS) are acute kidney injuries (AKI), electrolyte imbalance, or kidney stones. AKI is a factor caused by the progression of CKD, followed by end-stage renal disease, and death. Pre-existing CKD is, on the other hand, a potential risk to developing AKI. There are many case reports on these adverse events related to herbal medicine worldwide (Luyckx, 2012). However, some CAM modalities are more complex and employ more than one CAM, such as using herbal medicine together with acupuncture, so it is difficult to identify which element caused any adverse effect. In addition, adulterants in unregistered herbal products may cause AKI, e.g. steroids and non-steroidal anti-inflammatory drugs, etc.

Patients with CKD or kidney transplant recipients, who use herbal medicines and/or dietary supplements often do so together with conventional medicine. As a result, HDS may interact with conventional medicines, and either decrease or increase the effect of them. Consequently, patients may experience ineffectiveness or toxicity from the conventional medicine. This issue will be discussed in Chapter 8. Not only can the health products cause such adverse events, but also their indirect effect may lead to worsening illnesses; for instance, through poor conventional medication adherence, and delaying diagnosis or treatment amongst CAM users.

Acute Kidney Injuries, Electrolyte Imbalance, and Kidney Stones

The current universally accepted definition of AKI as proposed by the Acute Kidney Injury Network (AKIN) in 2007 (Table 7) (Lopes et al., 2013).

Table 7. The classification of severity of acute kidney injury

Stage	Serum Creatinine (SCR)	Urine Output
1 (Risk stage)	1.5 times baseline OR increase in Scr ≥ 0.3 mg/dl	< 0.5 ml/kg/h for 6 hours
2 (Injury stage)	2.0 times baseline	< 0.5 ml/kg/h for > 12 hours
3 (Failure stage)	3.0 times baseline OR	< 0.3 ml/kg/h for 24 hours OR
	Increase in Scr ≥ 4.0 mg/dl	Anuria for 12 hours

With this definition, two serum creatinine evaluations within 48 hours of symptom onset are necessary for the diagnosis of AKI; dialysis should be considered for any patient with AKI stage 3 (failure stage).

Evaluation of Nephropathy Related to Herbal and Dietary Supplements

To assess HDS that may induce AKI, any herbal medicines or dietary supplements resulting in AKI would be identified as nephrotoxic agents, if there are no other causes related to AKI, such as dehydration or conventional medicines, i.e. non-steroidal anti-inflammatory drugs (NSAIDs) (Table 8) (Choudhury et al., 2006; Lameire et al., 2013).

The World Health Organisation's Uppsala Monitoring Center causality assessment is a validated general questionnaire to evaluate adverse effects of medication. Due to a lack of tools assessing causality of herbal medicine related to nephropathy, the WHO causality assessment is frequently used (Table 9) (Tangkiatkumjai et al., 2015; The Uppsala Monitoring Centre, 2015).

For instance, if an herbal medicine which may be associated with AKI is assessed by these criteria and falls into the category of 'certain', this means that it is definitely associated with AKI. The World Health Organization's Uppsala Monitoring Center causality assessment can also be used to evaluate any adverse effects, such as electrolyte imbalance and kidney stones, as it is designed based on a general concept of evaluating adverse effects. Its limitations are that it does not use quantitative causality assessment, so assessors need to judge the likelihood of the adverse effect being related to the herbal medicine themselves. The modified Naranjo algorithm has been proposed as a way to evaluate causal relationships of adverse events with HDS (Table 10) (Ide et al., 2015). The main problem with the Naranjo algorithm is that there is a lack of evidence to confirm that HDS is related to adverse

Table 8. Common causes of acute kidney injuries

Causes	Region
Bleeding, dehydration	Worldwide
Sepsis, shock	
Nephrotoxic medicines	
ACEIs/ ARBs	
Aminoglycosides	
Amphotericin B	
Cyclosporine, tacrolimus	
Indinavir	
NSAIDs	
COX-2 inhibitors	
Radiocontrast media	
Diarrhoea	Tropical countries
Snake bite	
Tropical infectious diseases	
Traditional medicines	

ACEIs = Angiotensin-converting enzyme inhibitors
ARBs = Angiotensin II receptor antagonists
NSAIDs = Non-steroidal anti-inflammatory drugs
COX-2 inhibitors = Cyclooxygenase-2 inhibitors

events. The modified Naranjo algorithm responded to this by requiring information from the label or package insert of the HDS. Ide et al. also used dose-dependence on the severity of an adverse event. There is a rating scale for the total: (1) highly probable is defined as the total score ≥ 9; (2) 5-8 are defined as probable; (3) scores of 3-4 are defined as highly possible; (4) 1-2 score(s) are defined as possible; and (5) ≤ 0 is defined as unlikely. The modified algorithm is therefore practical. The limitation of this tool is that some HDS may cause AKI associated with hypersensitivity, so question no. 6 (Table 10) is not applicable.

The pathogenesis of AKI is due to the involvement of various cellular responses including leukocyte infiltration and humoral responses with proinflammatory cytokines, which induces apoptotic activities, abnormalities in immune modulators, and growth factors in the repair response (Devarajan, 2006; Kellum et al., 2011; Sanoff et al., 2011). The knowledge of the pathogenetic mechanism has founded a basis of current therapeutic interventions. There are three main rationales for AKI therapies. First,

Table 9. Causality assessment of suspected adverse effects

Category	Assessment Criteria
Certain	• Event or laboratory test abnormality, with plausible time relationship to suspected products intake • Cannot be explained by disease or other drugs • Response to withdrawal plausible (pharmacologically, pathologically) • Event definitive pharmacologically or phenomenologically (i.e. an objective and specific medical disorder or a recognised pharmacological phenomenon) • Rechallenge satisfactory, if necessary
Probable/ likely	• Event or laboratory test abnormality, with reasonable time relationship to suspected products intake • Unlikely to be attributed to disease or other drugs • Response to withdrawal clinically reasonable • Rechallenge not required
Possible	• Event or laboratory test abnormality, with reasonable time relationship to suspected products intake • Could also be explained by disease or other drugs • Information on suspected product withdrawal may be lacking or unclear
Unlikely	• Event or laboratory test abnormality, with a time to suspected products that makes a relationship improbable (but not impossible) • Disease or other drugs provide plausible explanations

Table 10. The modified Naranjo algorithm adapted from Ide et al. (2015)

Question	Yes	No	Do Not Know
1. Is there any notification about the adverse event on the label or package insert of the HDS?	+1	0	0
2. Did the adverse event appear after the suspected HDS intake?	+2	-1	0
3. Did the adverse event improve when the suspected HDS was discontinued?	+2	0	0
4. Did the adverse event reappear when the HDS was retaken?	+3	-1	0
5. Are there any alternative causes (other than the suspected HDS) that could on their own have caused the event?	-1	+2	0
6. Was the event more severe when the dose was increased or less severe when the dose was decreased?	+1	0	0
7. Did the consumer have a similar event to the same or a similar HDS in any previous exposure?	+1	0	0
8. Was the adverse event confirmed by any objective evidence?	+2	0	0

increasing oxygen delivery to the injured renal tissues by improving renal blood flow or decreasing oxygen demand in the repairing of renal tubular tissues. Second, reducing inflammatory processes via the inhibition or elimination of proinflamatory cytokines, free radical oxygen species, apoptotic activities, expressions of adhesion molecules, or leukocyte function. Third, promoting tissue repair by enhancing renal tubular regeneration via growth factors or mesenchymal stem cell therapy. However, most clinical trials have failed to establish any significant specific treatments (Conger, 1995; Jo et al., 2007; Ronco et al., 2003) as many have focused on eliminating inflammatory responses alone, believing that inflammation is maladaptive. To definitively identify pathophysiological effects of AKI, a kidney biopsy is required which is suited for research rather than routine practice as it is costly and needs specialists to operate and interpret the results. Several case reports of AKI being caused by health products have not had a kidney biopsy, so there is lack of evidence on this issue.

Assessment of Herbal and Dietary Supplements Associated With Electrolyte Imbalance and Kidney Stones

Several herbal medicines or dietary supplements can cause electrolyte imbalance, and urolithiasis. Excessive intake of vitamin C or star fruits, increase urinary oxalate excretion thereby increasing the risk of obstructive nephropathy from calcium oxalate crystals, which are identified by urinalysis (Abeysekera et al., 2015; Ferraro et al., 2015). Nonetheless, ultrasonography or computed tomography (CT) is sometimes required to diagnose obstruction from urolithiasis. In the advanced CKD patient (stage 3 CKD ; eGFR $<$ 60 ml/min/1.73m^2), taking these herbal medicines or dietary supplements can cause a faster decline in GFR (called AKI on CKD) and can eventually progress to end stage renal disease (stage 5 CKD) (Palevsky et al., 2013). Electrolyte imbalances, particularly hyperkalemia (serum potassium $>$ 5.5 mmoL/L) (Hollander-Rodriquez et al., 2006), and hyperphosphatemia (serum phosphate $>$ 4.5 mg/dL) (Moretti et al., 2008) have been associated with herbal medicine usage. Individuals with advanced CKD, especially stage 5, are already susceptible to hyperkalemia and hyperphosphatemia and therefore the accumulative use of HDS may potentially lead to life-threatening conditions such as arrhythmias, cardiac arrest or coronary artery disease. Due to limited evidence from clinical studies, animal studies are a further information source relating to the issue of safety. In general, herbal medicines should be tested for organ-targeted toxicity, including kidneys, in animal models. Therefore, it is suggested that practitioners and consumers should avoid usage without clear evidence of benefits.

In summary, health care providers should regularly monitor serum creatinine, levels of potassium and phosphate, and urinalysis in patients with renal insufficiency in order to prevent nephropathy from using herbal medicines or dietary supplements. Due to a lack of evidence on renal adverse effects of these products, practitioners who discover products related to such effects should report them in order to build up such evidence.

Indirect Risks From CAM Use

Many studies of patients with CKD and hypertension report that CAM users are less likely to adhere to their conventional medications than non-users (Gohar et al., 2008; Krousel-Wood et al., 2010; Tangkiatkumjai et al., 2013). Medication non-adherence causes uncontrolled blood pressure in the population and may result in worsening kidney function. Reasons for CAM users having poor medication adherence may involve having negative attitudes towards conventional medicine, such as concern about their potential adverse effects. Health practitioners should acknowledge this issue, identify CAM users who may have poor conventional medication adherence, and tackle the problem. There are many methods to detect this problem such as self-report, medication records at the pharmacy, pill counts, electronic monitoring systems, or monitoring of serum drug levels. The Morisky Scale is widely used in evaluating medication adherence in CAM users and routine practice due to the instrument being simple, convenient, and short. This questionnaire has been translated into more than 10 languages, including Arabic, Chinese, French, German, Korean, Norwegian, Persian, Spanish, Thai, and Turkish. A limitation of this self-report tool is the likelihood of overestimates of medication adherence because of recall, and social desirability bias. The 8-item Morisky Medication Adherence Scale® (MMAS-8-Item®) is the latest version of this validated questionnaire and has been used in patients with CKD. Permission for using it is required, and a license fee depends on the purpose of use.

Another indirect risk from using CAM is that it may delay patients from being diagnosed and treated (Wardle et al., 2014). This is because patients may consult CAM practitioners about non-specific symptoms, i.e. anorexia, fatigue, swelling, weight loss and diarrhoea, which may be indicative of serious diseases, such as chronic kidney disease or cancer. Therefore, CAM practitioners should be aware of this problem and refer patients to a doctor when they have symptoms that could indicate serious illnesses. Additionally, some CAM users refuse to disclose their use to their doctor because of concerns about disapproval from their doctor. As a result, interactions between

CAM and conventional medicines may not be recognised by health care providers, and patients may suffer from adverse effects or ineffectiveness of conventional medicines.

FUTURE RESEARCH DIRECTIONS

A high number of the validated questionnaires measure the humanistic outcomes of conventional medicine, and some of these questionnaires have been employed by CAM researchers or practitioners. Meanwhile, there is the lack of questionnaires which assess nephropathy due to using herbal medicines. The World Health Organisation's Uppsala Monitoring Center causality assessment is a general questionnaire to evaluate adverse effects from conventional medicines and is widely used. However, it needs a skillful assessor to evaluate adverse effects from using herbal medicines due to the questionnaire not including a quantitative causality assessment. To use this tool effectively requires knowledge about evaluating AKI, time to onset of AKI related to HDS, and other risk factors of AKI. The Naranjo algorithm is also a quantitative causality assessment model and is commonly used. Neither of these causality assessment instruments are disease-specific nor validated in patients who suffer from nephrotoxicity related to herbal medicines. Further research therefore needs to develop and validate a disease-specific tool to assess causality of nephropathy related to herbal medicine. The MYMOP has been widely used in measuring the improvement of any symptoms due to CAM, but it has not been tested in patients with kidney diseases. Therefore, the validity and reliability of this questionnaire in this population is required. There is also a lack of validated questionnaires to assess patient satisfaction with their lives related to CAM in these populations.

CONCLUSION

This chapter proposes methods for evaluating the benefits and risks of using CAM in CKD, dialysis therapy, kidney transplantation or urolithiasis. The target outcomes of CAM in these diseases are slowing the progression of CKD, alleviating symptoms in patients receiving dialysis, and a decrease in renal allograft rejection. Serum creatinine and eGFR are the markers employed to assess kidney function and AKI from both CAM or conventional medicine. These parameters are appropriate for a short-term follow-up, such as 6-12 months. Meanwhile, ESRD could be a long-term outcome of an intervention but requires 3-5 years. There are several validated questionnaires to evaluate symptoms, particularly in patients receiving dialysis. The Human Activity Profile measures the energy expenditure required to perform tasks and has been used with CKD, haemodialysis, and kidney transplant patients. This questionnaire may be used in evaluating the improvement of symptoms due to CAM. The MYMOP is widely used in evaluating alleviation of symptoms due to using CAM. The clinical outcomes of kidney transplantation and urolithiasis require a nephrologist to evaluate and interpret findings from renal biopsies, urinalysis or CT scans.

Some CAMs may improve a person's the health-related quality of life (HRQoL) rather than physiological changes, so validated questionnaires should be used in measuring this outcome. The SF-36 is frequently used in evaluating the HRQoL in CKD, dialysis therapy, kidney transplantation, urolithiasis, and CAM research.

CAM could cause both direct, and indirect, risks to health in patients with kidney diseases. Regarding the direct risks caused by active ingredients or adulterants in health products, AKI, electrolyte imbalance, or urolithiasis are the most common nephrotoxicity resulting from using HDS. Due to the lack of a disease-specific tool to evaluate nephropathy due to these products, the World Health Organisation's Uppsala Monitoring Center causality assessment, and the modified Naranjo algorithm have been proposed for evaluating causal relationships of nephropathy related to CAM and HDS, respectively. The potential indirect risks to the health of CAM users are poor adherence to conventional medicine, and a delay in diagnosis or treatment of a kidney disease. The next chapter will explain how to search, appraise, and make a clinical decisions based on robust evidence.

REFERENCES

Abeysekera, R. A., Wijetunge, S., Nanayakkara, N., Wazil, A. W., Ratnatunga, N. V., Jayalath, T., & Medagama, A. (2015). Star fruit toxicity: a cause of both acute kidney injury and chronic kidney disease: a report of two cases. *BMC Research Notes*, *8*(1), 796. doi:10.1186/s13104-015-1640-8 PMID:26680759

Badal, S. S., & Danesh, F. R. (2015). Diabetic nephropathy: Emerging biomarkers for risk assessment. *Diabetes*, *64*(9), 3063–3065. doi:10.2337/db15-0738 PMID:26294427

Barbadoro, P., Chiatti, C., D'Errico, M. M., Minelli, A., Pennacchietti, L., Ponzio, E., & Prospero, E. (2011). Complementary and alternative medicine (CAM) among adults in Italy: Use and related satisfaction. *European Journal of Internal Medicine*, *3*, e325–e332.

Barotfi, S., Molnar, M. Z., Almasi, C., Kovacs, A. Z., Remport, A., Szeifert, L., & Mucsi, I. et al. (2006). Validation of the kidney disease quality of life-short form questionnaire in kidney transplant patients. *Journal of Psychosomatic Research*, *60*(5), 495–504. doi:10.1016/j.jpsychores.2005.09.009 PMID:16650590

Bellomo, R., Ronco, C., Kellum, J. A., Mehta, R. L., & Palevsky, P. & Acute Dialysis Quality Initiative Workshop (2004). Acute renal failure - definition, outcome measures, animal models, fluid therapy and information technology needs: The Second International Consensus Conference of the Acute Dialysis Quality Initiative (ADQI) Group. *Crit Care, 8*(4), R204-212.

Bensalah, K., Tuncel, A., Gupta, A., Raman, J. D., Pearle, M. S., & Lotan, Y. (2008). Determinants of quality of life for patients with kidney stones. *The Journal of Urology*, *179*(6), 2238–2243. doi:10.1016/j.juro.2008.01.116 PMID:18423704

Bergner, M., Bobbitt, R. A., Carter, W. B., & Gilson, B. S. (1981). The sickness impact profile: Development and final revision of a health status measure. *Medical Care*, *19*(8), 787–805. doi:10.1097/00005650-198108000-00001 PMID:7278416

Bhowmik, D. M., Dinda, A. K., Mahanta, P., & Agarwal, S. K. (2010). The evolution of the Banff classification schema for diagnosing renal allograft rejection and its implications for clinicians. *Indian J Nephrol*, *20*(1), 2–8. doi:10.4103/0971-4065.62086 PMID:20535263

Busija, L., Pausenberger, E., Haines, T. P., Haymes, S., Buchbinder, R., & Osborne, R. H. (2011). Adult measures of general health and health-related quality of life. *Arthritis Care & Research (Hoboken)*, *63*(S11), S383–S412. doi:10.1002/acr.20541 PMID:22588759

Butt, Z., Yount, S. E., Caicedo, J. C., Abecassis, M. M., & Cella, D. (2008). Quality of life assessment in renal transplant: Review and future directions. *Clinical Transplantation*, *22*(3), 292–303. doi:10.1111/j.1399-0012.2007.00784.x PMID:18482050

Chiou, C. P. (1998). Development and psychometric assessment of the Physical Symptom Distress Scale. *Journal of Pain and Symptom Management*, *16*(2), 87–95. doi:10.1016/S0885-3924(98)00036-0 PMID:9737099

Chisholm-Burns, M. A., Erickson, S. R., Spivey, C. A., Gruessner, R. W. G., & Kaplan, B. (2011). Concurrent validity of kidney transplant questionnaire in US renal transplant recipients. *Patient Prefer Adherence*, *5*, 517–522. doi:10.2147/PPA.S24261 PMID:22114465

Choudhury, D., & Ahmed, Z. (2006). Drug-associated renal dysfunction and injury. *Nature Clinical Practice. Nephrology*, *2*(2), 80–91. doi:10.1038/ncpneph0076 PMID:16932399

Chuku, C. L., Valdez, J. R., & Ajonuma, L. C. (2010). Is Nottingham Health Profile a reliable tool to measure quality of life of Filipinos with chronic kidney diseases undergoing hemodialysis. *East African Journal of Public Health*, *7*(4), 286–288. PMID:22066322

Chung, V. C. H., Wong, V. C. W., Lau, C. H., Hui, H., Lam, T. H., Zhong, L. X., & Griffiths, S. M. et al. (2010). Using Chinese version of MYMOP in Chinese medicine evaluation: Validity, responsiveness and minimally important change. *Health and Quality of Life Outcomes*, *8*(111). PMID:20920284

Cirillo, M. (2010). Evaluation of Glomerular Filtration Rate and of Albuminuria/Proteinuria. *Journal of Nephrology*, *23*(2), 125–132. PMID:20213606

Conger, J. D. (1995). Interventions in clinical acute renal failure: What are the data? *American Journal of Kidney Diseases*, *26*(4), 565–576. doi:10.1016/0272-6386(95)90590-1 PMID:7573008

Coons, S. J., Rao, S., Keininger, D. L., & Hays, R. D. (2000). A comparative review of generic quality-of-life instruments. *PharmacoEconomics*, *17*(1), 13–35. doi:10.2165/00019053-200017010-00002 PMID:10747763

Cravedi, P., Ruggenenti, P., & Remuzzi, G. (2012). Proteinuria should be used as a surrogate in CKD. *Nature Reviews. Nephrology*, *8*(5), 301–306. doi:10.1038/nrneph.2012.42 PMID:22391456

DAgati, V. D. (2008). The spectrum of focal segmental glomerulosclerosis: New insights. *Current Opinion in Nephrology and Hypertension*, *17*(3), 271–281. doi:10.1097/MNH.0b013e3282f94a96 PMID:18408478

Davison, S. N., Jhangri, G. S., & Johnson, J. A. (2006). Cross-sectional validity of a modified Edmonton symptom assessment system in dialysis patients: A simple assessment of symptom burden. *Kidney International*, *69*(9), 1621–1625. doi:10.1038/sj.ki.5000184 PMID:16672923

Devarajan, P. (2006). Update on mechanisms of ischemic acute kidney injury. *Journal of the American Society of Nephrology*, *17*(6), 1503–1520. doi:10.1681/ASN.2006010017 PMID:16707563

Dobbels, F., Moons, P., Abraham, I., Larsen, C. P., Dupont, L., & De Geest, S. (2008). Measuring symptom experience of side effects of immunosuppresive drugs: The Modified Transplant Symptom Occurrence and Distress Scale. *Transplant International*, *21*(8), 764–773. doi:10.1111/j.1432-2277.2008.00674.x PMID:18435683

Earley, A., Miskulin, D., Lamb, E. J., Levey, A. S., & Uhlig, K. (2012). Estimating equations for glomerular filtration rate in the era of creatinine standardization: A systematic review. *Annals of Internal Medicine*, *156*(11), 785–795. doi:10.7326/0003-4819-156-11-201203200-00391 PMID:22312131

Edgell, E. T., Coons, S. J., Carter, W. B., Kallich, J. D., Mapes, D. L., Damush, T. M., & Hays, R. D. (1996). A review of health-related quality of life measures used in end-stage renal disease. *Clinical Therapeutics*, *18*(5), 887–938. doi:10.1016/S0149-2918(96)80049-X PMID:8930432

Edwards, I. R., & Aronson, J. K. (2000). Adverse drug reactions: Definitions, diagnosis, and management. *Lancet*, *356*(9237), 1255–1259. doi:10.1016/S0140-6736(00)02799-9 PMID:11072960

Ferraro, P. M., Curhan, G. C., Gambaro, G., & Taylor, E. N. (2015). Total, dietary, and supplemental vitamin C intake and risk of incident kidney stones. *American Journal of Kidney Diseases*, *67*(3), 400–407. doi:10.1053/j.ajkd.2015.09.005 PMID:26463139

Flythe, J. E., Powell, J. D., Poulton, C. J., Westreich, K. D., Handler, L., Reeve, B. B., & Carey, T. S. (2015). Patient-reported outcome instruments for physical symptoms among patients receiving maintenance dialysis: A systematic review. *American Journal of Kidney Diseases*, *66*(6), 1033–1046. doi:10.1053/j.ajkd.2015.05.020 PMID:26210069

Franke, G. H., Reimer, J., Kohnle, M., Luetkes, P., Maehner, N., & Heemann, U. (1999). Quality of life in end-stage renal disease patients after successful kidney transplantation: Development of the ESRD Symptom Checklist - Transplantation Module. *Nephron*, *83*(1), 31–39. doi:10.1159/000045470 PMID:10461033

Gohar, F., Greenfield, S. M., Beevers, D. G., Lip, G. Y. H., & Jolly, K. (2008). Self-care and adherence to medication: A survey in the hypertension outpatient clinic. *BMC Complementary and Alternative Medicine*, *8*(8), 4–12. doi:10.1186/1472-6882-8-4 PMID:18261219

Gu, X., & Itoh, K. (2015). Factors behind dialysis patient satisfaction: Exploring their effects on overall satisfaction. *Therapeutic Apheresis and Dialysis*, *19*(2), 162–170. doi:10.1111/1744-9987.12246 PMID:25363874

Hart, L. G., & Evans, R. W. (1987). The functional status of ESRD patients as measured by the sickness impact profile. *Journal of Chronic Diseases*, *40*(Suppl 1), 117S–136S. doi:10.1016/S0021-9681(87)80041-3 PMID:3298302

Hays, R. D., Kallich, J., Mapes, D. L., Coons, S. J., Amin, N., Carter, W. B., & Kamberg, C. J. (1997). *Kidney Disease Quality of Life Short Form (KDQOL-SF™) version 1.3: A manual for use and scoring*. Santa Monica, CA: Rand.

Hays, R. D., Kallich, J. D., Mapes, D. L., Coons, S. J., & Carter, W. B. (1994). Development of the kidney disease quality of life (KDQOL) instrument. *Quality of Life Research: An International Journal of Quality of Life Aspects of Treatment, Care and Rehabilitation*, *3*(5), 329–338. doi:10.1007/BF00451725 PMID:7841967

Hedayat, A. S., Wang, J., & Xu, T. (2015). Minimum clinically important difference in medical studies. *Biometrics*, *71*(1), 33–41. doi:10.1111/biom.12251 PMID:25327276

Heerspink, H. J. L., Tighiouart, H., Sang, Y., Ballew, S., Mondal, H., & Matsushita, K. et al.. (2014). GFR decline and subsequent risk of established kidney outcomes: A meta-analysis of 37 randomized controlled trials. *American Journal of Kidney Diseases*, *64*(6), 860–866. doi:10.1053/j.ajkd.2014.08.018 PMID:25441439

Hollander-Rodriquez, J. C., & Calvert, J. F. J. (2006). Hyperkalemia. *American Family Physician*, *73*(2), 283–290. PMID:16445274

Hull, S. K., Page, C. P., Skinner, B. D., Linville, J. C., & Coeytaux, R. R. (2006). Exploring outcomes associated with acupuncture. *Journal of Alternative and Complementary Medicine (New York, N.Y.)*, *12*(3), 247–254. doi:10.1089/acm.2006.12.247 PMID:16646723

Ide, K., Yamada, H., Kitagawa, M., Kawasaki, Y., Buno, Y., Matsushita, K., & Umegaki, K. et al. (2015). Methods for estimating causal relationships of adverse events with dietary supplements. *BMJ Open*, *5*(11), e009038. doi:10.1136/bmjopen-2015-009038 PMID:26608636

IN-CAM. (2014). *Framework of health outcome domains*. Retrieved from www.incamresearch.ca/content/browse-domain

Jo, S. K., Rosner, M. H., & Okusa, M. D. (2007). Pharmacologic treatment of acute kidney injury: Why drugs havent worked and what is on the horizon. *Clinical Journal of the American Society of Nephrology; CJASN*, *2*(2), 356–365. doi:10.2215/CJN.03280906 PMID:17699435

Johansen, K. L., Painter, P., Kent-Braun, J. A., Ng, A. V., Carey, S., Da Silva, M., & Chertow, G. M. (2001). Validation of questionnaires to estimate physical activity and functioning in end-stage renal disease. *Kidney International*, *59*(3), 1121–1127. doi:10.1046/j.1523-1755.2001.0590031121.x PMID:11231369

Kang, G. W., Lee, I. H., Ahn, K. S., Lee, J., Ji, Y., & Woo, J. (2015). Clinical and psychosocial factors predicting helth-related quality of life in hemodialysis patients. *Hemodialysis International. International Symposium on Home Hemodialysis*, *19*(3), 439–446. doi:10.1111/hdi.12271 PMID:25643587

Kellum, J. A., Unruh, M. L., & Murugan, R. (2011). Acute kidney injury. *BMJ Clin Evid*, *28*, 2011. PMID:21443811

Kempen, G. I. J. M., van Sonderen, E., & Sanderman, R. (1997). Measuring health status with the Dartmouth COOP charts in low-functioning elderly. Do the illustrations affect the outcomes? *Quality of Life Research: An International Journal of Quality of Life Aspects of Treatment, Care and Rehabilitation*, *6*(4), 323–328. doi:10.1023/A:1018427225299 PMID:9248314

Kidney Disease; Improving Global Outcome (KDIGO) CKD Work Group. (2012a). KDIGO 2012 clinical practice guideline for the evaluation and management of chronic kidney disease. *Kidney International. Supplement*, *3*(1), 34.

Kidney Disease; Improving Global Outcome (KDIGO) CKD Work Group. (2012b). KDIGO 2012 clinical practice guideline for the evaluation and management of chronic kidney disease. *Kidney International. Supplement, 3*(1), 1–150.

Kirchgessner, J., Perera-Chang, M., Klinkner, G., Soley, I., Marcelli, D., Arkossy, O., & Kimmel, P. L. et al. (2006). Satisfaction with care in peritoneal dialysis patients. *Kidney International, 70*(7), 1325–1331. doi:10.1038/sj.ki.5001755 PMID:16900092

Krousel-Wood, M. A., Muntner, P., Joyce, C. J., Islam, T., Stanley, E., Holt, E. W., & Webber, L. S. et al. (2010). Adverse effects of complementary and alternative medicine on antihypertensive medication adherence: Findings from the cohort study of medication adherence among older adults. *Journal of the American Geriatrics Society, 58*(1), 54–61. doi:10.1111/j.1532-5415.2009.02639.x PMID:20122040

Lamb, E. J., Stevens, P. E., & Deeks, J. J. (2015). What is the best glomerular filtration marker to identify people with chronic kidney disease most likely to have poor outcomes? *BMJ (Clinical Research Ed.), 350*(g7667). PMID:25583704

Lameire, N. H., Bagga, A., Cruz, D., De Maeseneer, J., Endre, Z., Kellum, J. A., & Vanholder, R. et al. (2013). Acute kidney injury: An increasing global concern. *Lancet, 382*(13), 170–179. doi:10.1016/S0140-6736(13)60647-9 PMID:23727171

Laupacis, A., Muirhead, N., Keown, P., & Wong, C. (1992). A disease-specific questionnaire for assessing quality of life in patients on hemodialysis. *Nephron, 60*(3), 302–306. doi:10.1159/000186769 PMID:1565182

Laupacis, A., Pus, N., Muirhead, N., Wong, C., Ferguson, B., & Keown, P. (1993). Disease-specific questionnaire for patients with a renal transplant. *Nephron, 64*(2), 226–231. doi:10.1159/000187318 PMID:8321355

Levey, A. S., Inker, L. A., Matsushita, K., Greene, T., Willis, K., Lewis, E., & Coresh, J. et al. (2014). GFR decline as an end point for clinical trials in CKD: A scientific workshop sponsored by the National Kidney Foundation and the US Food and Drug Administration. *American Journal of Kidney Diseases, 64*(6), 821–835. doi:10.1053/j.ajkd.2014.07.030 PMID:25441437

Lin, M. Y., Chiu, Y. W., Chang, J. S., Lin, H. L., Lee, C. T. C., & Chiu, G. F. et al.. (2015). Association of prescribed Chinese herbal medicine use with risk of end-stage renal disease in patients with chronic kidney disease. *Kidney International*, 5. PMID:26244923

Lopes, J. A., & Jorge, S. (2013). The RIFLE and AKIN classifications for acute kidney injury: A critical and comprehensive review. *Clin Kidney J*, *6*(1), 8–14. doi:10.1093/ckj/sfs160 PMID:27818745

Luyckx, V. A. (2012). Nephrotoxicity of alternative medicine practice. *Advances in Chronic Kidney Disease*, *19*(3), 129–141. doi:10.1053/j.ackd.2012.04.005 PMID:22578672

Merkus, M. P., Jager, K. J., Dekker, F. W., Boeschoten, E. W., Stevens, P., & Krediet, R. T. (1997). Quality of life in patients on chronic dialysis: Self-assessment 3 months after the start of treatment. *American Journal of Kidney Diseases*, *29*(4), 584–592. doi:10.1016/S0272-6386(97)90342-5 PMID:9100049

Miller, N. L., & Lingeman, J. E. (2007). Management of kidney stones. *BMJ (Clinical Research Ed.)*, *334*(7591), 468–472. doi:10.1136/bmj.39113.480185.80 PMID:17332586

Moreiras-Plaza, M., Blanco-Garcia, R., Cossio-Aranibar, C. R., & Rodriguez-Goyanes, G. (2011). Assessment of health-related quality of life: The cinderella of peritoneal dialysis. *International Journal of Nephrology*, *2011*, 528685. doi:10.4061/2011/528685 PMID:21808736

Moretti, E., & Funk, D. (2008). Endocrine and electrolyte disorders. In M. Newman, L. Fleisher, & M. Fink (Eds.), *Perioperative Medicine: Managing for outcome* (pp. 627–648). Philadelphia: Saunders.

Murphy, E. L., Murtagh, F. E., Carey, I., & Sheerin, N. S. (2009). Understanding symptoms in patients with advanced chronic kidney disease managed without dialysis: Use of a short patient-completed assessment tool. *Nephron. Clinical Practice*, *111*(1), c74–c80. doi:10.1159/000183177 PMID:19088482

Murtagh, F. E. M., Addington-Hall, J., & Higginson, I. J. (2007). The prevalence of symptoms in end-stage renal disease: A systematic review. *American Journal of Kidney Diseases*, *14*(1), 82–99. PMID:17200048

Naranjo, C. A., Busto, U., Sellers, E. M., Sandor, P., Ruiz, I., Roberts, E. A., & Greenblatt, D. et al. (1981). A method for estimating the probability of adverse drug reactions. *Clinical Pharmacology and Therapeutics*, *30*(2), 239–245. doi:10.1038/clpt.1981.154 PMID:7249508

National Kidney Foundation. (2002). Evaluation of laboratory measurements for clinical assessment of kidney disease. *American Journal of Kidney Diseases*, *39*(2suppl 1), S76–S110. doi:10.1053/ajkd.2002.30944

Ogutmen, B., Yildirim, A., Sever, M. S., Bozfakioglu, S., Ataman, R., Erek, E., & Emel, A. et al. (2006). Health-related quality of life after kidney transplantation in comparison intermittent hemodialysis, peritoneal dialysis, and normal controls. *Transplantation Proceedings*, *38*(2), 419–421. doi:10.1016/j.transproceed.2006.01.016 PMID:16549136

Palevsky, P. M., Liu, K. D., Brophy, P. D., Chawla, L. S., Parikh, C. R., Thakar, C. V., & Weisbord, S. D. et al. (2013). KDOQI US commentary on the 2012 KDIGO clinical practice guideline for acute kidney injury. *American Journal of Kidney Diseases*, *61*(5), 649–672. doi:10.1053/j.ajkd.2013.02.349 PMID:23499048

Palliative Care Outcome Scale. (2012). *IPOS-Renal*. Retrieved from http://pos-pal.org/maix/ipos-renal-in-english.php

Paterson, C. (1996). Measuring outcomes in primary care: A patient generated measure, MYMOP, compared with the SF-36 health survey. *BMJ (Clinical Research Ed.)*, *312*(7037), 1016–1020. doi:10.1136/bmj.312.7037.1016 PMID:8616351

Paterson, C., & Britten, N. (2000). In oursuit of patient-centered outcomes: A qualitative evaluation of the Meausre Yourself Medical Outcome Profile. *Journal of Health Services Research & Policy*, *5*(1), 27–36. doi:10.1177/135581960000500108 PMID:10787584

Penniston, K. L., & Nakada, S. Y. (2013). Development of an instrument to assess the health related quality of life of kidney stone formers. *The Journal of Urology*, *189*(3), 921–930. doi:10.1016/j.juro.2012.08.247 PMID:23017521

Polus, B. I., Kimpton, A. J., & Walsh, M. J. (2011). Use of the measure your medical outcome profile (MYMOP2) and W-BQ12 (Well-Being) outcomes measures to evaluate chiropractic treatment: An observational study. *Chiropr Man Therap*, *19*(1), 7. doi:10.1186/2045-709X-19-7 PMID:21418608

Rabin, R., & de Charro, F. (2001). EQ-5D: A measure of health status from the EuroQol Group. *Annals of Medicine*, *33*(5), 337–343. doi:10.3109/07853890109002087 PMID:11491192

Raja, A., ONeill, C., Joshi, H. B., & Salek, S. (2014). Re: development of an instrument to assess the health related quality of life of kidney stone formers: K.L. Penniston and S.Y. Nakada J Urol 2013;189:921930. *The Journal of Urology*, *192*(1), 280–281. doi:10.1016/j.juro.2014.01.112 PMID:24742763

RAND Health. (2015). *Dialysis patient satisfaction survey (DPSS)*. Retrieved from www.rand.org/health/surveys_tools/dpss.html

Refolo, P., Minacori, R., Mele, V., Sacchini, D., & Spagnolo, A. G. (2012). Patient-reorted outcomes (PROs): The significance of using humanistic measures in clinical trial and clinical practice. *European Review for Medical and Pharmacological Sciences*, *16*(10), 1319–1323. PMID:23104647

Rettig, R. A., Sadler, J. H., Meyer, K. B., Wasson, J. H., Parkerson, G. R. Jr, Kantz, B., & Patrick, D. L. et al. (1997). Assessing health and quality of life outcomes in dialysis: A report on an institute of medicine workshop. *American Journal of Kidney Diseases*, *30*(1), 140–155. doi:10.1016/S0272-6386(97)90578-3 PMID:9214415

Revicki, D., Hays, R. D., Cella, D., & Sloan, J. (2008). Recommended methods for determining responsiveness and minimally important differences for patient-reported outcomes. *Journal of Clinical Epidemiology*, *61*(2), 102–109. doi:10.1016/j.jclinepi.2007.03.012 PMID:18177782

Robinson-Cohen, C., Littman, A. J., Duncan, G. E., Roshanravan, B., Ikizler, T. A., Himmelfarb, J., & Kestenbaum, B. R. (2013). Assessment of physical activity in chronic kidney disease. *Journal of Renal Nutrition*, *23*(2), 123–131. doi:10.1053/j.jrn.2012.04.008 PMID:22739659

Ronco, C., & Bellomo, R. (2003). Prevention of acute renal failure in the critically ill. *Nephron. Clinical Practice*, *93*(1), c13–c20. doi:10.1159/000066646 PMID:12411754

Rubin, H. R., Jenckes, M., Fink, N. E., Meyer, K., Wu, A. W., Bass, E. B., & Powe, N. R. et al. (1997). Patients view of dialysis care: Development of a taxonomy and rating of importance of different aspects of care. *American Journal of Kidney Diseases*, *30*(6), 793–801. doi:10.1016/S0272-6386(97)90084-6 PMID:9398123

Sakthong, P., & Kasemsup, V. (2012). Health utility measured with EQ-5D in Thai patients undergoing peritoneal dialysis. *Value in Health*, *15*(1Suppl), S79–S84. doi:10.1016/j.jval.2011.11.005 PMID:22265072

Sanoff, S., & Okusa, M. (2011). *Possible prevention and therapy of postischemic acute tubular necrosis*. Retrieved from www.uptodate.com/contents/possible-prevention-and-therapy-of-postischemic-ischemic-acute-tubular-necrosis

Sathvik, B. S., Parthasarathi, G., Narahari, M. G., & Gurudev, K. C. (2008). An assessment of the quality of life in hemodialysis patients using the WHOQoL-BREF questionnaire. *Indian J Nephrol*, *18*(4), 141–149. doi:10.4103/0971-4065.45288 PMID:20142925

Schena, F. P. (2000). Epidemiology of end-stage renal disease: International comparison of renal replacement therapy. *Kidney International*, *57*(Suppl 74), S39–S45. doi:10.1046/j.1523-1755.2000.07407.x

Skevington, S. M., Lotfy, M., & OConnell, K. A. (2004). The World Health Organizations WHOQOL-BREF quality of life assessment: Psychometric properties and results of the internationl field trial. A report from the WHOQOL group. *Quality of Life Research: An International Journal of Quality of Life Aspects of Treatment, Care and Rehabilitation*, *13*(2), 299–310. doi:10.1023/B:QURE.0000018486.91360.00 PMID:15085902

Spiegel, D. M., Evans, R. W., Gitlin, M., & Mayne, T. J. (2009). Psychometric evaluation of the National Kidney Dialysis and Kidney Transplantation Study symptom checklist: Reliability and validity. *Nephrology, Dialysis, Transplantation*, *24*(2), 619–625. doi:10.1093/ndt/gfn523 PMID:18799605

Tangkiatkumjai, M., Boardman, H., Praditpornsilpa, K., & Walker, D.-M. (2013). Prevalence of herbal and dietary supplement usage in Thai outpatients with chronic kidney disease: A cross-sectional survey. *BMC Complementary and Alternative Medicine*, *13*(1), 153. doi:10.1186/1472-6882-13-153 PMID:23815983

Tangkiatkumjai, M., Boardman, H., Praditpornsilpa, K., & Walker, D.-M. (2015). Association of herbal and dietary supplements with progression and complications of chronic kidney disease: A prospective cohort study. *Nephrology (Carlton, Vic.)*, *20*(10), 679–687. doi:10.1111/nep.12531 PMID:26040915

Teo, B. W., Xu, H., Wang, D., Li, J., Sinha, A. K., Shuter, B., & Lee, E. J. C. et al. (2011). GFR estimating equations in a multiethnic Asian population. *American Journal of Kidney Diseases*, *58*(1), 56–63. doi:10.1053/j.ajkd.2011.02.393 PMID:21601325

The National Collaborating Centre for Chronic Conditions (Great Britain). (2008). *Chronic kidney disease: national clinical guideline for early identification and management in adults in primary and secondary care* (1st ed.). London: Royal College of Physicians.

The Nephrology Society of Thailand. (2009). *Clinical practice guidelines for pre-dialysis patients in 2009* (1st ed.). Bangkok: The Nephrology Society of Thailand.

The Uppsala Monitoring Centre. (2015). *The use of the WHO-UMC system for standardised case causality assessment*. Retrieved from http://who-umc.org/Graphics/24734.pdf

The WHOQoL Group. (1995). The World Health Organization Quality of Life assessment (WHOQoL): Position paper from the World Health Organization. *Social Science & Medicine*, *41*(10), 1403–1409. doi:10.1016/0277-9536(95)00112-K PMID:8560308

Travers, K., Martin, A., Khankhel, Z., Boye, K. S., & Lee, L. J. (2013). Burden and management of chronic kidney disease in Japan: Systematic review of the literature. *Int J Nephrol Renovasc Dis*, *6*, 1–13. doi:10.2147/IJNRD.S30894 PMID:23319870

Tsai, S. Y., Tseng, H. F., Tan, H. F., Chien, Y. S., & Chang, C. C. (2009). End-stage renal disease in Taiwan: A case-control study. *Journal of Epidemiology*, *19*(4), 169–176. doi:10.2188/jea.JE20080099 PMID:19542686

Tsutsui, H., Ohkubo, T., Tsuruta, Y., Kato, S., Yasuda, Y., & Oshida, Y. (2014). Development and validation of a short-version checklist for patients undergoing hemodialysis based on the International Classification of Functioning, Disability and Health. *Clinical and Experimental Nephrology*, 28. PMID:25543186

Tsutsui, H., Ojima, T., Tsuruta, Y., Kato, S., Yasuda, Y., & Oshida, Y. (2014). Validity of a checklist for hemodialysis patients based on the International Classification of Functioning, Disability and Health. *Therapeutic Apheresis and Dialysis*, *18*(5), 473–480. doi:10.1111/1744-9987.12163 PMID:25195794

Unruh, M., Yan, G., Radeva, M., Hays, R. D., Benz, R., & Athienites, N. V. et al.. (2003). Bias in assessment of health-related quality of life in a hemodialysis population: A comparison of self-administered and interview-administered surveys in the HEMO study. *Journal of the American Society of Nephrology*, *14*(8), 2132–2141. doi:10.1097/01.ASN.0000076076.88336.B1 PMID:12874468

Verhoef, M. J., Vanderheyden, L. C., Dryden, T., Mallory, D., & Ware, M. A. (2006). Evaluating complementary and alternative medicine interventions: In search of appropriate patient-centered outcome measures. *BMC Complementary and Alternative Medicine*, *6*(1), 38. doi:10.1186/1472-6882-6-38 PMID:17118197

Wakefield, M. L. (2014). Case report: The effects of massage therapy on a woman with thoracic outlet syndrome. *Int J Ther Massage Bodywork*, *7*(4), 7–14. PMID:25452819

Wardle, J. J. L., & Adams, J. (2014). Indirect and non-health risks associated with complementary and alternative medicine use: An integrative review. *European Journal of Internal Medicine*, *6*(4), 409–422.

Ware, J. E., & Sherbourne, C. D. (1992). The MOS 36-item short-form helth survey (SF-36). I. Conceptual framework and item selection. *Medical Care*, *30*(6), 473–483. doi:10.1097/00005650-199206000-00002 PMID:1593914

Wasserfallen, J. B., Moinat, M., Halabi, G., Saudan, P., Perneger, T., Feldman, H. I., & Wauters, J. P. et al. (2006). Satisfaction of patients on chronic haemodialysis and peritoneal dialysis. *Swiss Medical Weekly*, *136*(13-14), 210–217. PMID:16633970

Weisbord, S. D., Fried, L. F., Arnold, R. M., Rotondi, A. J., Fine, M. J., Levenson, D. J., & Switzer, G. E. (2004). Development of a symptom assessment instrument for chronic hemodialysis patients: The Dialysis Symptom Index. *Journal of Pain and Symptom Management*, *27*(3), 226–240. doi:10.1016/j.jpainsymman.2003.07.004 PMID:15010101

Wiklund, I. (1990). The Nottingham Health Profile - a measure of health-related quality of life. *Scandinavian Journal of Primary Health Care. Supplement*, *1*, 15–18. PMID:2100359

Wu, A. W., Fink, N. E., Cagney, K. A., Bass, E. B., Rubin, H. R., Meyer, K. B., & Powe, N. R. et al. (2001). Developing a health-related quality of life measure for end-stage renal disease: The CHOICE Health Experience Questionnaire. *American Journal of Kidney Diseases*, *37*(1), 11–21. PMID:11136162

Wyld, M., Morton, R. L., Hayen, A., Howard, K., & Webster, A. C. (2012). A systematic review and meta-analysis of utility-based quality of life in chronic kidney disease. *PLoS Medicine*, *9*(9), e1001307. doi:10.1371/journal.pmed.1001307 PMID:22984353

Yang, F., Lau, T., Lee, E., Vathsala, A., Chia, K. S., & Luo, N. (2015). Comparison of the preference-based EQ-5D-5L and SF-6D in patients with end-stage renal disease (ESRD). *The European Journal of Health Economics*, *16*(9), 1019–1026. doi:10.1007/s10198-014-0664-7 PMID:25519850

Zyoud, S. H., Daraghmeh, D. N., Mezyed, D. O., Khdeir, R. L., Sawafta, M. N., Ayaseh, N. A., & Al-Jabi, S. W. et al. (2016). Factors affecting quality of life in patients on haemodialysis: A cross-sectional study from Palestine. *BMC Nephrology*, *17*(1), 44. doi:10.1186/s12882-016-0257-z PMID:27117687

KEY TERMS AND DEFINITIONS

Acute Kidney Injury: A decline in kidney function within less than 3 months.

Clinical Outcome: A positive outcome of intervention which alters the physiological status and is measured by a laboratory test or physical examination.

Electrolyte Imbalance: An abnormality of a serum level of electrolytes which may be increased or decreased from their normal value.

Estimated Glomerular Filtration Rate: A standard parameter of the measurement of kidney function.

Health-Related Quality of Life: A perception of an individual in terms of their physical, mental and social well-being which is influenced by their health status.

Humanistic Outcome: A positive outcome of intervention which alters the quality of life, symptoms, and the patient's satisfaction with health care.

Indirect Risk: An unwanted harm which does not directly result from an exposure.

Progression of Chronic Kidney Disease: A constant decline in kidney function among people with chronic kidney disease.

Proteinuria: A parameter which is measured by amounts of protein in urine and indicates the progression of kidney diseases.

Renal Adverse Effect: An unwanted effect of renal problems which may be associated with either conventional or alternative medicine.

Chapter 5
How to Search and Critique Scientific Evidence for Decision-Making

Mayuree Tangkiatkumjai
Srinakharinwirot University, Thailand

Win Winit-Watjana
International Medical University, Malaysia

Li-Chia Chen
The University of Manchester, UK

ABSTRACT

A clinical decision on the use of complementary and alternative medicine (CAM) should be made based on evidence-based medicine (EBM) together with practitioner's knowledge and experiences. This chapter describes the process of EBM, including how to address a clinical question, do a systematic search for appropriate evidence with key search terms, appraise the evidence and make a clinical decision on CAM applications. An effective literature search should be performed by using a structured search strategy in searching biomedical and CAM databases, such as the National Center for Complementary and Alternative Medicine (CAM Citation Index). Few standard tools are recommended to evaluate the quality of CAM studies, i.e. the CONSORT extension for herbal interventions and STRICTA for RCTs of acupuncture. Additionally, some guidelines for designing RCTs in Chinese herbal medicine (CHM) can also be adopted to critique CAM literature. A clinical decision on choosing optimal CAM for patient care should be based on the current best evidence emerged from the EBM process.

DOI: 10.4018/978-1-5225-2882-1.ch005

INTRODUCTION

Decision-making on optimising the use of complementary and alternative medicine (CAM) is challenged for clinical practitioners due to a lack of robust clinical evidence. Therefore alternative approaches such as anecdotes or recommendations from others, may be used to rationalise clinical decisions. However, the evidence-based medicine (EBM) process which is employed in western or conventional medicine to facilitate clinical decision making, is an appropriate approach to making a decisions whether to use CAM. Three key components, i.e. clinical expertise, patient's values and preferences, and the best research evidence, should be integrated into the EBM decision-making process to ensure optimum health outcomes in terms of therapeutic, economic or humanistic impacts.

According to Sackett and team (1996) EBM refers to the conscientious, explicit and judicious use of current best evidence in making decisions about individual patient care. Another definition is 'the 'systematic reviewing, critically appraising and using results from clinical studies in order to provide optimal patient care' (Rosenberg, et al., 1995). The correct concept of evidence source and quality, together with the relevant skills required to retrieve, appraise and apply the best current evidence is the foundation for making an evidence-based clinical decision when choosing CAM. This chapter outlines these processes.

Prior knowledge of best current evidence is the cornerstone to implementing EBM into clinical decision-making. Evidence is generally referred to as a fact or information obtained from clinical or scientific studies using appropriate methodologies, however the quality of evidence varies. Several organisations, e.g. Oxford Centre for Evidence-Based Medicine, or the Scottish Intercollegiate Guidelines Network (SIGN), have endeavoured to categorise the levels of evidence for judging the causal relationship of clinical interventions, i.e. from the highest to the lowest, based on the quality of the clinical studies. To facilitate decision-making when choosing CAM, the category proposed by National Health and Medical Research Council (2009) is often used (Table 1).

A systematic review of randomized controlled trials (RCTs), including meta-analysis, is the strongest evidence level, followed by RCTs, non-RCTs, observational studies (e.g. cohort or case-control studies), and cross-sectional research for judging causality. The RCT is an experimental design aimed to minimise bias and control confounding factors. RCTs provide more rigorous

Table 1. Levels of evidence (National Health and Medical Research Council, 2009)

Level	Study Design
I	Systematic reviews of level II studies
II	Randomised controlled trials (RCTs)
III	Non-RCTs, observational studies, cross-sectional studies
IV	Case series, case reports, expert opinions
V	Animal studies

evidence than observational studies or other study types as can infer causality between interventions and outcomes. In contrast, case reports, together with expert opinions, and animal studies, are regarded as weak levels of evidence for causality. On the whole, if a systematic review or RCT is currently available, it should be chosen as the best evidence to support clinical decision making. If no such study exists, the decision may be based on a weaker level of evidence. A clinical judgement might be changed at a later date if new evidence at a stronger level emerges. Although results derived from RCTs are deemed the 'gold standard' of evidence for evaluating efficacy and safety of CAM, and conventional medicine in the management of kidney disorders, it is a challenge to carry out an RCT on CAM. Currently, there have been few systematic reviews and meta-analyses on the efficacy or safety of CAM in kidney diseases (Chapter 7). Most CAM studies are small in scale and non-RCT. A large number of studies in herbal medicines are conducted in animals in order to prove their biological and toxic effects. Thus, the results of animal studies are likely to be extrapolated by clinical decision makers to support the efficacy and safety of herbal medicines used in humans. In reality, CAM has been used in daily life for hundreds of years and people choose CAM based on their own experiences or knowledge.

In general, the process of EBM is categorised into five steps, called the "5 A's", including; asking an answerable question, finding an article (or evidence), critically appraising the evidence, applying the evidence, and assessing the outcome, Figure 1 (Straus, et al., 2010).

Figure 1. Five steps of evidence-based medicine for complementary and alternative medicine

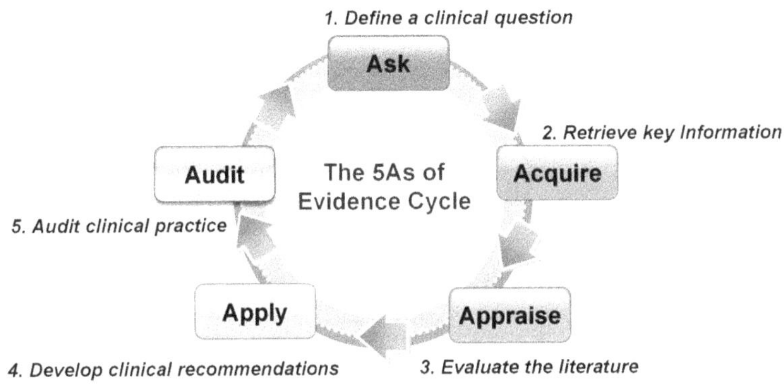

ADDRESSING QUESTIONS AND CREATING KEY SEARCH TERMS

First and foremost, a focused clinical question about CAM must be identified. However, it is often difficult to translate a clinical problem into a question that can be answered. Therefore, a 'PICO' framework, i.e. the population (or patient), intervention (or indicator), comparator (or control) and outcome, is recommended to guide defining a clinical question (Wilson, et al., 2002). For instance, the question, 'Can vitamin C reduce cardiovascular events in adult patients with chronic kidney disease at stages 3 – 5?' can be constructed using PICO as:

- **Population:** Adult patients with stages 3 – 5 chronic kidney disease.
- **Intervention:** Vitamin C given to the patients.
- **Comparator:** Either a placebo or standard treatment.
- **Outcome:** Cardiovascular events that may include direct and surrogate outcomes, such as all-cause mortality, length of stay, etc.

The PICO framework is applicable to defining different types of CAM questions. Flower, et al. (2014) categorised ten types of questions related to CAM (Table 2). The most common one is about how to manage a disease or condition, which is sometimes called an 'intervention' question. It should be noted that not all question types requires all of the PICO elements. For example, in a qualitative approach to explore an experience the question may only require the 'P' and 'O' elements.

Table 2. Questions related to CAM adapted from Flower et al. (2014)

Type	Question
1. Treatment/intervention	What is the efficacy of CAM for a specific disease/condition?
2. Treatment/intervention	What is the effectiveness of CAM in practice?
3. Risk/safety	Are there any adverse effects from CAM?
4. Health promotion	How effective is CAM to promote/boost health?
5. Disease prevention or protection	How effective is CAM to prevent a disease/condition?
6. Health rehabilitation	How effective is CAM for the rehabilitation?
7. Experience	What is the patient's experience of using CAM?
8. Indication/prediction	Which conditions seem to respond well to CAM?
9. Prognosis	When (or how long) will CAM have an effect?
10. Component	What are the active ingredients of a particular herbal medicine?

SEARCHING MEDICAL DATABASES

To answer a focused CAM question, appropriate evidence is needed, hence a systematic literature search is recommended. This process includes identifying key search terms, selecting suitable databases (or information sources), searching for pertinent literature, and keeping search records. Initially, either 'narrow' or 'broad' search terms can be applied to the literature search. Considering the example above, the narrow terms may be adult patients, advanced chronic kidney disease, vitamin C, and cardiovascular events. If the search terms only render limited records, broader terms, e.g. antioxidant therapy, kidney diseases, etc., may be used. Alternatively, we can make use of the keywords provided by several databases or previous systematic reviews as search terms.

If CAM terminologies are not consistently indexed by standard subject headings among various databases, a wide range of search terms should be tried to identify all relevant evidence, such as different CAM modalities, e.g. homeopathy, meditation, etc. (Pilkington, 2007). For example, if you wished to find the evidence for meditation to help relieve the complications of chronic kidney disease. The key search terms of the intervention, i.e. meditation, mind-body therapy, mind-body medicine, relaxation therapy, and relaxation techniques may be applied. Moreover, if we need to search for CAM efficacy in clinical outcomes, 'slow progression of chronic kidney disease', may also be used as a key search term. Pharmacological or biological effects of CAM, such as diuretic effects and inhibition of angiotensin-converting enzyme, may also be applicable.

Regarding the information sources, practitioners can choose a wide range of biomedical and CAM databases that may be general or specific to CAM related issues. The online general databases for literature include the Medical Literature Analysis and Retrieval System Online (MEDLINE), Excerpta Medica Database (EMBASE), and Scopus. Whilst Cochrane Collaboration is a good resource for finding systematic reviews. Table 3 shows the advantages and disadvantages of the biomedical databases (Coelho et al., 2007).

Examples of specific CAM databases are the National Center for Complementary and Alternative Medicine (CAM Citation Index), and Research Council for Complementary Medicine (CISCOM). A list of comprehensive databases for primary CAM literature is shown in Table 4.

With respect to Ayurveda medicine, practitioners have to access Indian databases, i.e. the Central Council for Research in Ayurveda and Sidha (CCRAS), IndMed, Annotated Bibliography of Indian Medicine (ABIM), or the National Institute of Science Communication and Information Resources (NISCAIR). IndMed, ABIM, and NISCAIR provides free access to full-texts of Indian journals of CAM (Table 5). To make their publications available for locals and save on the cost of publication, Indian researchers are likely to publish their work in Indian journals rather than Western ones (Aleem, et al., 2009). Likewise, relevant literature on Chinese herbal medicine and acupuncture are often provided by Chinese databases, i.e. Chinese BioMedical Literature Database (CBM), Chinese Medical Current Contents (CMCC), Traditional Chinese Medical Literature Analysis and Retrieval System (TCMLARS), Chinese Dissertation database, China Medical Academic Conference, Chinese National Knowledge Infrastructure databases, and Index to Taiwan Periodical Literature. Subscriptions to these databases is required.

A structured-literature search strategy is constructed by using key search terms either alone or with general or CAM database specific search operators. For example, the Boolean 'and', 'or', 'not', wild cards for single characters (?), or strings (*), and field restrictions for tags (e.g. title, abstract and year of publication) are commonly used operators. Applying CAM database specific operators usually retrieves more eligible hits than using general operators.

Table 3. Biomedical databases

Database	Produced by	Advantages	Disadvantages
CINAHL	EBSCO	■ The largest nursing research database ■ Coverage in complementary and alternative medicine, Traditional Chinese Medicine, herbs & medicinal plants and chiropractic medicine ■ Indexing more than 5,400 journals	Subscription required
EMBASE®	Elsevier	■ Strong coverage in pharmaceutical and pharmacological topics ■ Including all MEDLINE records ■ Including conference abstracts since 2009 ■ Indexing more than 8,500 journals published worldwide ■ Journal origins: 33.8% from North America and 49.7% from Europe ■ Updated weekly	Subscription required
MEDLINE®	The U.S. National Library of Medicine	■ Provides the core clinical literature of biomedicine, e.g. pharmacy, nursing and allied health ■ Indexing 5,600 journal citations and abstracts worldwide ■ Journal origins: 40.5% from North America and 48.5% from Europe ■ Free access ■ Updated daily ■ Easier to search than OVID®	■ Limited coverage in basic sciences, e.g. phytochemistry, biology and chemistry ■ Does not include book chapters
OVID®	Ovid Technologies	■ Searches MEDLINE database ■ Includes textbooks ■ Provides more relevant research than MEDLINE®	■ Subscription required ■ 7-days less up-to-date than MEDLINE®
Scopus	Elsevier	■ Searches both MEDLINE and EMBASE databases ■ Coverage in all health sciences Indexes 12,850 journals ■ Includes textbooks ■ Updated 1-2 times weekly	Subscription required
The Cochrane Library	The Cochrane Collaboration	■ Contains 6 databases: Cochrane Database of Systematic Reviews, Cochrane Central Register of Controlled Trials, Cochrane Methodology Register, Database of Abstracts of Reviews of Effects, Health Technology Assessment Database, and NHS Economic Evaluation Database ■ Contains systematic reviews and meta-analyses of biomedical literature ■ Mostly free to access	■ The secondary literature ■ Update every two years
PsynINFO®	APA PsycNET®	■ Coverage in behavioural and social science research worldwide ■ Included abstracts and all dissertation records ■ Indexing 2,500 journals ■ Updated weekly	Subscription required

CINAHL = the Cumulative Index of Nursing and Allied Health Literature

Table 4. Comprehensive databases regarding CAM

Database	Produced by	Information	Available
HerbalMed	Nonprofit Alternative Medicine Foundation	Effectiveness, adverse events and product preparations of the most commonly used herbal medicines in the US, e.g. black cohosh, horse chestnut, garlic, aloe vera, Hawthorn, Echinacea, Eleuthero (formerly Siberian ginseng), ginkgo, St. John's wort, olive, Asian ginseng, kava, elderberry, saw palmetto, milk thistle, stinging nettle, cranberry, bilberry, valerian and ginger	www.herbmed.org/index.html#param.wapp?sw_page=herblist%3Fletter%3DA [last accessed 26/03/17]
Natural Medicines	Therapeutic Research Center	Effectiveness and adverse effects of herbal medicines and dietary supplements, including drug-herbs/supplement interactions	https://naturalmedicines.therapeuticresearch.com/ [last accessed 26/03/17] (subscription required)
AMED*	Health Care Information Service of the British Library	Bibliographic records of CAM, and Allied Health Professional research, e.g. occupational therapy, physiotherapy, etc.	www.ebscohost.com/academic/AMED-The-Allied-and-Complementary-Medicine-Database [last accessed 26/03/17] (subscription required)
Alt HealthWatch	EBSCOhost	Full-texts of CAM studies from relevant journals, e.g. American J. Chinese Medicine, European J. Clinical Hypnosis, etc.	www.ebscohost.com/academic/alt-healthwatch [last accessed 26/03/17] (subscription required)
CAMbase	Chair of Medical Theory and Complementary Medicine	Bibliographic records of CAM	http://cambase.dmz.uni-wh.de/opencam/index_en.html [last accessed 26/03/17]

* The Allied and Complementary Medicine Database

Table 5. Indian databases regarding CAM

Database	Produced by	Information	Available
ABIM	Jan Meulenbeld	▪ Coverage of Indian Medical Literature ▪ Contains 50,000 articles and textbooks. ▪ Free access	http://indianmedicine.eldoc.ub.rug.nl/index.php?Search=&pSearch=Zoeken [last accessed 26/03/17]
CCRAS	Ministry of AYUSH, Government of India	▪ Focus on Ayurvedic sciences ▪ Coverage of 3 journals, i.e. *J. Res. Ayurvedic Sciences, J. Drug R. Ayurvedic Sciences, J. Indian Medical Heritage* ▪ Abstracts and textbooks but poor availability of full-texts	www.ccras.nic.in/mainpublication.html [last accessed 26/03/17]
IndMed	National Informatics Centre	▪ Contains 100 peer reviewed Indian medical journals ▪ Free access	http://indmed.nic.in/ [last accessed 26/03/17]
NISCAIR	Government of India	▪ Natural products repository ▪ Free access	http://nopr.niscair.res.in/handle/123456789/7305 [last accessed 26/03/17]

However, some of the CAM databases requires a subscription, which can be costly. The HerbMed database is suitable for users, particularly in the US. The Cochrane CAM group includes the systematic reviews of RCTs on CAM and the benefits and safety of several CAM modalities in various conditions, such as stroke, dementia, diabetes, liver or kidney diseases. From 2011 to 2015, the Cochrane CAM group has published the most systematic reviews for herbal medicines or acupuncture for rheumatological treatment. A few systematic reviews of CAM for kidney diseases are included, such as Astragalus for treating chronic kidney disease (CKD) (Zhang, et al., 2014), *Rheum officinale* for preventing CKD progression (Wang, et al., 2012), *Cordyceps sinensis* for CKD management (Zhang, et al., 2014), and fish oil for kidney transplant recipients (Lim, et al., 2007). Details of these findings are described in Chapter 7.

Overall, an effective searching method for CAM is to search different sources, i.e. generic and specific databases. After retrieving all relevant articles, the abstracts or full-texts will then be screened for their relevance. It is also recommended to keep articles which are eligible for reviewing in a personal database or reference management software, e.g. Reference Manager™, EndNote™ or Zotero™ (free software from Firefox). They are then ready for the next step of critical appraisal.

PRINCIPLES OF APPRAISING EVIDENCE

Critical appraisal in EBM refers to the process of systematically examining research evidence in terms of its validity, impact, and applicability before using the evidence for decision-making in practice (Sackett, et al., 1996). To achieve the objectives, various checklists have been investigated. However, the easiest way is to ask seven questions:

1. What are the research questions or objectives?
2. What are the study variables or outcomes?
3. Is the study designed to minimise biases and control confounders?
4. How about the study design in terms of study type, population and samples, study instrument and procedure?
5. Is the statistical analysis appropriate?
6. Do the results answer the research questions or objectives?
7. Are the findings beneficial to your work?

The critical appraisal of an original article starts with assessing whether a research question is aligned with PICO. The evaluation of research methods is regarding the study design, population and sample (plus sampling procedure), study instrument, data collection, and data analysis. Study designs embrace descriptive, analytical (or associational) or intervention studies. Strengths and weaknesses of different study designs are summarised in Table 6.

The most relevant study design should be used to address specific CAM research questions (Table 7). Take the previous question "Can vitamin C reduce cardiovascular events in adult patients with chronic kidney disease at stages 3 – 5?" as an example. To assess the efficacy of vitamin C, the most appropriate study design would be a RCT. Another example is, if practitioners would like to check whether senna (a mild laxative) can be safely used in patients with CKD. When there are no RCTs or any observation studies available, a case report may be a better information source. Some research questions are too complex to be answered by only one type of study design or one level of

Table 6. Strengths and weaknesses of study designs

Study Design	Strength	Weakness
Systematic review	▪ More reliable than discrete studies ▪ Minimises bias ▪ Inexpensive	May be difficult to synthesise evidence due to heterogeneity
Randomised controlled trial	▪ Provides efficacy of interventions ▪ Internal validity ▪ Minimises bias	▪ Not pragmatic (external validity) ▪ Expensive and time-consuming
Prospective cohort studies	▪ Establishes causality between exposure and outcome ▪ Investigates real circumstances ▪ Provides incidence of outcomes ▪ Can measure several outcomes for one exposure	▪ Requires large sample sizes ▪ Risk for confounding ▪ Inappropriate for rare diseases or outcomes ▪ Expensive ▪ Requires long periods of follow-up
Case-control studies	▪ Useful for rare diseases/outcomes ▪ Short period of study ▪ Inexpensive ▪ Can measure several risk factors for a single outcome	▪ High confounding and bias such as recall bias ▪ Cannot fully establish causality between exposure and outcome
Cross-sectional studies	▪ Provides prevalence of outcomes ▪ Short period of study ▪ Inexpensive	▪ High confounding and bias ▪ Cannot establish causality between exposure and outcome ▪ Inappropriate for rare diseases
Case series and case reports	▪ Provides rare diseases or adverse events of exposure ▪ Simple and inexpensive	Cannot establish prevalence or incidence
Animal studies	Provides biological and toxic effects of intervention	▪ Poor extrapolating from laboratory animals to humans ▪ Expensive and time-consuming

Table 7. Research questions and respective study designs adapted from Flower et al. (2014)

Research Question	Study Design
What is the efficacy of CAM for a specific disease/condition?	Randomised controlled trial
What is the effectiveness of CAM in practice?	Pragmatic randomised trials
Are there adverse effects from CAM?	Observational studies and case reports
How effective is CAM to promote/boost health?	Pragmatic randomised trials and observational studies
How effective is CAM to prevent a disease/condition?	Pragmatic randomised trials and observational studies
How effective is CAM for the rehabilitation?	Pragmatic randomised trials and observational studies
What is the patient's experience of using CAM?	Qualitative research
Which conditions seem to respond well to CAM?	Cross-sectional surveys of CAM practitioners
What are the active ingredients of a particular herbal medicine?	Laboratory experiments

evidence. As a result, a wide range of evidence, such as clinical trials together with qualitative studies, may be exploited to provide an optimal solution.

Some CAM interventions, such as the combination of acupuncture and herbal medicine, may not be appropriate for an RCT. Instead, pragmatic clinical trials (PCTs) are used to investigate the effectiveness of the complex CAM modalities in a real world practice. PCTs normally have three salient features, including recruitment of participants with characteristics similar to actual practice (e.g. older patients with renal insufficiency), performing more than one intervention as is in practice, and providing patient-centred outcomes, such as quality of life or patient satisfaction (Elm, et al., 2007). Details of PCTs are described in Chapter 10. Observational studies and case reports are more useful in providing evidence about adverse events of CAM rather than efficacy, whilst, cross-sectional surveys of CAM practitioners may elicit expert opinion regarding what CAM modalities are appropriate for a particular condition with what expected outcomes. Regarding herbal medicines, evidence from animal studies has been used when human studies are not available, such as nephrotoxicity, liver toxicity and teratogenicity of herbal medicines. This evidence informs us which herbal products are likely to cause adverse events in humans. Laboratory experiments usually reveal various active ingredients that could probably have a biological effect on a certain condition. This evidence may support the benefits of herbal medicines. When a high level of evidence is not available, traditional knowledge or expert opinions may be employed to support the use of CAM, as CAMs have been used for self-care, especially among Asian people, for generations.

APPRAISING EVIDENCE DERIVED FROM DIFFERENT STUDY DESIGNS

As mentioned above, the critical appraisal of evidence includes the evaluation of research questions, methods, and findings. There are some standard tools for assessing studies with diverse designs (Table 8).

Table 8. Standard tools for the critical appraisal of study designs adapted from EQUATOR (www.equator-network.org)

Study Design	Assessment Tool	Key Assessment Item
Randomised controlled trials	CONSORT 2010 Explanation and Elaboration	▪ Specific objectives ▪ Methods: study design, participants, interventions, outcomes, sample size, randomisation, blinding, and statistical methods ▪ Results: participant flow, baseline data, numbers analysed, outcomes and estimation, harms ▪ Discussion: limitations, generalisability, and interpretation
	Dalhousie Assessment Instrument for natural products	▪ Intervention - Genus and species, the raw material, and the process of preparing the product - Products derived from a plant, microorganism or animal: active ingredients - Commercial products: the brand name, manufacturer, lot or batch numbers, and active ingredients - Qualitative and quantitative analysis of active ingredients - Dosage form and daily dose - Placebo and comparison treatments should be matched in terms of taste, smell and/or appearance, and dosage regimen
	Revised STRICTA 2010 for acupuncture	▪ Similar to the CONSORT as stated above, except the intervention - Style of acupuncture: traditional Chinese medicine (TCM), Japanese, Korean, Western medical, etc. - Details of needling - Treatment regimen - Other components of treatment, e.g. moxibustion, cupping, herbs, exercise, lifestyle advice - Practitioner background - Comparator interventions
Pragmatic clinical trials	Extension of the CONSORT statement 2008	▪ The main items of assessment are similar to the CONSORT ▪ The extension includes: - Describing eligible participants who match typical patients in practice - Describing details of an intervention in order to implement the intervention - Explaining the rationale behind the measurement of outcomes - Calculating sample size based on the minimally important difference of the outcomes - Explaining generalisation in terms of various settings, health service organisations, and practitioners

continued on following page

Table 8. Continued

Study Design	Assessment Tool	Key Assessment Item
Cohort studies Case-control studies Cross-sectional studies	STROBE	▪ Specific objectives ▪ Methods: study design, participants, definitions of variables, measurement/data sources, bias, study size, and statistical methods ▪ Results: participant flow, characteristics of participants, exposures, confounders, and outcomes ▪ Discussion: limitations, generalisability, and interpretation
Case reports	Guidelines for submitting adverse event reports for Publication endorsed by ISPE and ISoP	▪ Patient: demographics, current health status, medical history, physical examination, patient's outcome ▪ Herbal medicine: - Latin binomial of herbal ingredients, plant part(s), type of preparation, proprietary name and name of producer for manufactured products - Dosage regimen - Therapy duration before the adverse event - Concomitant therapies ▪ Adverse events
Animal studies	ARRIVE Guidelines for Reporting Animal Research 2010	▪ Objectives or specific hypotheses being tested ▪ Methods: study design, experimental procedures, details of animals used, housing and husbandry, sample size, allocating animals to experimental groups, outcomes, and statistical methods ▪ Results: baseline data, numbers analysed, outcomes and estimation, adverse events ▪ Discussion: interpretation/ scientific implications, generalisability/translation

Note: ISPE = International Society for Pharmacoepidemiology
ISoP = International Society of Pharmacovigilance

Randomised and Pragmatic Controlled Trials

The Consolidated Standards of Reporting Trials (CONSORT) statement has been proposed for improving the quality of reporting of RCTs since 1996, updated in 2010 (Moher, et al., 2010). The CONSORT is a generic tool for assessing the reporting of RCTs and several tools have been further developed based on CONSORT to evaluate pragmatic trials (Elm, et al., 2007) and RCTs in CAM. Three specific tools have been developed for evaluating clinical trials of herbal medicine and acupuncture, including the CONSORT extension for herbal interventions in 2006, the Dalhousie Assessment Instrument for Critical Appraisal of RCTs of Natural Products, and the revised STRICTA for assessing clinical trials of acupuncture.

The CONSORT extension for herbal interventions was developed by expert consensus to extend the CONSORT with details of herbal interventions (Gagnier, et al., 2006). It includes herbal product name, characteristics of the product, such as the parts of plant used, type of product, dosage regimen, qualitative testing, i.e. standardisation of the product, and practitioner background. Jurgens, et al. (2009) further developed and validated the

CONSORT extension for herbal interventions, i.e. Dalhousie Assessment Instrument for Critical Appraisal of RCTs of Natural Products. The key principles in the Dalhousie Assessment Instrument are similar to the CONSORT for herbal interventions, but Jurgens' tool precisely describes a wide range of types of natural products (Table 8).

The STRICTA was developed from the CONSORT with added details for acupuncture, such as style of acupuncture, details of needling, and practitioner's background (MacPherson, et al., 2010). These items describe specific interventions which allows practitioners to use an intervention if the findings show positive effects of acupuncture. Therefore, the STRICTA has been recommended for evaluating the evidence for acupuncture.

Other CAMs have a lack of specific guidelines to assess their RCTs. The extension of the CONSORT for pragmatic trials is able to assess PCTs of these CAMs although the details of interventions and outcomes of the CAMs should be defined in the light of CAM knowledge. For instance, to answer the question 'Can acupressure improve depression or anxiety in patients who have received haemodialysis?' a literature search found one relevant RCT which was conducted in Malaysia (Hmwe, et al., 2015). This trial aimed to assess the efficacy of acupressure on depression, anxiety, stress, and general psychological distress in patients who have received haemodialysis. The researchers recruited 108 patients who had received haemodialysis, and who had either depression or anxiety, or did not have either. This study seems to match the clinical question. The study design of this research was an open-label RCT, which may affect the outcome. This study was not blind as this is a challenge in CAM research. The sample size had been calculated and was sufficient. The intervention during dialysis therapy was well defined by the protocol, including how to press on acupoints, the defined acupoints, defined the precision of acupressure, and the duration of acupressure session. The control group received usual care with routine haemodialysis treatment. The target outcomes in Hmwe's study were measured by a validated questionnaire, which was the Depression, Anxiety Stress Scales (DASS-21). Although this questionnaire is acceptable to measure symptoms of depression and anxiety, it is a self-report instrument for measuring subjective outcomes, therefore more likely to be biased than objective outcome measures. There was no difference in baseline characteristics between the intervention and control groups, which indicates minimal selection bias. The findings of this RCT found no difference in scores of depression and anxiety between the intervention and control groups. Meanwhile, a small number of the participants suffered from hypotension due to dialysis therapy and acupressure. This evidence shows the adverse effects outweighs the benefits, so this CAM is not currently recommend for relieving depression and anxiety.

Observational Studies

The Strengthening the Reporting of Observational Studies in Epidemiology (STROBE) statement was developed to improve the reporting of observational studies (Patsopoulos, 2011). This statement could guide critiquing observational studies, including cohort studies, case-control studies, and cross-sectional studies. These studies aim to observe the associations between an exposure and outcomes in real circumstances; however, research findings may be influenced by confounding factors. There are three key items in the STROBE that differ from the CONSORT, i.e. 'Are there clearly defined exposures, potential confounding factors, and outcomes?', 'Did authors describe potential sources of bias?', and 'Did they describe an effect size between unadjusted and confounder-adjusted estimates?' The STROBE could be applied to assess the quality of observation studies in CAM. It is important to be mindful that exposure, confounders, and outcomes in CAM studies may be difficult to define and measure due to a variation of exposure and ambiguous outcomes. This is the same challenge found in evaluating RCTs in CAM. For example, to answer the question 'Does Chinese herbal medicine (CHM) harm kidney function in patients with advanced chronic kidney disease?' a literature search of the biomedical databases found one retrospective cohort study from Taiwan (Lin, et al., 2015). The hypothesis of this study was that the use of CHM increases end-stage renal disease (ESRD) risk in patients with CKD, so this study would match the question. The study included patients with stage 3-5 CKD as identified by the International Classification of Diseases, Ninth Revision, Clinical Modification (ICD-9-CM), which is related to the population in the question. The exclusion criteria are well defined; older patients, having cancer, and/or using Chinese medicine before recruitment. Therefore, this may influence the application of the research results. Exposure (prescribed CHMs within one year before dialysis initiation), and outcome (patients receiving dialysis) was clearly defined. The baseline characteristics of both exposed and unexposed groups were not statistically different, thus indicating minimal confounding factors. The effects of other potential confounding factors on the outcomes were adjusted by statistical analysis, and cause-specific hazard ratios and adjusted- cause-specific hazard ratios are presented. The findings of this study revealed that two formulas of CHM, i.e. dampness-dispelling, and purgative formulas, are associated with an increase in the risk of ESRD. Overall, the evidence from this study seems to be reliable, so it may be used for answering the research question.

Case Reports

For both conventional medicines and CAM, case reports of adverse events provide evidence of potential harm. The guidelines for submitting adverse event reports for publication has been proposed and endorsed by the International Society for Pharmacoepidemiology (ISPE) and the International Society of Pharmacovigilance (ISoP) (Kelly, et al., 2007). These guidelines suggest standard reporting for adverse drug events, and adverse events from herbal medicine, and these could also be adopted for the evaluation of case reports in CAM. The key items of assessing the case reports are patient's status, exposure, therapy duration before the adverse event, and concomitant therapies. Theoretically, to establish the causual relationship of a CAM related adverse event, patients should be exposed before the adverse event occurs, and there should be no other factors (such as medical history or concomitant conventional medicines) associated with the adverse event. For example, Greene, et al. (2014) reported that an energy drink had induced an acute kidney injury. A 40-year-old man with well controlled diabetes and hypertension, drank 100-120 oz of energy drink daily over the prior 2-3 weeks before being admitted to hospital. His serum creatinine had increased 6 times compared with his baseline measurements. This indicated acute kidney injury (AKI). After he stopped using the energy drink, his serum creatinine returned to his baseline within two weeks. He rarely used medications related to AKI (i.e. ibuprofen). One of his concomitant medications, Lisinopril, is an angiotensin-converting enzyme inhibitor (ACEI) that may cause AKI; however, the patient had taken this medication over one year and had no prior incident of AKI. In addition, his co-morbidities, e.g. having well controlled diabetes, are not likely to cause AKI. The authors clearly described the patient's condition and the exposure, and reported the causality between the energy drink and AKI using the Naranjo algorithm. This showed there was a probable relationship between the exposure and AKI. This can also be confirmed by the previous literature. However, there is an unknown mechanism underlying energy drink induced

AKI. In short, the causality in this case report is reliable. Therefore, a middle aged man with diabetes and hypertension should be recommended not drink a high amount of energy drink.

Animal Studies

Animal studies are likely to provide information about the efficacy and safety of herbal medicines. The Animals in Research: Reporing *In Vivo* Experiments (ARRIVE) has been developed from the CONSORT statement in order to provide guidelines for reporting animal research (Kilkenny, et al., 2010). The ARRIVE could be used for assessing the quality of reporting animal studies as well. The main items recommended for reporting an animal study are similar to the CONSORT (Table 8), but are more specific to animal research. For example, the experimental unit should be described as a single animal, group, or cage of animals. Details of the animals used, including species, strain, sex, developmental stage (e.g. mean or median age plus age range), and weight should be clearly described. In addition, the housing (e.g. the type of facility, type of cage, bedding material, and number of cage companions), and husbandry conditions (e.g. breeding programme, light/dark cycle, temperature, type of food, and environmental enrichment) should all be reported. If the methods of the reported study show minimum bias and appropriate outcome measures, the research findings should be acceptable. It is important to keep in mind that the results from animal studies could provide evidence for benefits and adverse effects of CAM; however human studies are still required to confirm the efficacy and safety of CAM.

Information From the Internet

There are four key steps to evaluate information sources from the internet: (1) identifying who wrote the website; (2) balance of information between the benefits and adverse effects; (3) up-to-date evidence; and (4) reliable references. Web sites or social media which represent companies of health products are likely to promote their products and provide the benefits of their products outweighing the adverse effects. These websites sometimes employ conventional practitioners to endorse the benefits of the products using their own opinion rather than using EBM approaches. Therefore, customers should avoid using information from such websites. There are trusted websites owned by governments, health organizations, such as WHO and Food and Drug

Administration, and education sectors. These websites are likely to provide accurate information.

Customers should also consider when the websites were updated. Ideally, it should be updated every year as CAM research emerges regularly. If the information on the websites is not up-to-date, it would be unreliable and the information may not be accurate. Finally, information should be based on scientific evidence, particularly human studies, that is published in acceptable journals, such as the BMC Complementary and Alternative Medicine, or the Journal of Alternative and Complementary Medicine, Evidence-Based Complementary and Alternative Medicine. Evidence from animal studies should be used with great caution.

On the whole, few valid and reliable tools are available for appraising CAM evidence. Researchers who are interested in CAM should work on developing an appropriate tool to evaluate observational CAM studies, particularly acupuncture, herbal medicine or Chinese herbal medicine. Observational studies are comparatively easy to carry out compared with RCTs, so there is a greater need for appraising observational studies. In addition to the tools for critical appraisal, it is vital to construct and validate a pragmatic instrument for clinical decision-making regarding CAM.

MAKING A DECISION ABOUT CAM USE

Making clinical decisions based on the current best evidence is the final EBM step to providing proper care for patients. Ideally, decision-making should also take account of practitioner's knowledge and experience, and patient's needs. Whether to use CAM in patients with kidney diseases is quite a challenging decision to make due to the limited quality of evidence, especially for the efficacy and safety of CAM. Some CAM modalities may satisfy patient's needs, such as improving their quality of life, but their adverse effects may be unknown and the CAM may be costly. Therefore, clinicians often face a dilemma whether to suggest using CAM. To translate EBM knowledge to clinical practice, the decision about choosing CAM for individual patients needs to be made based on the patient's factors (e.g. conditions and constraints), practitioner's factors (e.g. best current evidence, knowledge and experience), and health care system (e.g. CAM availability and costs) (Mills, et al., 2002), as listed in Table 9.

The decision-making on CAM use is a complex process. Practitioners may make use of a conventional approach with three steps to reach a clinical

Table 9. Factors affecting clinical decision-making in CAM

Factors	Example
Patient	▪ Demographic characteristics, e.g. age, sex, etc. ▪ Prognosis of disease ▪ Co-morbidities, e.g. renal impairment, etc. ▪ Constrains, e.g. financial problems, etc. ▪ Non-adherence to medicines ▪ Patient's needs
Practitioner	▪ Evidence ▪ Guidelines ▪ Knowledge ▪ Experience ▪ Clinical skills, particularly acupuncture or massage
Health care system	▪ Availability of alternative medicines ▪ Costs

decision, including: (1) searching for evidence and using it together with their own knowledge and experience; (2) weighing up the benefits and risks of CAM based on patient's factors; and (3) providing the best option for their patients. The National Health and Medical Research Council in Australia suggests how to grade evidence in order to aid decision-making on CAM use based on levels and consistency of evidence, clinical impact, and generalisability (Table 10). This is sometimes quite challenging as one CAM may have great benefits but also more side effects; whilst another therapy may provide few benefits but have less adverse effects. Therefore, practitioners may contemplate more than one modality and discuss the choices with their patients in order to help patients select the best option. This approach will encourage the patient-centred use of CAM. Chapter 6 will offer more practical recommendations for clinical decision making based on risk versus efficacy.

This traditional decision making method may not suit inexperienced practitioners, and an alternative may be needed. Aleem, et al (2009) proposed a clinical decision analysis of conventional medicine that incorporates the evidence into the patient's needs. A decision tree that is the main component of this analysis seems to be applicable to the decision-making in CAM also. Each branch of the tree gives the probability of each possible choice of treatment, linked to the desired outcomes of the patient. The probability of each treatment is calculated using the findings of current best evidence. There are still some limitations of this tool for CAM. If the CAM modalities have no evidence, it would not be feasible to use this tool in practice. Moreover, the tool is more complex and time-consuming than the conventional approach as mentioned earlier.

Table 10. Decision-making based on evidence (National Health and Medical Research Council, 2009)

Decision-making	Strongly recommendation	Recommendation	Probable recommendation	No recommendation
Evidence				
Systematic review of RCTs or	≥ 1 systematic review with a low risk of bias		Systematic review with a moderate risk of bias	Systematic review with a high risk of bias
RCTs or	Several RCTs with a low risk of bias	One or two RCTs with a low risk of bias	RCTs with a moderate risk of bias	RCTs with a high risk of bias
Non-RCTs, observational studies, cross-sectional studies or		Several studies with a low risk of bias	One or two studies with a low risk of bias	One or two studies with a high risk of bias
Case series, case reports, expert opinions				Several studies
Consistency of the evidence	All studies consistent	Most studies consistent and inconsistency may be explained	Some inconsistency reflecting genuine uncertainty around clinical question	Evidence is inconsistent
Clinical impact	Very large	Substantial	Moderate	Slight or restricted
Generalisability	The target population is similar to the study population		The study population differs from the target population, but it is clinically sensible to apply this evidence to target population	The study population differs from the target population and hard to judge whether it is sensible to generalise to target population

CONCLUSION

The evidence-based approach plays an important role in CAM as well as conventional medicine. The five steps of EBM should be utilised in clinical practice, i.e. addressing a clinical question, searching and retrieving the appropriate evidence, appraising the evidence, making a clinical decision, and assessing the outcome. Decision-making in using CAM should take account of three factors, i.e. patients, practitioners, and health care system, into consideration. These embrace patient's preference, best current evidence, practitioner's knowledge and experience, and CAM availability. In addition, evidence with a low level of causality are sometimes accepted and used in decision making when there is no evidence from RCTs or PCTs available. Overall, the EBM approach should inform clinical decisions about CAM use in patients with chronic kidney disease. The next chapter will elaborate on the types of CAM modalities recommended by standard guidelines for chronic illnesses.

REFERENCES

Aleem, I. S., Jalal, H., Aleem, I. S., Sheikh, A. A., & Bhandari, M. (2009). Clinical decision analysis: Incorporating the evidence with patient preferences. *Patient Prefer Adherence*, *3*, 21–24. PMID:19936141

Coelho, H. F., Pittler, M. H., & Ernst, E. (2007). An investigation of the contents of complementary and alternative medicine journals. *Alternative Therapies in Health and Medicine*, *13*(4), 40–44. PMID:17658121

Elm, E., Altman, D. G., Pocock, S. J., Gotzsche, P. C., Vandenbroucke, J. P., & Initiative, S. (2007). Strengthening the Reporting of Observational Studies in Epidemiology (STROBE) statement: Guidelines for reporting observational studies. *BMJ (Clinical Research Ed.)*, *335*(7624), 806–808. doi:10.1136/bmj.39335.541782.AD PMID:17947786

Gagnier, J. J., Boon, H., Rochon, P., Moher, D., Barnes, J., & Bombardier, C. (2006). Reporting randomised, controlled trials of herbal interventions: An elaborated CONSORT statement. *Annals of Internal Medicine*, *144*(5), 364–367. doi:10.7326/0003-4819-144-5-200603070-00013 PMID:16520478

Greene, E., Oman, K., & Lefler, M. (2014). Energy drink-induced acute kidney injury. *The Annals of Pharmacotherapy*, *48*(10), 1366–1370. doi:10.1177/1060028014541997 PMID:24986632

Hmwe, N. T. T., Subramanian, P., Tan, L. P., & Chong, W. K. (2015). The effects of acupressure on depression, anxiety and stress in patients with hemodialysis: A randomized controlled trial. *International Journal of Nursing Studies*, *52*(2), 509–518. doi:10.1016/j.ijnurstu.2014.11.002 PMID:25468282

Jurgens, T., Whelan, A. M., MacDonald, M., & Lord, L. (2009). Development and evaluation of an instrument for the critical appraisal of randomized controlled trials of natural products. *BMC Complementary and Alternative Medicine*, *9*(11). PMID:19389240

Kelly, W. N., Arellano, F. M., Barnes, J., Bergman, U., Edwards, R. I., Fernandez, A. M., & Wise, R. P. et al. (2007). Guidelines for submitting adverse event reports for publication. *Drug Safety*, *30*(5), 367–373. doi:10.2165/00002018-200730050-00001 PMID:17472416

Kilkenny, C., Browne, W. J., Cuthill, I. C., Emerson, M., & Altman, D. G. (2010). Improving bioscience research reporting: The ARRIVE guidelines for reporting animal research. *PLoS Biology*, *8*(6), e1000412. doi:10.1371/journal.pbio.1000412 PMID:20613859

Lim, A. K. H., Manley, K. J., Roberts, M. A., & Fraenkel, M. B. (2007). Fish oil for kidney transplant recipients. *Cochrane Database of Systematic Reviews*, *2*, CD005282. PMID:17443580

Lin, M. Y., Chiu, Y. W., Chang, J. S., Lin, H. L., Lee, C. T. C., & Chiu, G. F. et al.. (2015). Association of prescribed Chinese herbal medicine use with risk of end-stage renal disease in patients with chronic kidney disease. *Kidney International*, 5. PMID:26244923

MacPherson, H., Altman, D. G., Hammerschlag, R., Youping, L., Taixiang, W., White, A., & Moher, D. (2010). Revised standards for reporting interventions in clinical trials of acupuncture (STRICTA): Extending the CONSORT statement. *PLoS Medicine*, *7*(6), e1000261. doi:10.1371/journal.pmed.1000261 PMID:20543992

Mills, E. J., Hollyer, T., Guyatt, G., Ross, C. P., Saranchuk, R., & Wilson, K.Evidence-Based Complementary and Alternative Medicine Working Group. (2002). Teaching evidence-based complementary and alternative medicine: 1. A learning structure for clinical decision changes. *Journal of Alternative and Complementary Medicine (New York, N.Y.)*, *8*(2), 207–214. doi:10.1089/107555302317371514 PMID:12006129

Moher, D., Hopewell, S., Schulz, K. F., Montori, V., Gotzsche, P. C., Devereaux, P. J., & Altman, D. G. et al. (2010). CONSORT 2010 explanation and elaboration: Updated guidelines for reporting parallel group randomised trials. *BMJ (Clinical Research Ed.)*, *340*(c869), c869. doi:10.1136/bmj.c869 PMID:20332511

National Health and Medical Research Council. (2009). *NHMRC additional levels of evidence and grades for recommendations for developers of guidelines*. Retrieved from www.nhmrc.gov.au/guidelines-publications/information-guideline-developers/resources-guideline-developers

Patsopoulos, N. A. (2011). A pragmatic view on pragmatic trials. *Dialogues in Clinical Neuroscience*, *13*(2), 217–224. PMID:21842619

Pilkington, K. (2007). Searching for CAM evidence: An evaluation of therapy-specific search strategies. *Journal of Alternative and Complementary Medicine (New York, N.Y.)*, *13*(4), 451–459. doi:10.1089/acm.2007.6308 PMID:17532740

Rosenberg, W., & Anna, D. (1995). Evidence based medicine: An approach to clinical problem-solving. *BMJ (Clinical Research Ed.)*, *310*(6987), 1122–1126. doi:10.1136/bmj.310.6987.1122 PMID:7742682

Sackett, D. L., Rosenberg, W. M. C., Gray, J. A. M., Haynes, R. B., & Richardson, W. S. (1996). Evidence based medicine: What it is and what it isn't. *BMJ (Clinical Research Ed.)*, *312*(7023), 71–72. doi:10.1136/bmj.312.7023.71 PMID:8555924

Straus, S. E., Glasziou, P., Richardson, W. S., & Haynes, R. B. (2010). *Evidence-based medicine: how to practice and teach it* (4th ed.). London: Churchill Livingstone.

Wang, H., Song, H., Yue, J., Li, J., Hou, Y. B., & Deng, J. L. (2012). Rheum officinale (a traditional Chinese medicine) for chronic kidney disease. *Cochrane Database of Systematic Reviews*, *7*, CD008000. PMID:22786510

Wilson, K., McGowan, J., Guyatt, G., & Mills, E. J. (2002). Teaching evidence-based complementary and alternative medicine: 3. Asking the quesions and identifying the information. *Journal of Alternative and Complementary Medicine (New York, N.Y.)*, *8*(4), 499–506. doi:10.1089/107555302760253702 PMID:12230911

Zhang, H. W., Lin, Z. X., Tung, Y. S., Kwan, T. H., Mok, C. K., Leung, C., & Chan, L. S. (2014). Cordyceps sinensis (a traditional Chinese medicine) for treating chronic kidney disease. *Cochrane Database of Systematic Reviews*, *12*, CD008353. PMID:25519252

Zhang, H. W., Lin, Z. X., Xu, C., Leung, C., & Chan, L. S. (2014). Astragalus (a traditional Chinese medicine) for treating chronic kidney disease. *Cochrane Database of Systematic Reviews*, *10*, CD008369. PMID:25335553

KEY TERMS AND DEFINITIONS

Clinical Decision-Making: A process of providing optimal care for an individual patient using scientific knowledge and practitioners' expertise.

Critical Appraisal: A process of evaluating objectives, methods and findings of scientific studies in order to accept or discard them.

Database: A systemic set of data from medical research is gathered on the internet or hardcopy.

Evidence-Based Medicine: A process of systematic searching, critical appraisal, and making a clinical decision.

Key Search Term: A key word is used for searching information.

Pragmatic Clinical Trial: A human study represents participants, interventions and outcomes in practice.

Systematic Searching: A process of searching through all eligible databases.

Chapter 6
CAM Recommended by Standard Guidelines for Chronic Illnesses

Annalisa Casarin
The NIHR Research Design Service East of England, UK

ABSTRACT

This chapter will focus on guidelines for clinical practice that mention a range of Complementary and Alternative Medicine (CAM) techniques. After exploring the definition and grading of clinical practice guidelines as a decision-making tool, the CAM methods included in the review will be described. A definition of chronic diseases will be provided and an overview of the current clinical practice guidelines on a number of prevalent conditions will be presented. Guidelines released by several international regulatory organisations will be compared in order to detect which CAM techniques have been or not been recommended for chronic illnesses in different countries. The challenges in implementing and appraising guidelines will be finally discussed.

INTRODUCTION

Decision making in medicine is the process of selecting actions in order to make diagnosis and plan treatment. Clinical judgement based upon experience and knowledge was fundamental to decision making for a long time until the scientific revolution had an impact on the healthcare sector. In the late 1960s, acknowledgement of bias within clinical reasoning came to light,

DOI: 10.4018/978-1-5225-2882-1.ch006

after which a call for the introduction of evidence based medicine was made. Since then, healthcare professionals should be applying research findings into practice in a systematic way (Feinstein, 1967). The amount of research output is continuously growing and it is almost impossible for a clinician to keep abreast of this new knowledge. Knowledge translation into practice needs to be quick and effective when a healthcare practitioner needs to manage a disease. Guidelines can offer easily accessible information on which interventions have been properly tested and can be safely adopted in managing patients. Moreover, the interest in quality regulation in medical practice and the efforts to standardise clinical practice, relies mainly upon guidelines (Weisz et al., 2007). Specialist associations and medical societies are usually the creators of guiding principles and typically investigate management of a single disease. Recently, several Complementary and Alternative Medicine (CAM) techniques have been included in guidelines. This is due to conventional medicine experts having to take into account the patients' decision of looking for other solutions when their conventional treatment fails or it not holistic enough to cover all of their concerns. It is the duty of healthcare professionals to know, and provide, information on all possible treatments available to their patients (Catto et al., 2014) even if complementary or alternative. It is important to understand what it is considered CAM as opposed to conventional or western medicine as its definition may differ among countries. A guideline published in the West may identify CAM as a technique that is considered conventional in the East. In this chapter these CAM definition discrepancies will be explored and several common chronic disease guidelines will be presented. For each illness, the recommendations of different international organisations on the use of CAM will be summarised.

BACKGROUND

The Quality of Clinical Practice Guidelines

The main definition of guidelines was proposed by the American Institute of Medicine in 1990. Clinical Practice Guidelines (CPG) are "statements systematically developed in order to assist practitioners and the public to make decisions, to determine a course of action." (American Institute of Medicine, 1990, p.38). Therefore, CPGs are commonly used to support the implementation of best practice and should assist providers and patients to make informed decisions. Although the first mention of CPG was in 1947, they flourished in the 1980s with three main purposes: to evaluate the cost-effectiveness of interventions, to offer protection to the medical population, and to assure regulation. From diagnosis to treatment, all of the steps of patients' care have been since put under scrutiny by expert clinicians in order to recommend the best available practice based on evidence. Lack of good quality research can make this process difficult, and professionals may not trust a guiding principle based on weak evidence. Critical appraisal of guidelines is supported by a grading system of the strength of recommendations and the quality of evidence supporting the guideline. Giving a grade highlights the strengths and weaknesses of the guideline. Stakeholders are then able to decide if the guideline is worth following or whether further research is needed. The most commonly used system of grading recommendations is called GRADE: Grading of Recommendations Assessment, Development and Evaluation (Guyatt, et al., 2008). In GRADE, recommendations are divided into two categories, strong and weak, based on the balance between risks, benefits, and costs. The quality of the supporting evidence is defined as high, moderate or low according to the design of the research studies underpinning the guideline (Table 1).

Other organisations, such as the Oxford Centre of Evidence Based Medicine (OCEBM), propose additional tools to evaluate the level of evidence. The OCEBM system provides a hierarchy for studies from 1 to 5 (where 1 is the

Table 1. Grading system for Clinical Practice Guidelines

Grade	Strength of Recommendation	Quality of Supporting Evidence	Implications
1a	Strong	High (Randomised Control Trials [RCTs], good quality studies)	Can be applied to most patients in most circumstances
1b	Strong	Moderate (RCTs with limitations, other robust research designs)	Can be applied to most patients
1c	Strong	Low (observational studies, clinical experience)	Can be applied to most patients, but some evidence is of low quality
2a	Weak	High (Randomised Control Trials, good quality studies)	There may be a better option depending on patients and circumstances
2b	Weak	Moderate (RCTs with limitations, other research designs)	Alternative approaches are likely to be better
2c	Weak	Low (observational studies, clinical experience)	Very weak recommendation

(Data source: www.uptodate.com/home/grading-guide [last accessed 26.03.17])

best and 5 is the weakest kind of evidence) in order to grade recommendations from A (derived from level 1 studies) to D (using level 5 studies). When the grade is available, clinicians can recognise which kind of studies were used to create the guideline and can decide whether to accept it or not (Oxford Centre for Evidence-based Medicine, 2009). Moreover, the procedures used to develop CPGs can also be assessed using an instrument developed by an international group of CPG developers and researchers known as the AGREE Collaboration (Appraisal of Guidelines, Research and Evaluation) (Brouwers, et al., 2010). The process of regulating the creation of guidelines and their reporting guarantees the standardisation of CPG development. Only studies reported in a certain way and presenting research conducted with robust methods are considered as good evidence. Usually, when quality data are available, a guideline recommends a particular pathway; if not enough evidence is available, the guideline may make suggestions for further research.

Offering research based options to meet standards of care, CPGs can be used as a clinical indicator to monitor quality of care and control costs. CPGs are widely recognised as a tool for regulating healthcare standards and to translate knowledge into practice. In order to use them properly, many countries have created guideline bodies that maintain catalogues of CPGs which avoids developing duplications. An important aspect of CPGs is the liability of professionals when they decide not to follow practice recommendations. Guidelines are usually not mandatory and should not be enforced on clinicians, but professionals must know of them in order to decide whether to implement them or not (Page and Casarin, 2016). The legal implications of this decision depend on the country where the clinician works. In the United Kingdom (UK), Italy, USA, and Germany, for example, there are no consequences if CPGs are not followed. In France in 1993 they were imposed by law in order to control costs and improve care, but with not much success. Whilst in China they are undertaking a major health reform but still lack capacity for transparent evidence based guideline development and coordination (Yang, et al., 2013). It appears that in China, a misconception exists between the role of CPGs in assisting practitioners or providing regulation. Regardless of country however, in general, clinical judgement can overrule CPGs. This is especially important when a treatment is not recommended as often happens when CAM techniques are involved. Before exploring CPGs disseminated by regulatory organisations around the world that mention CAMs, the CAM term itself needs to be defined.

THE OPERATIONAL DEFINITION OF CAM

Complementary, alternative, integrative, traditional, and holistic are only some of the expressions used to define interventions that are different from conventional medicine which can be also called allopathic, mainstream, orthodox, Western or biomedicine. These terms are objects of controversy internationally. A description that defies time and geographical borders does not currently exist; too many professional associations and traditional beliefs are involved. From a Western perspective, 'conventional' is the medicine practiced by graduates of medical schools while 'complementary' refers to therapies used in combination with conventional medicine. If a technique is used in place of a conventional treatment then it is called 'alternative'. From an Eastern perspective however, conventional refers to traditional medicine. Therefore, conventional care in China can include a technique considered complementary in the UK. Moreover, the definition of CAM is linked to the context in which it is used: a complementary method in one speciality can be seen as alternative in another one. For example, acupuncture can be used as complementary treatment for infertility, while it is often used as alternative to physiotherapy in cases of low back pain. As Kaniklidis wrote on a popular researchers' website: "...boundaries within CAM, and borders between the CAM domain and that of conventional medicine, are neither consistently clear nor constant, and these boundaries and borders change and are shaped over time across a continuum of gradually increasing acceptance and integration with conventional medicine." (Kaniklidis, 2013). Integrative is actually another way of describing a combination of conventional medicine and CAM and often results in a positive and effective interaction between the two. Different definitions of CAM by several international organisations were presented in Chapter 1.

Among CPG providers, the Cochrane Collaboration is a global, independent network established to ensure that up-to-date, accurate information about the effects of healthcare interventions is readily available. The Cochrane Collaboration defines CAM as a "broad domain of healing resources that encompasses all health systems, modalities, and practices and their accompanying theories and beliefs, other than those intrinsic to the politically dominant health system of a particular society or culture in a given historical period." (Wieland et al., 2011). When developing this operational definition of CAM, the authors listed all the techniques that can be considered as CAM (Table 2). The Cochrane Collaboration is renowned worldwide for its freely

Table 2. Therapies included within the Cochrane Collaboration CAM definition (data from Wieland et al., 2011)

Acupressure	Hypnosis
Acupuncture (needle acupuncture, electroacupuncture, etc.)	Imagery/visualization techniques
Alexander technique	Light therapy/phototherapy
Aromatherapy	Magnetic field therapy (e.g. transcranial magnetic stimulation)
Arts therapy (dance therapy, drama therapy, music therapy…)	Massage
Ayurvedic traditional medicine	Meditation
Balneotherapy	Morita therapy
Bee products (honey, pollen, propolis, etc.)	Moxibustion
Biofeedback	Naturopathy
Chelation therapy	Osteopathic manipulation
Chinese traditional medicine	Ozone therapy
Chiropractic/spinal manipulation	Play therapy
Color therapy/chromotherapy	Prolotherapy
Craniosacral manipulation	Qi gong
Dietary supplements (non-herbal) as vitamins, hormones, amino acids	Reflexology
Diet therapy	Reiki therapy
Distant healing	Relaxation techniques
Electric stimulation therapy as transcutaneous electrical nerve stimulation	Snoezelen
Electromagnetic therapy	Speleotherapy
Eye Movement Desensitization and Reprocessing	Spiritual healing through e.g. prayer
Feldenkrais method	Tai chi
Herbal supplements	Therapeutic touch
Homeopathy	Traditional healers and healing practices (other than Chinese): Kampo, Shamanism, etc.
Hydrotherapy	Tuina
Hyperbaric oxygenation	Ultrasonic therapy
	Yoga

accessible guidelines database. In the UK, CPGs for conventional medicine and CAM are provided by the National Institute for Health and Clinical Excellence (NICE). NICE is part of the UK's Department of Health and develops CPGs to ensure consistent, high quality evidence based care to the population. It also assesses health technologies and gives guidance on public health promotions and social care services (National Institute for Health and Clinical Excellence, 2016). NICE is internationally considered as a role model for the creation of CPG. NHS Scotland has its own guidelines provider, the Scottish Intercollegiate Network (SIGN). Its aim is similar to NICE's: to reduce variation in practice and outcomes through the dissemination of CPGs developed from high quality systematic reviews (Scottish Intercollegiate Guidelines Network, 2016).

All countries who are members of WHO are determined to regulate the treatments offered to the public, whether they are conventional, complementary or alternative. WHO mentioned guidelines in the Traditional Medicine Strategy 2014–2023 as key performance indicators for the Member States and fifty countries disclosed a great need of involving WHO in developing CPGs on CAM (World Health Organisation, 2013). The following paragraphs will discuss international CPGs. It will contain the definition of chronic illnesses, the selection of the most common ones and, for each one, the CPG that mentions CAM methods.

GUIDELINES FOR CHRONIC ILLNESSES THAT MENTION CAM

The WHO definition of chronic illnesses is 'non-communicable diseases'. (World Health Organization, 2015). The four main types of chronic diseases in the developed countries are cardiovascular, respiratory, cancer, and diabetes. These are joined with high incidence conditions: dementia, multiple sclerosis, epilepsy, depression, kidney diseases, obesity, arthritis, lower back pain and headaches. They are characterised by a duration of more than three months, and in some cases, have a slow progression, and are the cause of avoidable, premature deaths (42% of non-communicable diseases affected patients die before the age of 70, 82% of whom are in low or middle-income countries) (World Health Organization, 2015). Unhealthy habits like smoking, lack of exercise, and poor diet are major contributors to the development of chronic diseases. Moreover, these illnesses tend to become more frequent with ageing.

CAM is sought by patients affected with these conditions because of a failure of conventional treatment or because they want to prevent future recurrences or complications, or by those who embrace a more proactive approach to their health (EuroCAM, 2014). Patients may seek advice from their general practitioner or other conventional healthcare providers. Where these professionals are not informed regarding CAM, it can negatively affect their relationship with the patient. The patient can feel a lack of trust when they perceive that the professional is distant or indifferent to their search for better care (Deng, et al., 2009). Therefore, healthcare practitioners who want to provide patients with holistic care should find evidence regarding CAM summarised in CPGs. In 2010, Ernst counted the CPGs created by NICE that mentioned CAM. He found 14 guidelines of the 65 assessed did (Ernst, 2010). In 2013, in an attempt to update the first review, Lorenc at al. (2014) evaluated further the NICE and SIGN databases retrieving 36 guidelines from NICE and 7 from SIGN. Table 3 shows the list of conditions for which NICE and SIGN mention CAM as listed in the two reviews. The increasing number of guidelines between 2010 and 2013 shows the growing interest of healthcare organisations in providing information on CAM to providers and receivers of care. In some cases, CAM was included for the first time after 2010, but for some diseases, CPGs were updated and the organisations removed the mention of CAM. This is the case for anxiety, chronic fatigue syndrome, diabetes type II, drug addiction, hypercholesterolemia, irritable bowel syndrome, multiple sclerosis, and obesity. Possibly more evidence was available for the review of the CPG, but data were not convincing enough to recommend CAM. Ernst (2010) mentioned that sometimes NICE omitted CAM therapies for conditions even if enough evidence was present. This happened for diabetes type I, hypertension, and stroke. This was rectified for stroke a few years later. This shows that even a rigorous organisation such as NICE, demonstrates some inconsistency in evaluating evidence and reporting findings. Moreover, Lorenc et al.'s review (2014) demonstrated that NICE

Table 3. Conditions for which NICE and SIGN guidelines mention CAM as listed in Ernst et al. (2010) and Lorenc et al. (2014). Where different aspects of a disease were analysed, the condition is considered just once

	Ernst, 2010	**Lorenc et al., 2014**		**Ernst, 2010**	**Lorenc et al., 2014**
Alcohol Dependence		X	Mood, perinatal		X
Angina, stable		X	Multiple Sclerosis	X	
Anxiety	X		Multiple Pregnancies		X
Asthma		X	Neonatal Jaundice		X
Cesarean section		X	Nocturnal Enuresis		X
Chronic Fatigue Syndrome	X		Obesity	X	
Chronic Heart Failure	X	X	Osteoarthritis	X	X
Depression	X	X	Psoriasis		X
Diabetes type II	X		Psychosis, adults and children		X
Drug Misuse	X		Pulmonary fibrosis		X
Eczema, atopic		X	Rheumatoid Arthritis	X	X
Hypercholesterolaemia	X		Sickle cell, acute episode		X
Headaches - Migraine		X	Sedation in children		X
Hepatitis B and C		X	Stroke		X
Intra Partum Care - Labour	X	X	Thrombosis, prophylaxis		X
Irritable Bowel Syndrome	X		Urinary tract infection		X
Low Back Pain, non-specific	X	X	Weight Management (pregnancy)		X

CPGs are not always known to CAM practitioners. Better communication between CPG providers and professionals in order to disseminate CPGs is therefore needed.

Chronic Diseases and CAM Recommendations

A selection of chronic diseases for which guidelines mention one or more of the most commonly used CAMs is presented in alphabetical order: asthma, cancer, chronic lower back pain, depression, headache, irritable bowel syndrome, and stroke. Some of these may affect chronic kidney disease (CKD) patients. Bronchial asthma, for example, can increase the risk of developing CKD possibly because of exercise limitation and inflammation due to the respiratory condition (Huang, et al., 2014). Likewise, CKD patients commonly suffer from depression, with a prevalence of 20% (Bautovich, et al., 2014). Stroke, and cancer are also conditions with high prevalence in renal patients since CKD is one of the risk factors for both (Masson, et al., 2015; Wong, at el., 2016). Acupuncture; chiropractic and spinal manipulation/mobilisation; herbal medicine; homeopathy; massage; meditation; osteopathy; and yoga are considered. The guidelines are listed, starting from the most recent, and when available, the strength of recommendation and the grade of evidence. Guidelines not published in English have been excluded (Table 4).

Asthma

SIGN published in 2014 the British Guideline on the Management of Asthma by the British Thoracic Society. Acupuncture took a paragraph in the context of secondary prevention. It mentioned reviews involving a total of 32 studies whose methodology were criticised. The conclusion was that there was no evidence of clinical benefit. In the section on non-pharmacological management, the experts mentioned two studies: an Italian study on the use of homeopathy, acupuncture, and herbal medicine by teenagers; and a US trial on the management of asthma symptoms with rubs, herbal teas, prayer, and massage. The panel concluded that professionals should be aware of the use of CAM not only to complement, but also to substitute normal treatment (SIGN, 2014).

In China, the Asthma Workgroup of the Chinese Thoracic Society and the Chinese Society of General Practitioners published the Chinese guideline for the prevention and management of bronchial asthma (2013). There was no mention of acupuncture. The use of aetiology-based recipes of traditional Chinese medicine was suggested for their potential of being effective on symptoms during remission. The main point raised by the panel was that clinicians and patients should be aware of the corticosteroids content of some common recipes such as empirical formula and *ancestral arcanum*. These recipes are potentially able to give temporary relief, but whilst creating steroid dependency and dangerous interaction with other medications (Asthma Workgroup, 2013).

The USA National Heart, Lung, and Blood Institute published the Guidelines for the Diagnosis and Management of Asthma which includes an overview of CAMs (2007). One of the key points drawn by the panel was that clinicians should always enquire about all medications and treatments used by the patient and should remind patients that CAM is not a substitute for conventional management. The guidelines then describe a review of acupuncture, chiropractic, homeopathy, herbal medicine, breathing and relaxation techniques, and yoga. Regarding acupuncture, the expert panel mentioned two Cochrane reviews and one meta-analysis, concluding that they didn't recommend its use (evidence B). For chiropractic, homeopathy or herbal medicine the panel concluded there was insufficient evidence, although they declared that some benefits were seen with chiropractic. Many studies on breathing techniques were found and these showed perceived and documented benefits for patients, but the evidence was not good quality. The only study the panel found on Yoga showed no significant effects (National Heart, Lung, and Blood Institute, 2007).

Cancer Related Symptoms and Integrative Oncology

Integrative oncology is part of the treatment for cancer related symptoms in which complementary medicine is widely accepted for its adjunctive role in the multidisciplinary approach to cancer patients worldwide. The idea of focusing on the patient as a whole person derives from a CAM holistic view which has recently been embraced by conventional medicine (Deng et al., 2009). Pain and other comorbid symptoms that reduce the quality of life of patients affected with cancer is an area where CAM can excel. In 2013, the American College of Chest Physicians published the Complementary Therapies and Integrative Medicine chapter in the Lung Cancer Diagnosis and Management of Lung Cancer Evidence-Based Clinical Practice Guidelines. The guidelines start by stating that alternative methods are unproven and misleading and that complementary care is rational, evidence based and helpful. The panel noted that cancer patients often ask for advice on CAM from their clinicians who need to expand their knowledge on these methods. The guidelines were written to address this gap. Mind and body modalities were the most cited ones as helpful in managing symptoms like anxiety, mood, and sleep disturbances, chemotherapy induced nausea and vomiting, and pain. Yoga, massage and acupuncture were suggested for improving overall quality of life and to benefit patients in the peri-operative stages. The experts concluded that several CAM therapies can be helpful in improving the overall care of patients with lung cancer (Deng et al., 2013).

Regarding cancer pain management, the China Guidelines on cancer pain management (2011) mentions acupuncture as a supplement to analgesics. The panel stated that when the two modalities are integrated, the efficacy of the pharmacological treatment can be enhanced. The SIGN guidelines on cancer pain control (2008) describe the efficacy of complementary therapies. Massage and acupuncture were included with a number of other mind and body modalities. Despite giving psychological comfort and short-term effect, massage was not suggested as a long-term treatment option and only auricular acupuncture showed some lasting beneficial effects (SIGN, 2008). The Society for Integrative Oncology (SIO) published a CPG (2009) for the application of integrative oncology. Authors from the USA and Canada summarized the evidence around the use of mind and body techniques, massage, physical activity, energy therapy, acupuncture, and nutrition. Massage was indicated as helpful for pain and anxiety (grade 1C), avoiding deep compression around cancer lesions, enlarged lymph nodes, radiation areas or in patients with bleeding risk (grade 2b). Acupuncture was recommended for pain control, chemotherapy or anaesthesia induced nausea and vomiting (grade 1a), or can be considered for xerostomia from radiation (grade 1b); menopausal hot flashes (grade 1b); or for stopping smoking (grade 2c) (SIO, 2009).

Chronic Kidney Diseases

In 2012, the Kidney Disease: Improving Global Outcomes organization updated their CPG to clarify the definition and classification system of CKDs (see Chapter 4), and to develop appropriate guidance for the management of patients. The experts comment that herbal remedies are not to be recommended in patients with CKD. This is because herbs that need to be excreted via kidneys filtration may accelerate the progression of CKD or induce acute on chronic kidney failure. The Asian Forum for Chronic Kidney Disease Initiatives (AFCKDI) best practice recommendations for early detection of CKD were published in 2011. The only statement made on CAM was that herbs can be nephrotoxic, especially the ones containing aristolochic acid. Patients from Asian populations showed a higher risk of developing CKD because of the tradition of using herbal medicine. For example, a study in Taiwan demonstrated that regular users of herbal medicines had a quarter higher risk of developing CKD than non-users. The panel therefore suggested the need for a screening procedure among these populations (AFCKDI, 2011).

Chronic Low Back Pain

The NICE perspective on CAM for low back pain (LBP) has been a positive, but criticized one. In 2009, an expert panel stated that patients suffering from persistent, nonspecific low back pain should be offered one of the following treatment options, taking into account patient preference: an exercise programme (10 sessions over a period of 12 weeks), a course of manual therapy that includes spinal manipulation, or a course of acupuncture (Savigny et al., 2009). Therefore, NICE includes acupuncture as a recommended treatment for chronic low back pain (more than 6 weeks).

The statements on acupuncture aroused controversy among scientific societies, i.e. The British Pain Society and the Royal College of Anaesthetists. The Studies on acupuncture that were analysed were lacking in quality and NICE were criticised for the interpretation of the evidence. In 2013, NICE accepted the remit of the Department of Health to update the guidelines in which they conducted a consultation in order to include all stakeholders' comments, especially patients'. In the new draft, greater importance is given to exercise, massage, and psychological support, whilst acupuncture is excluded because the evidence is not enough to support its recommendation. Herbal remedies such as *Harpagophytum Procumbens, Salix Alba,* and *Capsicum Frutescens* were not recommended because of a paucity of evidence (NICE, 2015).

The Philippine Academy of Rehabilitation Medicine (PARM) published guidelines for the management of LBP. In their recommendations, the authors include acupuncture for acute, sub-acute and chronic LBP. Massage and spinal mobilization are endorsed for non-complicated chronic LBP, while spinal manipulation is described as a possible option. Manipulation and mobilization are not recommended in the case of spinal stability or scoliosis (PARM,

2012). In 2007, the American College of Physicians and the American Pain Society published a CPG on the management of LBP. The CAMs mentioned were herbal therapies, acupuncture and acupressure, yoga, massage, spinal manipulation, and mind and body techniques. They suggest that clinicians should consider non-pharmacological interventions for patients who do not improve. Acupuncture, massage, yoga and spinal manipulation are defined as moderately effective. Herbal therapy such as devil's claw, willow bark, and capsicum were considered safe for acute exacerbations of LBP, with small to moderate benefits. The Italian CPG on LBP management dates back to 2006. The authors exclude acupuncture for chronic LBP because of a lack of evidence (evidence B). Massage and manipulation/mobilization are mentioned as pain relievers (evidence A) even in cases of disk herniation (evidence C).

Depression

Recently, the Institute for Clinical Systems Improvement, a USA organisation of medical groups and hospitals, provided the seventeenth edition of the Health Care Guideline for Depression in Primary Care. The authors mention integrative medicine in the form of acupuncture, yoga, and herbs because of the evidence base, and also that they are commonly used. The authors state that the use of acupuncture is supported in pregnancy-linked depression, and that it is as effective as counselling in improving symptoms. Yoga is suggested for decreasing symptom severity, and studies showed that herbs (St John's Wort/Hypericum, and Saffron) have indications for mild to moderate depression. The guidelines remind professionals that St John's Wort interacts with many drugs, like other antidepressants, warfarin, oral contraceptives, antiretroviral, anti-cancer, and anti-rejection drugs. Therefore safety, tolerability and dosage of herbal treatment require further analysis (Trangle et al., 2016).

The Scottish Intercollegiate Guidelines Network published in 2010 the CPG on non-pharmaceutical management of depression in adults. One cited study found that massage is less effective than acupuncture in symptom relief, while all trials on yoga reported positive effects. Despite promising results, the authors stated that there is insufficient evidence on acupuncture, homeopathy, massage or yoga to inform recommendation. St John's Wort/Hypericum, Ginkgo, and Ginseng were mentioned, but the CPG advises professionals not to suggest their use (Scottish Intercollegiate Guidelines Network, 2010). In 2009, NICE issued guidelines for the management of depression in adults. The authors suggest that professionals should advise patients to take regular physical exercise. Moreover, they recommend not prescribing St John's Wort/ Hypericum "...because of uncertainty about appropriate doses, persistence of effect, variation in the nature of preparations and potential serious interactions with other drugs (including oral contraceptives, anticoagulants and anticonvulsants)." Importantly, the CPG recommends practitioners to be informed and advise patients on these issues (NICE, 2009).

Headache

The Japanese Society of Neurology and the Japanese Headache Society jointly reviewed their guidelines in 2013. Acupuncture was listed among the therapies and said it to be effective even if the trials that verified it were of poor quality (recommendation b). Chiropractic and spinal manipulation divided the experts because of the risks involved in the procedures (recommendation c). Massage, when in combination with relaxation (including meditation) and an exercise program, was deemed effective for tension type headache relief. Feverfew was reported as effective in migraines (recommendation b). The Italian guidelines for primary headaches (2012) argued that non-pharmacological therapies were valid in cases of migraines, tension type or cluster headaches. Studies were mentioned which compared acupuncture with Sumatriptan or Flunarizine (medications used for migraines). The evidence demonstrated a similar effect between pharmacological and non-pharmacological treatments (evidence 1a in case of acupuncture for tension type headaches). The authors stated that acupuncture should not be used in cases of coagulopathies, cardiac pacemakers, cardiac arrhythmias, or epilepsy. Spinal manipulation and mobilisation were included in the review as helpful in migraine prevention, but with a low strength recommendation. Osteopathic, chiropractic and massage protocols were found useful for tension type headache prevention, but requires further research to determine efficacy. Herbal remedies like Butterbur Root extract at the dose of 150mg/day proved to be effective, while *Tanacetum Parthenium* gave conflicting results (Sarchielli et al., 2012).

Herbal therapy is the only CAM method mentioned by the Canadian Headache Society guideline for migraine prophylaxis (2012). Butterbur was recommended in the dose of 75mg twice daily (evidence 1b), even if the benefit may be small, while the authors were against suggesting feverfew as it is no better than placebo (Canadian Headache Society, 2012).

In the same year, NICE published the guidelines on diagnosis and management of headaches in those aged over 12s. Ten sessions of acupuncture over 5 to 8 weeks are suggested as treatment for chronic tension headaches, or for when pharmacological treatment fails to prevent migraine (NICE, 2012).

The British Association for the Study of Headache disseminated a CPG on the diagnosis and management of migraine, tension type, or cluster headaches, and the associated medication overuse (2010). The authors listed acupuncture as potentially providing additional benefit to conventional care. They furthermore state that even if its role is not proven, acupuncture may be used as an alternative when no other options are effective. Homeopathy effects are deemed as unknown. For tension type headaches, massage and manipulation are recommended since this condition is most common in sedentary people. Yoga and meditation are suggested for patients as a source of relaxation (British Association for the Study of Headache, 2010).

SIGN published in 2008 a national clinical guideline on the diagnosis and management of headaches in adults. Although there was good quality evidence that massage has a positive effect in a multidisciplinary approach to migraine, the authors state that specific evidence on massage is not sufficient. Spinal manipulation is suggested for cervicogenics headaches. The interpretation of acupuncture studies is difficult because of faults in the research methods. The authors mention a Cochrane review that has no conclusive evidence, but recognises the possibility of positive effects. A well conducted randomised controlled trial on acupuncture in migraine found that needling is effective in reducing headache scores when compared to usual care. Therefore, the SIGN panel concluded that acupuncture can be used as a preventive measure for migraine (evidence B), and for reducing the frequency of episodes. Homeopathy was not recommended because of studies showing that its efficacy is no better than placebo (SIGN, 2008). The German Headache Society guidelines mention acupuncture. Unfortunately, the guidelines are in German and only summaries are available in English (German Headache Society, 2007-2008).

Irritable Bowel Syndrome in Adults

The World Gastroenterology Organisation disseminated a Global Guideline in 2015. The experts state that in India and China, herbal therapy is widely used, but its efficacy and safety depends on the concentration of active ingredients, not easy to quantify and study. The American College of Gastroenterology Task Force analysed studies on Chinese herbal formulas, concluding that they show some benefits, but carry potential toxic effects like liver failure.

Regarding acupuncture, more evidence is needed (World Gastroenterology Organisation 2015). NICE updated its guidance on Irritable Bowel Syndrome in adults in 2015. The panel states that acupuncture and reflexology should not be encouraged. Herbal products, such as herbal teas, are mentioned only as a source of daily fluid (NICE, 2015). In the Inflammatory Bowel Disease guidelines published in 2013 by the Australian Gastroenterological Society, a number of CAM methods are mentioned. Herbal remedies are acknowledged as commonly used for symptoms like abdominal pain, constipation or diarrhea, but with limited and poor-quality evidence. On the other hand, a few studies supported the use of peppermint oil, considered a safe approach for symptoms. Acupuncture is recognised by the authors as having a positive effect on patients but with no convincing evidence. Other therapies, like meditation and yoga, were considered as not being well studied yet, even if their use is declared common (Gastroenterological Society of Australia, 2013).

Stroke

Stroke is a cardiovascular disease that causes high mortality and morbidity. For this reason, many countries develop their own guidelines addressing treatment of the stroke itself or its consequences. The website www.treatmentguideline.com provides a guidelines database organised by illness in which 41 files are found under stroke. Australia, Brazil, Canada, Europe, India, Japan, Malaysia, New Zealand, South Africa, UK, and USA have all issued guidelines on this second highest cause of death worldwide (WHO, 2014). Regarding CAM, recently, the American Heart Association/American Stroke Association reported that all patients showed functional gains when acupuncture was compared to physiotherapy, but no additional advantage was seen when the two treatments were delivered together. When offered as adjuvant for the treatment of hemiplegic shoulder pain, acupuncture showed effectiveness, even though the number of trials available is limited. Moreover, acupuncture may be considered in cases of dysphagia, motor cooridination or walking rehabilitation. However, it is not recommended for the treatment of the upper extremities. The other CAM method considered by the authors is yoga. Inconsistent conclusions were found in balance and ataxia studies (American Heart Association/American Stroke Association, 2016).

The Intercollegiate Stroke Working Party in UK prepared the National Clinical Guideline for Stroke. The experts' opinion was that during rehabilitation stroke patients should not be offered acupuncture until the quality of evidence is more robust. No other forms of CAM were discussed (Intercollegiate Stroke Working Party, 2012). In 2011, the Philippine Academy of Rehabilitation Medicine mentioned transcutaneous electrical stimulation effectiveness for improving functional recovery, but only one study was found on the stimulation applied to acupuncture points. Among the other CAM methods under scrutiny, the guidelines recommended only massage for pain control (Philippine Academy of Rehabilitation Medicine, 2011). The Australian National Stroke Foundation stated in 2010 that acupuncture and traditional Chinese herbal medicine are not recommended either in acute management or in rehabilitation. There was insufficient evidence around acupuncture benefits and although Chinese herbs could improve symptoms, they have potential harmful drug interactions. Importantly, the authors recognised the necessity for conventional medicine practitioners to being sensitive and willing to discuss CAM with the patient, especially for pain relief (National Stroke Foundation, 2010).

GUIDELINES LIFESPAN AND IMPLEMENTATION CONTROVERSIES

The listing of different CPGs for chronic conditions demonstrates a large variability among countries in discussing and recommending CAM interventions. The CPGs are published in different years therefore the underpinning articles may have differed between them. CPGs are generally developed in order to disseminate knowledge, improve communication, reduce variability in clinical practice, and provide standard of care. Since CPGs offer recommendations on the best possible disease management, they are based on evidence. Research findings, that are the foundations of evidence, are produced daily. Sometimes research studies explore new topics; other times replace previous findings with new conclusions. In this case, a guideline becomes obsolete but cannot be replaced or updated straight away. A long process of consultation among stakeholders is needed around the new evidence. This new supply of knowledge is therefore responsible of the short lifespan of CPGs. Practitioners must be aware that new evidence can emerge daily, since every study published may provide a piece of information that challenges current evidence based medicine. Therefore, organisations in charge of producing CPGs provide regular updates to them. The validity of guidelines relies on these updates. A recent Spanish study on this topic showed that 1 out of 5

Table 4. Chronic conditions and CAM interventions as recommended by international organisations (see text for details)

Chronic Condition	Cam Intervention	Specifics of Recommendation
Asthma	Acupuncture Specific herbal recipes Chiropractic Breathing techniques Yoga	No evidence of clinical benefit Potentially efficacious Some benefits Documented benefit No effects
Cancer related symptoms	Mind & Body techniques Yoga, massage and acupuncture Acupuncture Auricular acupuncture Massage	Helpful in anxiety, pain, nausea-vomit Increase quality of life As supplement for pain management Long lasting effects on pain Efficacious for pain and anxiety
Chronic Kidney Diseases	Herbal remedies	Not recommended (toxicity)
Chronic Low Back Pain	Exercise Manual therapy Herbal therapy Acupuncture	To be offered To be recommended, with caution Controversy, depend on organisation Controversy, depend on organisation
Depression	Acupuncture Yoga Herbal remedies Massage	Recommended in pregnancy related depr. Recommended Caution, risk of drugs interactions Low efficacy
Headache	Acupuncture Spinal manipulation Herbal remedies Massage	Widely supported, sometime in prevention Recommended, with caution Butterbur, supported Efficacious in cervicogenic headache
Irritable Bowel Syndrome	Herbal remedies Acupuncture Reflexology Yoga	Some benefit, but risk of toxicity No convincing evidence available Not recommended Not well studied
Stroke	Acupuncture Yoga massage	Recommended for pain, rehabilitation (conflicting opinions among societies) Inconclusive evidence Recommended for pain

recommendations is out of date after 3 years (Martinez Garcia, et al., 2014). Unfortunately, there are several obstacles to keep CPGs up to date. Many professionals think that often the importance of new studies is not sufficient to call for a change in the recommendations, such as when the quality of the new evidence is not adequate enough to call for an update (Garcia et al., 2014). Moreover, many countries publish articles in their native languages and this makes a review of the evidence very difficult, especially when the CPGs are produced in countries where the use of CAM is widely accepted like Germany or Thailand. These countries maintain CPG databases, but their valuable recommendations are not accessible to an international audience because of the language barrier faced by foreign readers. Another cause of delay in updating CPGs is the misuse of evidence. There are conditions and treatments for which no guidelines exist even if there is evidence (Ernst, 2010), or where guidelines are available, they may not be traceable in literature searches (Lorenc et al., 2015). Again, consistency in reviewing evidence and better communication are advocated in order to maintain accessible and up to date databases of CPGs.

Despite these obstacles, guideline providers endeavour to maintain their databases up to date, revise their CPGs regularly, and to disseminate them to professionals and patients. Still, users may struggle in implementing them. Studies conducted on the use of CPGs showed that most of the time guidelines are not applied, which leads to about 30-40% of patients not benefiting from an evidence based cure (Grol & Grimshaw, 2003). Furthermore, 20-25% of therapies may be unnecessary and sometimes harmful (Grol & Grimshaw, 2003). It appears that guideline's implementation by professionals depends on several factors: the lack of knowledge of their existence for a specific condition or treatment; the lack of agreement with the recommendations; and the lack of personal motivation in updating practice. In other cases, the professionals may not have the resources needed to make changes in their daily activity or the cost effectiveness ratio of implementing the CPG seems unsatisfactory (Maue et al., 2004). The time needed for reading and critically appraising the guidelines, plus the time spent for learning a new approach are with liability and organisational factors other barriers mentioned by practitioners (Saillour-Glénisson et al., 2008). The reasons why patients don't follow guidelines are linked with patients' characteristics (age and education for example), the disease (especially if the condition is chronic), the treatment (in the case of complex therapeutic regimes), and the doctor-patient relationship. Trusting the practitioners and their disposition to listening and providing information are related to high adherence to guidelines (Majani, 1991). Professional bodies still regard guidelines as the standard of care and, even if many barriers exist to their proper use, many patients and professionals still rely on them as source of information for a conditions' management.

TOOLS FOR GUIDELINES APPRAISAL

Guidelines disseminated by professional bodies may be consensus based instead of evidence based. Moreover, guidelines may not be developed appropriately. For example, controversy has arisen regarding the rigour used by NICE in developing CPGs which include CAM. Experts argue that when analysing CAM studies, NICE reviewers are not always consistent and that not all reviews are comprehensive (Ernst & Terry, 2009). Moreover, comparison among studies is not always appropriate. In the economic analyses of acupuncture for osteoarthritis and low back pain for example, different treatment comparators were used, resulting in opposite outcomes in effectiveness and a call for new evidence (Latimer, et al., 2012). It has therefore been suggested that NICE should evaluate CAM by the same standards as conventional medicine (Ernst & Terry, 2009). The appraisal of CPGs can be accomplished using the GRADE or AGREE checklists as previously mentioned (Guyatt et al., 2008; Brouwers, et al., 2010). When an organisation recommends a therapy or a management pathway in their CPG, generally the authors indicate the strength of the recommendation and the quality of the evidence from which the suggestion arose in order to inform readers of the validity of data. When these quality indicators are not enough for a professional to trust the recommendation, other approaches are available to critically appraise a guideline. The first was adapted from the *Users' Guide to the Medical Literature* (Table 5) (Hayward et al., 1995):

- Are the guideline recommendations valid?
- Were all relevant outcomes considered?
- Was the inclusion of appropriate studies complete?
- Who developed the guideline?
- How was conflict of interest managed?

Table 5. Criteria for critical appraisal of Clinical Practice Guidelines (Hayward et al., 1995)

Are the Recommendations Valid?
• Were all important options and outcomes clearly specified? • Was an explicit and sensible process used to identify, select, and combine evidence? • Was an explicit and sensible process used to consider the relative value of different outcomes? • Is the guideline likely to account for important recent developments? • Has the guideline been subject to peer review and testing?
What Were the Recommendations?
• Are practical, clinically important, recommendations made? • How strong are the recommendations? • What is the impact of uncertainty associated with the evidence and values used in the guidelines?
Will the Recommendations Help me in Caring for Your Patients?
• Is the primary objective of the guideline consistent with your objective? • Are the recommendations applicable to your patients?

- What were the methods of assessing the quality of evidence?
- Has the guideline been subjected to peer review?
- What are the recommendations?
- How strong are the recommendations?
- Are the recommendations pragmatic?
- Are the recommendations applicable to your patient?

At the end of the appraisal, practitioners should be confident in applying the recommendations to their daily practice and could discuss the findings with their patients (Clubb & Dahm, 2011). A second approach considers the safety and efficacy of a procedure or treatment. If the safety and efficacy showed in a study are strong, there is no problem in recommending the treatment. But if the evidence is weak, it is reasonable for the professional to offer to patients a better option. Unfortunately, the evidence on CAM methods is limited or mixed. Therefore, good clinical judgment is needed when a patient wants to use a CAM approach (Table 6). The health care provider should assess the risk of potential harm by examining the safety evidence first. Then they should estimate the efficacy of the treatment. The financial impact should also be considered in order to help the patient in making a decision on a treatment.

Table 6. Clinical decision making based on risk vs. efficacy (Deng, et al., 2009)

Treatment			**Recommendations**
Safety inconclusive, Efficacious	EFFICACY	SAFETY	Consider tolerating, encourage caution, closely monitor safety
Safe, Efficacious			Recommend and continue to monitor
Safe, Efficacy inconclusive			Tolerate, encourage caution, closely monitor effectiveness
If not efficacious, with serious risk: Avoid and actively discourage			

FUTURE RESEARCH DIRECTIONS

Research in CAM is a recent, emerging discipline. Since healthcare stakeholders realised that patients are attracted to CAM, this research area has been developing in priority (Fischer, et al., 2014) (see Chapter 10). The main area of interest is the integration of CAM and conventional medicine. Integrating CAM into health systems has been suggested among the WHO's key points of their strategy for traditional medicine 2014-2023 (World Health Organisation, 2013). Recognising that many Member States accept the contribution that CAM approaches can make to health, the organisation advocates appropriate integration, regulation and supervision. The WHO mission is to support countries in developing policies to facilitate the integration of CAM techniques, regulate their use, and in researching safety and effectiveness. In Europe, the research group CAMbrella, a pan-European research network for CAM, identified clinical and epidemiological key areas in need of analyses (as discussed in Chapter 10). Moreover, the CAMbrella group mentions the need of using appropriate research methods for specific queries (Fischer, et al., 2014). As demonstrated by several CPGs mentioned, one of the main concerns of professionals is the lack of good quality studies on CAM. A fault in the methodology is often the reason. Clinical trials, especially when randomisation and blinding are used, seem to be the preferred and advocated research method in all reviews, followed by surveys and interviews. Systematic reviews and meta-analysis are the gold standard CPG design, but reviewers can only compare results and reliably suggest efficacy when outcomes are standardised. Therefore, research studies should aim to use the same patient reported outcomes in order to allow cross-study comparison and statistical meta- analysis. This approach will lead to more informative evidence based guidelines (Eton, et al. 2011). Reporting outcome measures have been the target of the COMET (Core Outcome Measures in Effectiveness Trials) Initiative. This organisation's aim is to promote the development of an agreed, standardised set of outcomes, known as 'core outcome sets' (COS), for each disorder. These sets represent the minimum that should be measured and reported in all clinical trials of a specific condition (Williamson, et al., 2012). There is therefore, an expectation that in future studies, these sets are collected among other outcomes of choice, and are asked for by funding bodies such as the Health Technology Assessment Programme of the UK National Institute of Health Research (COMET endorsement, 2016). Through this practice, guideline validity will be enhanced because using COS will improve studies' comparisons and promote quality of evidence.

Focusing on topics rather than methodologies, several high priority research domains have been proposed by CAM professionals. Within integrative oncology, for example, researchers from the USA and Canada suggest focussing research efforts on CAM implementation features: the symptoms and conditions for which current conventional treatment may not be adequate and where CAM interventions may succeed; CAM mechanisms using modern biomedical science techniques; the creation of a database of drug and supplement interactions; and the design of oncology therapies derived from natural products in order to assess their potential as cancer treatment with synergistic effects (Deng, et al., 2009). At the end of every published review or guideline researchers tend to suggest future directions within the topic. In the case of acupuncture and dry-needling for low back pain, the Cochrane review's authors suggest that future publications report means and standard deviations for continuous measures, or number of events and total patients analysed for dichotomous measures. Future research should focus on areas where there are few trials and use large sample sizes, and provide data on both short and long term follow up. The authors also suggested that trials report the proportion of subjects who obtain a clinically important improvement to facilitate judgment about the treatment, and that research assesses cost-effectiveness of acupuncture compared to other treatments (Furlan, et al., 2005). Since much detailed information is given to researching clinicians on methods and topics, hopefully CAM practitioners and users will see, in time, well-designed studies that will inform guideline makers.

CONCLUSION

This chapter focused on guidelines for clinical practice addressing chronic conditions. The proportion of CPGs considering CAM methods is growing, but the evidence is still not strong enough to recommend them for a number of symptoms for which CAM techniques are frequently advocated by patients. Practitioners need to routinely inquire about the use of CAM in the evaluation of patients. Open communication, and being able to provide information on CAM interventions, will gain the patient's trust in the practitioner. Also, clinical decision making should be shared between healthcare providers and patients using CPGs when available. Remembering that guidelines have a short lifespan, professionals have several tools to assess CPG's strength and quality in order to implement evidence based CAM techniques and avoid gaps in patient-practitioner communications.

REFERENCES

American Heart Association/American Stroke Association. (2016). Guidelines for Adult Stroke Rehabilitation and Recovery. *Stroke, 47*.

American Institute of Medicine Committee to Advise the Public Health Service on Clinical Practice Guidelines. (1990). *Clinical Practice Guidelines: Directions for a new program*. Washington, DC: National Academy Press.

Asthma Workgroup, Chinese Thoracic Society, and Chinese Society of General Practitioners. (2013). Chinese guideline for the prevention and management of bronchial asthma (Primary Health Care Version). *Journal of Thoracic Disease*, *5*(5), 667–677. PMID:24255781

Bautovich, A., Katz, I., Smith, M., Loo, C. K., & Harvey, S. B. (2014). Depression and chronic kidney disease: A review for clinicians. *The Australian and New Zealand Journal of Psychiatry*, *48*(6), 530–541. doi:10.1177/0004867414528589 PMID:24658294

British Association for the Study of Headache. (2010). *Guidelines for All Healthcare Professionals in the Diagnosis and Management of Migraine, Tension-Type, Cluster and Medication-Overuse Headache*. Retrieved from www.bash.org.uk

Broom, A., & Adams, J. (2007). Current issues and future directions in complementary and alternative medicine (CAM) research. *Complementary Therapies in Medicine*, *15*(3), 217–220. doi:10.1016/j.ctim.2006.08.001 PMID:17709067

Brouwers, M., Kho, M. E., Browman, G. P., Burgers, J. S., Cluzeau, F., Feder, G., & Zitzelsberger, L et al.. (2010). AGREE II: Advancing guideline development, reporting and evaluation in health care. *Canadian Medical Association Journal*, *182*(18), E839–E842. doi:10.1503/cmaj.090449 PMID:20603348

Canadian Headache Society. (2012). Guideline for Migraine Prophylaxis. *The Canadian Journal of Neurological Sciences*, *39*(Suppl. 2). PMID:22683887

Cancer Pain Management Expert Panel of the Chinese Ministry of Health. (2013). Guidelines on cancer pain management (2011 Edition). *Annals of Palliative Medicine*, *2*(1). PMID:25841739

Catto, G., Cork, N., & Williams, G. (2014). Should medical students be taught alternative medicine? *British Medical Journal, 348*, g2417. doi:10.1136/bmj.g2417 PMID:24682533

Chou, R., Qaseem, A., Snow, V., Casey, D., Cross, J. T. Jr, Shekelle, P., & Owens, D. K. (2007). Diagnosis and Treatment of Low Back Pain: A Joint Clinical Practice Guideline from the American College of Physicians and the American Pain Society. *Annals of Internal Medicine, 147*(7), 478–491. doi:10.7326/0003-4819-147-7-200710020-00006 PMID:17909209

Clubb, A. B., & Dahm, P. (2011). How to critically appraise a clinical practice guideline. *Indian Journal of Urology, 27*(4), 498–502. doi:10.4103/0970-1591.91441 PMID:22279318

COMET Endorsement. (2016). Retrieved from www.comet-initiative.org/about/COMETendorsement

Deng, G. E., Frenkel, M., Cohen, L., Cassileth, B. R., Abrams, D. I., Capodice, J. L., & Sagar, S et al.. (2009). Evidence-Based Clinical Practice Guidelines for Integrative Oncology: Complementary Therapies and Botanicals. *Journal of the Society for Integrative Oncology, 7*(3), 85–120. PMID:19706235

Deng, G. E., Rausch, S. M., Jones, L. W., Gulati, A., Kumar, N. B., Greenlee, H., . . . Cassileth, B. R. (2013). Complementary Therapies and Integrative Medicine in Lung Cancer. In Diagnosis and Management of Lung Cancer (3rd ed.). American College of Chest Physicians.

Ernst, E. (2010). Assessments of Complementary and Alternative Medicine: The Clinical Guidelines from NICE. *International Journal of Clinical Practice, 64*(10), 1350–1358. doi:10.1111/j.1742-1241.2010.02453.x PMID:20716143

Ernst, E., & Terry, R. (2009). NICE guidelines on complementary/alternative medicine: More consistency and rigour are needed. *The British Journal of General Practice, 59*(566), 695. doi:10.3399/bjgp09X454232 PMID:19761673

Eton, D. T., Bauer, B. A., Sood, A., Yost, K. J., & Sloan, J. A. (2011). Patient-reported outcomes in studies of complementary and alternative medicine: Problems, solutions, and future directions. *Explore (New York, N.Y.), 7*(5), 314–319. doi:10.1016/j.explore.2011.06.002 PMID:21907154

EuroCAM. (2014). *CAM 2020: The contribution of Complementary and Alternative Medicine to sustainable healthcare in Europe*. Retrieved from www.camdoc.eu/Pdf/CAM%202020%20final.pdf

Falkenberg, T., Lewith, G., Roberti di Sarsina, P., von Ammon, K., Santos-Rey, K., Hök, J., & Uehleke, B. et al. (2012). Towards a Pan-European Definition of Complementary and Alternative Medicine – a Realistic Ambition? *Forschende Komplementarmedizin, 19*(s2), 6–8. doi:10.1159/000343812 PMID:23883939

Feinstein, A. R. (1967). *Clinical Judgement.* Williams & Wilkins.

Fischer, F., Lewith, G., Witt, C. M., Linde, K., von Ammon, K., Cardini, F., & Brinkhaus, B. et al. (2014). A research roadmap for complementary and alternative medicine - what we need to know by 2020. *Forschende Komplementarmedizin, 21*(2), e1–e16. doi:10.1159/000360744 PMID:24851850

Furlan, A.D., van Tulder, M.W., Cherkin, D., Tsukayama, H., Lao, L., Koes, B.W., Berman, B.M. (2005). Acupuncture and dry-needling for low back pain. *Cochrane Database of Systematic Reviews, 1.*

Gastroenterological Society of Australia. (2013). *Australian Guidelines for General Practitioners and Physicians: Inflammatory Bowel Disease.* Retrieved from http://www.gesa.org.au/content.asp?id=239

German Headache Society Guidelines. (2007-2008). Retrieved from http://www.ihs-headache.org/ichd-guidelines/national-society-guidelines

Grol, R., & Grimshaw, J. (2003). From best evidence to best practice: Effective implementation of change. *Lancet, 362*(9391), 1225–1230. doi:10.1016/S0140-6736(03)14546-1 PMID:14568747

Guyatt, G. H., Oxman, A. D., Vist, G. E., Kunz, R., Falck-Ytter, Y., Alonso-Coello, P., & Schünemann, H. J. (2008). GRADE: An emerging consensus on rating quality of evidence and strength of recommendations. *British Medical Journal, 336*(7650), 924–926. doi:10.1136/bmj.39489.470347.AD PMID:18436948

Hayward, R. S. A., Wilson, M. C., Tunis, S. R., Bass, E. B., & Guyatt, G. (1995). VIII. Users Guides to the medical literature. How to use Clinical Practice Guidelines. *Journal of the American Medical Association, 274*(7), 570. doi:10.1001/jama.1995.03530070068032 PMID:7629987

House of Lords. (2000). *Definitions of the Various CAM Therapies.* Retrieved from http://www.publications.parliament.uk/pa/ld199900/ldselect/ldsctech/123/12304.htm

Huang, H.-L., Ho, S.-Y., Li, C.-H., Chu, F.-Y., Ciou, L.-P., Lee, H.-C., & Tzeng, N.-S. et al. (2014). Bronchial asthma is associated with increased risk of chronic kidney disease. *BMC Pulmonary Medicine*, *14*(1), 80. doi:10.1186/1471-2466-14-80 PMID:24885269

Inker, L. A., Astor, B. C., Fox, C. H., Isakova, T., Lash, J. P., Peralta, C. A., & Feldman, H. I. et al. (2014). KDOQI US Commentary on the 2012 KDIGO Clinical Practice Guideline for the Evaluation and Management of CKD. *American Journal of Kidney Diseases*, *63*(5), 713–735. doi:10.1053/j.ajkd.2014.01.416 PMID:24647050

Intercollegiate Stroke Working Party. (2012). *National clinical guideline for stroke*. Retrieved from https://www.rcplondon.ac.uk/file/1299/download?token=mcyQFjEq

Kaniklidis, C. (n.d.). *What should be defined as complementary and alternative medicine?*. Retrieved from www.researchgate.net/post/What_should_be_defined_as_complementary_and_alternative_medicine

Latimer, N. R., Bhanu, A. C., & Whitehurst, D. G. T. (2012). Inconsistencies in NICE guidance for acupuncture: Reanalysis and discussion. *Acupuncture in Medicine*, *30*(3), 182–186. doi:10.1136/acupmed-2012-010152 PMID:22759903

Li, P. K. T., Chow, K. M., Matsuo, S., Yang, C. W., Jha, V., Becker, G., & Tsukamoto, Y. et al. (2011). Asian chronic kidney disease best practice recommendations: Positional statements for early detection of chronic kidney disease from Asian Forum for Chronic Kidney Disease Initiatives (AFCKDI). *Nephrology (Carlton, Vic.)*, *16*, 633–641. PMID:21771177

Lorenc, A., Leach, J., & Robinson, N. (2014). Clinical guidelines in the UK: Do they mention Complementary and alternative medicine (CAM) – Are CAM professional bodies aware? *European Journal of Internal Medicine*, *6*(2), 164–175. PMID:24373628

Majani, G. (1991). *Compliance, adhesion, adherence: critical points in the therapeutic relation*. Milano, Italy: McGraw-Hill.

Martínez García, L., Sanabria, A. J., García Alvarez, E., Trujillo-Martín, M. M., Etxeandia-Ikobaltzeta, I., Kotzeva, A., & Alonso-Coello, P et al.. (2014). The validity of recommendations from clinical guidelines: A survival analysis. *Canadian Medical Association Journal*, *186*(16), 1211–1219. doi:10.1503/cmaj.140547 PMID:25200758

Masson, P., Webster, A. C., Hong, M., Turner, R., Lindley, R. I., & Craig, J. C. (2015). Chronic kidney disease and the risk of stroke: A systematic review and meta-analysis. *Nephrology, Dialysis, Transplantation, 30*(7), 1162–1169. doi:10.1093/ndt/gfv009 PMID:25681099

Maue, S. K., Segal, R., Kimberlin, C. L., & Lipowski, E. E. (2004). Predicting physician guideline compliance: An assessment of motivators and perceived barriers. *The American Journal of Managed Care, 10*, 383–391. PMID:15209482

National Heart, Lung, and Blood Institute. (2007). *Expert Panel Report 3: the Guidelines for the Diagnosis and Management of Asthma*. Bethesda, MD: NHLBI Health Information Center.

National Institute for Health and Clinical Excellence. (2009). *Depression in adults: recognition and management.* Retrieved from https://www.nice.org.uk/guidance/cg90/chapter/1-Guidance

National Institute for Health and Clinical Excellence. (2015). *Back pain - low (without radiculopathy).* Retrieved from http://cks.nice.org.uk/back-pain-low-without-radiculopathy#!scenario:1

National Institute for Health and Clinical Excellence. (2016). Retrieved from http://www.nice.org.uk/about

National Institute for Health and Clinical Excellence Guidelines (CG150). (2010). *Headaches in over 12s: diagnosis and management.* Retrieved from https://www.nice.org.uk/guidance/cg150?unlid=898111992201621961431

National Institute for Health and Clinical Excellence Guidelines (CG61). (2015). *Irritable bowel syndrome in adults: diagnosis and management.* Retrieved from https://www.nice.org.uk/guidance/cg61?unlid=239638599201612264946

National Stroke Foundation. (2010). *Clinical Guidelines for Stroke Management.* Melbourne, Australia: Author.

Negrini, S., Giovannoni, S., Minozzi, S., Barneschi, G., Bonaiuti, D., Bussotti, A., & Violante, F. S. et al. (2006). Diagnostic therapeutic flow-charts for low back pain patients: The Italian clinical guidelines. *Europa Medicophysica, 42*(2), 151–170. PMID:16767064

Oxford Centre for Evidence-based Medicine. (2009). Retrieved from http://www.cebm.net/oxford-centre-evidence-based-medicine-levels-evidence-march-2009/

Page, V., & Casarin, A. (2016). The quality and lifespan of guidelines. *Minerva Anestesiologica, 82*(2), 157–159. PMID:26744267

Panel on Definition and Description. (1997). Defining and describing complementary and alternative medicine. *Proceedings of CAM Research Methodology Conference 1995*. Alternative Therapy Health Medicine.

Park, H., Lee, H., Shin, B., Liu, J., Shang, Q., Yamashita, H., & Lim, B. (2012). Traditional Medicine in China, Korea, and Japan: A Brief Introduction and Comparison. *Evidence-Based Complementary and Alternative Medicine, 24*, 429103. PMID:23133492

Philippine Academy of Rehabilitation Medicine. (2011). *Stroke rehabilitation guideline*. Retrieved from http://www.eparm.org/images/STROKE-Guideline.pdf

Philippine Academy of Rehabilitation Medicine. (2012). *Low back pain management guideline*. Retrieved from http://www.eparm.org

Research Council for Complementary Medicine (RCCM). (2013). *CISCOM thesaurus*. Retrieved from http://www.rccm.org.uk/node/229

Saillour-Glénisson, F., Domecq, S., Pouchadon, M. L., Jacques, B., & Sibé, M. (2008). Combined quantitative and qualitative methods to identify local facilitators of and barriers to physician's adherence to clinical practice guidelines. *Revue d'Epidemiologie et de Sante Publique*, *56*(Suppl. 3), 207–219. PMID:18550309

Sarchielli, P., Granella, F., Prudenzano, M. P., Pini, L. A., Guidetti, V., Bono, G., & Zanchin, G. et al. (2012). Italian guidelines for primary headaches: 2012 revised version. *The Journal of Headache and Pain*, *13*(S2), S31–S70. doi:10.1007/s10194-012-0437-6 PMID:22581120

Savigny, P., Watson, P., & Underwood, M. (2009). Early management of persistent non-specific low back pain: Summary of NICE guidance. *British Medical Journal*, *338*, 1441–1442. PMID:19502217

Scottish Intercollegiate Guidelines Network. (2016). Retrieved from http://www.sign.ac.uk/about/index.html

Scottish Intercollegiate Guidelines Network 106. (2008). *Control of pain in adults with cancer. A national clinical guideline.* Retrieved from http://www.sign.ac.uk/pdf/SIGN106.pdf

Scottish Intercollegiate Guidelines Network 107. (2008). *Diagnosis and management of headache in adults. A national clinical guideline*. Retrieved from http://www.sign.ac.uk/pdf/sign107.pdf

Scottish Intercollegiate Guidelines Network 114. (2010). *Non-pharmaceutical management of depression in adults. A national clinical guideline*. Retrieved from www.sign.ac.uk/pdf/sign114.pdf

Scottish Intercollegiate Guidelines Network 141. (2014). *British guideline on the management of asthma*. Retrieved from https://www.brit-thoracic.org.uk/document.../asthma/btssign-asthma-guideline-2014/

Scottish Intercollegiate Guidelines Network (SIGN). (n.d.). Retrieved from www.sign.ac.uk

The Japanese Society of Neurology and the Japanese Headache Society. (2013). *Clinical Practice Guideline for Chronic Headache 2013*. Retrieved from https://www.neurology-jp.org/guidelinem/ch/documents/guideline2013.pdf

Trangle, M., Gursky, J., Haight, R., Hardwig, J., Hinnenkamp, T., Kessler, D., . . . Myszkowski, M. (2016). *Institute for Clinical Systems Improvement. Adult Depression in Primary Care*. Retrieved from https://www.icsi.org/_asset/fnhdm3/Depr-Interactive0512b.pdf

Treatment Guideline. (n.d.). *Get all medical guidelines under one roof*. Retrieved from http://www.treatmentguideline.com/guidelines-by-disease.aspx?MSDID=18&CountryID=0

Wardle, J., Lui, C. W., & Adams, J. (2012). Complementary and Alternative Medicine in Rural communities: Current Research and Future Directions. *The Journal of Rural Health*, *28*(1), 101–112. doi:10.1111/j.1748-0361.2010.00348.x PMID:22236320

Weisz, G., Cambrosio, A., Keating, P., Knaapen, L., Schlich, T., & Tournay, V. J. (2007). The emergence of clinical practice guidelines. *The Milbank Quarterly*, *85*(4), 691–727. doi:10.1111/j.1468-0009.2007.00505.x PMID:18070334

Wieland, L. S., Manheimer, E., & Berman, B. M. (2011). Development and classification of an operational definition of complementary and alternative medicine for the Cochrane collaboration. *Alternative Therapies in Health and Medicine*, *17*(2), 50–59. PMID:21717826

Williamson, P. R., Altman, D. G., Blazeby, J. M., Clarke, M., Devane, D., Gargon, E., & Tugwell, P. (2012). Developing core outcome sets for clinical trials: Issues to consider. *Trials*, *13*(1), 132. doi:10.1186/1745-6215-13-132 PMID:22867278

Wong, G., Staplin, N., Emberson, J., Baigent, C., Turner, R., Chalmers, J., & Craig, J. (2016). Chronic kidney disease and the risk of cancer: An individual patient data meta-analysis of 32,057 participants from six prospective studies. *BMC Cancer*, *16*(1), 488. doi:10.1186/s12885-016-2532-6 PMID:27421889

World Gastroenterology Organisation Global Guidelines. (2015). *Irritable Bowel Syndrome: A Global Perspective*. Author.

World Health Organization. (2000). *Traditional Medicine: Definitions*. Retrieved from http://www.who.int/medicines/areas/traditional/definitions/en/

World Health Organization. (2013). *WHO Traditional Medicine Strategy 2014–2023*. Retrieved from http://www.who.int/medicines/publications/traditional/trm_strategy14_23/en/

World Health Organization. (2014). *The top 10 causes of death*. Retrieved from http://www.who.int/mediacentre/factsheets/fs310/en/

World Health Organization. (2015). *Non communicable diseases*. Retrieved from http://www.who.int/mediacentre/news/releases/2015/noncommunicable-diseases/en/

Yang, K., Chen, Y., Li, Y., & Schünemann, H. J. (2013). Editorial: Can China master the guideline challenge? *Health Research Policy and Systems*, *11*(1), 1. doi:10.1186/1478-4505-11-1 PMID:23302417

Zollman, C., & Vickers, A. (1999). What is complementary medicine? *British Medical Journal*, *319*(7211), 693–696. doi:10.1136/bmj.319.7211.693 PMID:10480829

KEY TERMS AND DEFINITIONS

CAM: Complementary and alternative medicine different from conventional practices.

Chronic Illness: A disease that is persistent or lasting more than 3 months.

Conventional Medicine: Diagnosis, treatment and prevention of disease that use medications, radiation and/or surgery to treat symptoms.

CPG: Clinical practice guidelines are communications that influence decision making in healthcare.

Evidence: Data provided by well-designed research that demonstrates a theory.

Holistic: A diagnostic system or treatment that considers the body as a whole and focus on the mental wellbeing as well.

Integrative Medicine: The integration between conventional and complementary medicine.

Recommendations: Instructions from an authoritative body on the best course of action.

Chapter 7
Efficacy and Safety of CAM in Kidney Diseases

Mayuree Tangkiatkumjai
Srinakharinwirot University, Thailand

Chatchai Kreepala
Srinakharinwirot University, Thailand

Li-Chia Chen
The University of Manchester, UK

ABSTRACT

The evidence of benefits and safety of complementary and alternative medicine for kidney diseases are still dubious to both practitioners and general public. Chinese herbal medicines are the main CAM in treating chronic kidney disease as an adjunctive therapy to conventional medicine. Several meta-analyses of randomised controlled trials assessing the efficacy of CHM reported that Astragalus and Cordyceps seem to have a beneficial effect on the kidneys. Acupuncture, yoga and aromatherapy may alleviate symptoms in patients with ESRD, such as pain, anxiety and pruritus. This evidence should be interpreted with caution due to several limitations of the RCTs of CAM, i.e., small sample sizes, unclear randomisation and blinding. Acute kidney injury is the common nephropathy caused by herbal and dietary supplements, e.g. aristolochic acid. Dietary supplements may induce uncontrolled hyperkalemia and hyperphosphatemia in patients with advanced CKD. Unregistered herbal products from India and China may be adulterated by conventional medicines and heavy metals, which could cause AKI.

DOI: 10.4018/978-1-5225-2882-1.ch007

INTRODUCTION

Patients with kidney diseases, particularly in Asian and African countries, are likely to seek complementary and alternative medicine (CAM) due to being disappointed with conventional medicine, suffering from adverse effects of conventional medicine, or not being able to access or afford standard therapy. In contrast, conventional practitioners often suggest avoiding using CAM on their patients due to the lack of scientific evidence for efficacy and safety of CAM. The Kidney Disease: Improving Global Outcomes organization in 2012 suggested avoiding the use of herbal medicine although patients with chronic kidney disease (CKD) are likely to use CAM and do not inform their doctor about CAM use.

In the literature, CAMs have been mainly used as an adjunctive therapy to conventional medicine in order to complement pharmacological effects of conventional medicines and reduce adverse effects of immunosuppresants in patients with glomerular disease and kidney transplantation. Recently, randomised controlled trials (RCTs) assessing the efficacy of CAM for treating kidney diseases have increased. Several RCTs report that CAM may delay the progression of CKD, and relieve symptoms in dialysis patients. However, the poor quality of these RCTs is the main obstacle to support the use of CAM to treat patients with renal disease. The key methodological concerns were small sample sizes, and unclear randomisation and allocation concealment. In addition, RCTs are more likely to examine short-term effects (less than one year) which jeopardises the external validity of trial results.

This chapter gives an overview of existing clinical evidence of the efficacy and safety of CAM for kidney diseases, dialysis and kidney transplantation to support clinical decision making. Evidence is described separately for Chinese herbal medicine (CHM) and other CAMs. The efficacy section for CHM focuses on herbal and dietary supplements (HDS), and the evidence is presented from the higher (meta-analyses or systematic reviews) to lower (observational studies) levels for inferencing causal relationship. Evidence on complications of end-stage renal disease (ESRD) is organised according to three common complications of ESRD and impacts on biomarkers.

For the safety of CAM, HDS related nephropathy is most frequently reported. However, as there is a lack of consistent and quality reporting of adverse events in RCTs, anecdotes (case reports or case series) are the main evidence source for signaling nephropathy of HDS (Luyckx, 2012).

Therefore, the safety section focuses on the nephropathy due to HDS, and describes pathology of nephropathy, acute kidney injury (AKI), electrolyte imbalance associated with HDS. In addition, adulteration and contamination as the adjunctive risk factor to HDS related nephropathy are also described. The authors also propose recommendations for preventing AKI from using HDS in practice. Other CAMs (e.g. acupuncture, message) are generally safe with no direct link to causing renal diseases based on current evidence.

EFFICACY OF HERBAL MEDICINES OR DIETARY SUPPLEMENTS FOR KIDNEY DISEASES

Synthesised evidence from systematic reviews for efficacy in different kidney diseases are summarised below including relevant RCTs which were not included in the existing systematic reviews, and observational studies.

Synthesised Evidence in Systematic Review and Meta-Analysis

Astragalus, Cordyceps, *Rheum officinale*, and *Tripterygium* have been frequently used as a combination CHM in China. Emerging evidence from systematic reviews and meta-analyses have demonstrated the efficacy and safety of CHM in treating CKD, antioxidants for reducing cardiovascular mortality in patients with kidney diseases, and fish oil used in kidney transplant recipients. RCTs included in the systematic reviews often lacked reported adverse events. Common limitations of the meta-analyses, were small number of RCTs included, and/or diverse samples (with various causes of CKD). This led to a high heterogeneity. Therefore, findings should be interpreted with caution and good quality RCTs are required to determine the efficacy and safety of herbal and dietary supplements (HDS), particularly Cordyceps, *Rheum officinale*, and *Tripterygium*. Chapter 10 will propose a new approach to improving the quality of RCTs in CAM research.

Astragalus for Treating CKD

Astragalus contains a high amount of flavonoids, which are rich in antioxidants. This may explain the possible mechanisms of Astragalus's effect in improving kidney function and proteinuria, including immunomodulatory, anti-inflammatory and renoprotective effects (Okuda et al., 2012; Zhang, et al., 2014a). Therefore, combining Astragalus with conventional therapy is likely to slow the progression of kidney function and decrease proteinuria in patients with various causes of CKD. The efficacy and safety of Astragalus for treating CKD have been assessed in two meta-analyses and one non-randomised controlled trial (Table 1). The poor quality of included RCTs in the meta-analyses and of clinical trials in Astragalus is due to unclear randomisation, unblinding, and a lack of reporting adverse effects.

The Cochrane group reviewed RCTs assessing the efficacy and safety of Astragalus injections together with conventional medicine for treating CKD and included 22 studies conducted in China (injection only available there) (Zhang, et al., 2014a). Most included RCTs assessed short-term effects ranging from 14 days to 3 months. This review and meta-analysis showed Astragalus significantly increased creatinine clearance (CrCl) in patients with chronic glomerulonephritis or CKD, compared with conventional treatment (mean difference [MD]: 5.75 ml/min; 95%CI: 3.16, 8.34; $I^2 = 0\%$). Astragalus injections combined with conventional medicine significantly decreased 24-hour proteinuria in patients with primary hypertension, CKD, IgA nephropathy, SLE with CKD, or chronic glomerulonephritis (MD: -0.53 g/24 hr; 95%CI: -0.79, -0.26, $I^2 = 90\%$). This finding should be interpreted with caution as there was high heterogeneity in the 10 small-scale studies.

Li, *et al.* (2011) conducted a systematic review and meta-analysis of Astragalus injections for associated diabetic nephropathy (DN) short term (2-8 weeks), and included 21 RCTs and 4 semi-randomised controlled trials conducted in China during 1999-2008. The sample, i.e. only patients with DN, differs from the Cochrane review. Li et al found that Astragalus injections combined with routine treatment significantly improved kidney function (Table 1). Although the authors evaluated the quality of the included studied based on Cochrane guidelines, they did not report the risk of bias, and did not appraise the quality of the RCTs in terms of incomplete outcome data and selective reporting. Two outcomes of this meta-analysis, i.e. measurement of serum creatinine and proteinuria, had high heterogeneity due to small sample sizes in the included studies, and variability in the control groups.

Okuda, *et al.* (2012) conducted a before and after non-randomised clinical trial to assess the effects of combining oral Astragalus with conventional therapy on improving kidney function and proteinuria in 35 Japanese patients with stages 4-5 CKD. This trial was not included in the Cochrane review as it was not an RCT. However, as it assessed the effects of Astragalus in the target study population, this Chapter also reviewed it. Instead of measuring

Table 1. Astralagus for chronic kidney disease

Authors	Number Of Studies	Sample Size And Blinding	Population	Intervention	Duration	Benefit	Adverse Effect
Zhang et al. (2014a)	MA; 21 RCTs and 1 quasi-RCT (n = 1323)	Most RCTs included ≤ 50 participants in each group Unblinding of all included studies	Adult patients with various stages of CKD, including those with haemodialysis Causes of CKD; chronic GN, DN, IgA nephropathy	Astragalus injection + conventional treatment vs. conventional treatment[a]	14 days to 3 months	**Increase in CrCl**: MD: 5.75 ml/min (95%CI: 3.16,8.34; I^2 = 0%) pooled from 4 trials (306 participants) **Decrease in Scr**: MD: -21.4 μmol/L (95%CI: -34.8, – 8; I^2 = 70%) pooled from 13 trials (775 participants)	70% of the included studies did not report. The remaining studies report no adverse effects.
			hypertension			**Decrease in 24 h proteinuria**: MD: -0.53 g/24 hr (95%CI: -0.79,-0.26; I^2 = 90%) pooled from 10 trials (640 participants)	
Li et al. (2011)	MA; 21 RCTs and 4 CCTs (n= 1804)	Most RCTs included ≤ 50 participants in each group Unblinding of all included studies	Patients with DN	Astragalus injection + routine treatment vs. routine treatment[b]	2-8 weeks	**Increase in CrCl:** WMD: 14.0 (95%CI: 12.5,15.6; I^2 = 53%) pooled from 2 RCTs and 1 CCT (219 participants) **Decrease in Scr**: WMD: -26.4 μmol/L (95%CI: -43.5, – 9.3; I^2 = 98%) pooled from 11 RCTs and 1 CCT (762 participants)	All included studied did not report.

continued on following page

Table 1. Continued

Authors	Number Of Studies	Sample Size And Blinding	Population	Intervention	Duration	Benefit	Adverse Effect
						Decrease in 24 h proteinuria: SMD: -1.78 g/24 hr (95%CI: -2.54,-1.02; $I^2 = 96\%$) pooled from 11 RCTs and 2 CCTs (958 participants)	
Okuda *et al.* (2012)	Before and after non-randomised clinical trial	35 participants Unblinding	Patients with stages 4-5 CKD	Astragalus 2.5 g twice a day + conventional treatment[c]	1 year	**Increase in mean eGFR**: 11.6±5.2 ml/min/1.73m^2 (before) vs. 13.9±6.1 ml/min/1.73m^2 (after) **Decrease in proteinuria**; 1.87±1.83 g/g Cr (before) vs. 1.38±1.29 g/g Cr (after)	Hypersensitivity GI symptoms in the first month

a Diet control, symptomatic treatment, i.e. maintaining water, electrolyte and acid-base balance, controlling blood pressure, and treating anaemia; b Diet control, exercise, controlling blood glucose; c treatment of CKD complications and 66% of participants received ACEIs/ARBs; CCT = Semi-randomised controlled trial; CKD = chronic kidney disease; CrCl = Creatinine clearance; DN = Diabetic nephropathy; GI = Gastrointestinal; GN = Glomerulonephritis; MA = Meta-analysis; MD = Mean difference; SMD = Standard mean difference; vs. = versus; WMD = Weight mean difference

serum creatinine and creatinine clearance this study measured eGFR, which is a more accurate estimate of kidney function and had a follow-up of one year. This trial found that oral Astragalus together with conventional medicines could delay initiation of dialysis therapy in patients with stage 4 CKD for one year, and decrease proteinuria despite no statistical significance due to the small sample size (Okuda, et al., 2012).

Cordyceps for Treating CKD

Cordyceps known as 'Chinese caterpillar fungus' significantly improves kidney function and slightly decreases proteinuria in patients with CKD according to a meta-analysis (Zhang et al., 2014b). The mechanisms suggested may be the immunostimulation, antioxidant, and anti-inflammatory effects (Zhang et al., 2014b). The Cochrane group reviewed 22 RCTs for assessing the efficacy of Cordyceps together with conventional medicine for treating CKD (Zhang et al., 2014b). The significant effects in increasing creatinine clearance and decreasing 24-hour proteinuria were observed in a short period of time (1 to 6 months). Two studies reported gastrointestinal problems associated with Cordyceps, such as nausea, abdominal discomfort, or constipation (Table 2). The limitations of this meta-analysis are similar to the previous meta-analyses of Astragalus, i.e. including RCTs with small and varied samples, unclear randomisation, and lack of blinding; leading to great heterogeneity.

Rheum officinale for Prevention of CKD Progression

Rheum officinale (Da Huang) contains rhein, emodin and aloemodin, which may slow the deterioration of kidney function by increasing excretion of waste production (such as ammonia) (Y.J.Wang, et al., 2012; Zhong, et al., 2013).

The Cochrane group have reviewed and analysed nine RCTs published until May 2015 which assessed the efficacy of *Rheum officinale* for the prevention of CKD progression (Wang, et al., 2012). Four of the nine included studies showed significant benefits of decreasing serum creatinine (Table 2). The dose of oral *Rheum officinale* for this indication ranged from 6 to 15 grams/day. However, two studies assessing the efficacy of *Rheum officinale* for improving proteinuria found no significant results. In addition, *Rheum officinale* could induce diarrhoea when the initial dose of CHM is greater than 3 grams/day.

All of the nine studies included in this Cochrane review had very small sample sizes, and did not report allocation methods or blinding. Due to the limitations and the small number of the included studies, further clinical trials are needed to examine the benefits of this medicine for CKD before any conclusion can be made.

Tripterygium Preparations for Treating CKD

Tripterygium contains triptolide which may treat CKD via its immunosuppressive, anti-inflammation, and antioxidant effects (Zhong et al., 2013). Zhu et al. (2013) reviewed 75 RCTs published before July 2012 that assessed the efficacy of Tripterygium preparations combined with usual treatment (e.g. ACEIs, ARBs, and prednisolone). This review found that Tripterygium significantly decreased proteinuria in patients with nephrotic syndrome, diabetic nephropathy, and IgA nephropathy in the short-term and slightly decreased serum creatinine (Table 3) (Zhu et al., 2013). Decreased

Table 2. Meta-analyses of CHMs for chronic kidney diseases

Authors	Number Of Studies	Sample Size And Blinding	Population	Intervention	Duration	Benefit	Adverse Effect
Zhang et al. (2014b)	21 RCTs and 1 quasi-RCT (n = 1746)	Most RCTs included ≤ 50 participants in each group 3 included RCTs reported blinding with unclear methods 19 included RCTs did not reported blinding information	Adult patients with various stages of CKD caused by chronic GN, DN, Arteriosclerosis, chronic pyelonephritis, hypertension	Cordyceps + conventional treatment[a] vs. Placebo, no treatment, or conventional treatment	1-6 months	**Increase in CrCl**: MD: 9.22 ml/min (95%CI: 3.10,15.34; $I^2 = 81\%$) pooled from 6 RCTs (362 participants) **Decrease in Scr**: MD: -60.8 μmol/L (95%CI: -85.8, – 35.7; $I^2 = 82\%$) pooled from 14 RCTs (987 participants) **Decrease in 24 h proteinuria**: MD: -0.15 g/24 hr (95%CI: -0.24, -0.05; $I^2 = 9\%$) pooled from 4 RCTs (211 participants)	15 included studies did not report. GI problems (N = 2) No AE (N = 5)
Wang et al. (2012)	9 RCTs (n = 682)	Most RCTs included ≤ 22 participants in each group All included RCTs did not reported blinding information	Adult patients with various stages of CKD	*Rheum officinale* + routine treatment[a] vs. Routine treatment (N = 7)	1-28 months	**Decrease in Scr**: MD: -87.5 μmol/L (95%CI: -139.2, – 35.7; $I^2 = 46\%$) pooled from 4 RCTs (196 participants) **Decrease in 24 h proteinuria**: MD: -0.35 g/24 hr (95%CI: -1.02, -0.31, $I^2 = 84\%$) pooled from 2 RCTs (181 participants)	One included study reported diarrhoea

[a]Dietary interventions, symptomatic treatment, i.e. maintaining water, electrolyte and acid-base balance, controlling blood pressure, and treating anaemia; AE = Adverse event; CrCl = Creatinine clearance; DN = Diabetic nephropathy; GI = Gastrointestinal; GN = Glomerulonephritis; MD = Mean differencen = Number of the population; Scr = Serum creatinine; vs. = versus

proteinuria is an important outcome in patients with nephropathy as kidney function is likely to improve after proteinuria decreases (Bakris, 2008). The included studies in this meta-analysis had the same issues as the prior meta-analyses, i.e. unclear randomisation and allocation concealment. These problems are common in CAM research as it is difficult to randomise patients who prefer to use CAM and may withdraw from a study if they know that they may receive placebo. Both outcomes; serum creatinine and proteinuria, reported high heterogeneity attributed to the various causes of CKD in the participants. In addition, this meta-analysis reported that Tripterygium was associated with increasing liver function tests (Relative risk [RR]: 4.03; 95%CI: 2.24,7.25), and altered menstruation due to ovarian injury (RR: 5.29; 95%CI 2.09,13.38) (Zhu et al., 2013). Health care providers should use Tripterygium with caution in patients with liver insufficiency and women of reproductive age. Moreover, another case report of adverse effects of Tripterygium signaled the potential risk of renal diseases. *Tripterygium wilfordii* is associated with hypovolemic shock, which consequently causes AKI (Chou et al., 1995).

Tripterygium Preparations for Treating Primary Nephrotic Syndrome

The Cochrane group reviewed 10 RCTs that assessed the efficacy and safety of Tripterygium combined with prednisolone and/or cyclophosphamide to treat primary nephrotic syndrome (Chen et al., 2013). Tripterygium used as an adjunctive therapy to conventional medicine increased complete remission rate of nephrotic syndrome when compared with the control group (RR: 1.46; 95%CI 1.18,1.80; $I^2 = 3\%$). However, there were no significant differences in complete remission when comparing Tripterygium against prednisolone or cyclophosphamide (Table 3). Limitations were small samples in the included RCTs and randomisation, blinding and allocation concealment was only vaguely described.

Antioxidants in Patients With Kidney Diseases

The Cochrane collaboration reviewed 10 RCTs of antioxidants for reducing cardiovascular mortality in patients with kidney diseases until 2011 (Jun et al., 2012). Comparing vitamin E 400-800 IU per day or N-acetyl cysteine 1,200 mg per day against placebo revealed no significant effect in reducing overall mortality (RR: 0.95; 95%CI: 0.70,1.27; $I^2 = 0\%$). Subgroup analysis

Table 3. Meta-analyses of Tripterygium for kidney diseases

Authors	Number of studies	Sample size and blinding	Population	Intervention	Duration	Benefit	Adverse effect
Zhu et al. (2013)	75 RCTs (n = 4386)	Most RCTs included ≤ 50 participants in each group Unblinding of all included studies	Adult patients with various stages of CKD caused by chronic GN, nephrotic syndrome, DN, IgA nephropathy	Tripterygium + usual treatment vs. Usual treatment	1-12 months	**Decrease in Scr**: WMD: -10.6 μmol/L (95%CI: -15.0, –5.3; I^2 = 93%) pooled from 32 RCTs (2150 participants) **Decrease in 24 h proteinuria**: WMD: -0.63 g/24 hr (95%CI: -0.74,-0.52; I^2 = 91%) (N = 37,2310 participants)	RR of LFTs abnormality = 4.03, 95%CI 2.24-7.25 RR of altered menstruation = 5.29, 95%CI 2.09-13.38
Chen et al. (2013)	10 RCTs (n = 630)	Most RCTs included ≤ 50 participants in each group All included studies did not report blinding methods	Adult patients with primary nephrotic syndrome	Tripterygium + usual treatment[a] vs. Usual treatment	3-16 months	**Complete remission**: Risk Ratio: 1.46 (95%CI: 1.18,1.80; I^2 = 3%) pooled from 4 RCTs (293 participants)	No serious AEs
				Tripterygium + no usual treatment or usual treatment[b] vs. Prednisolone	6-18 months	**Complete remission**: Risk Ratio: 1.09 (95%CI: 0.83,1.43; I^2 = 0% pooled from 4 RCTs (223 participants)	
				Tripterygium + Prednisolone vs. Cyclophosphamide + prednisolone	3-12 months	**Complete remission**: Risk Ratio: 1.06 (95%CI: 0.82,1.37; I^2=0%) pooled from 2 RCTs (114 participants)	

[a]Prednisolone and cyclophosphamide, or prednisolone alone;[b] Cyclosporine or prednisolone; AE = Adverse event; CrCl = Creatinine clearance; DN = Diabetic nephropathy; GI = Gastrointestinal; GN = Glomerulonephritis; n = Number of the population; RR = Relative risk; Scr = Serum creatinine; vs. = versus; WMD = Weight mean difference

of two RCTs in haemodialysis patients showed that antioxidants decrease cardiovascular events (RR: 0.57; 95%CI: 0.41, 0.80). This may be due to haemodialysis patients having a higher prevalence of cardiovascular disease and risk of cardiovascular mortality than patients with CKD (Table 4) (Cheung et al., 2004).

Fish Oil for Kidney Transplant Patients

Fifteen RCTs of fish oil for kidney transplant recipients were reviewed and analysed by Cochrane until March 2016 (Lim et al., 2016). Comparing fish oil against placebo, the authors reported no difference of graft loss or acute graft rejection. Four RCTs reported participants having GI upset from using fish oil (Table 4).

A Review of Randomised Controlled Trials

There are four RCTs conducted in China to assess the efficacy and safety of CHMs for early stage CKD which were not included in the previous meta-analyses (Table 5). CHM were used as either adjuvant or primary interventions. Abelmoschus manihot contains flavonoids which may have an immunosuppressive and anti-inflammatory effects (Zhong et al, 2015). Mixed CHM concoctions (Radix Astragali, Radix Angelicae Sinensis, Radix Saposhnikoviae, Rhizoma Atractylodis alba, Herba Leonuri, Radix Salviae Miltiorrhizae, Fructus Pyrrosia Sheareri, Radix Rehmanniae, Rhizoma Anemarrhenae, and Radix Glycyrrhizae) may stimulate immune system and decrease proteinuria (Qing et al., 2001). A variety of outcomes were reported (including serum creatinine, 24-hour proteinuria, eGFR, graft survival rates, acute renal allograft rejection rate, and recurrence rate of nephrotic syndrome). All of the RCTs reported adverse effects of CHMs.

Three out of four RCTs clearly clarified their randomisation methods (Qing et al., 2001; Wang et al., 2012; Zhang et al., 2014b). Two RCTs had sufficient power and the number in each arm ranged from 130 to 186 (Wang et al., 2012; Zhang et al., 2014b). However, three of the four did not report blinding procedures and only one was double-blinded (Wang et al., 2012). The quality of one RCT was poorer than others due to no report on their randomisation method, blinding procedure, or sample size calculation (Qing, et al., 2001). Therefore, Qing's results should be interpreted with caution.

Table 4. Meta-analyses of dietary supplements for reduced cardiovascular mortality in patients with kidney diseases and kidney transplant

Authors	Number of studies	Sample size and blinding	Population	Intervention	Duration	Benefit	Adverse effect
June et al. (2012)	10 RCTs (n=1979)	Most RCTs included > 500 participants in each group	Adult patients with various stages of CKD, including KT	Antioxidant therapy[a] vs. Placebo	1.2-1.4 years	**Reduced CV mortality**: RR: 0.95 (95%CI: 0.70,1.27; I^2 = 0% pooled from 3 RCTs (1323 participants)	**Serious AE**[e]: RR: 2.26 (95%CI: 0.74,6.95; I^2 = 57%) pooled from 3 RCTs (557 participants)
		Most included studies reported double-blinding	Subgroup analysis in patients with CKD	Antioxidant therapy[b] vs. Placebo	52 weeks	**CVD prevention**: RR: 1.06 (95%CI: 0.84,1.32; I^2 = 0% pooled from 2 RCTs (1220 participants)	
			Subgroup analysis in patients received haemodialysis	Antioxidant therapy[c] vs. Placebo	1.2-1.4 years	**CVD prevention**: RR: 0.57 (95%CI: 0.41,0.80; I^2 = 0%) pooled from 2 RCTs (330 participants)	
Lim et al. (2016)	15 RCTs (n = 733)	Most RCTs included < 50 participants in each group	Adult kidney transplant recipients	Fish oil[d] vs. Placebo	1-12 months	**Graft loss**: RR: 0.91 (95% CI: 0.51,1.63; I^2 = 0%) pooled from 12 RCTs (640 participants)	GI upset reported in 4 RCTs
		53% of the included studies were blind				**Acute rejection**: RR: 1.00 (95%CI: 0.80,1.25; I^2 = 0%) pooled from 8 RCTs (482 participants)	

[a]Vitamin E 400-800 IU/day or acetylcysteine 60 mg twice a day;[b] Vitamin E 400 IU/day or bardoxolone methyl; [c] Vitamin E 800 IU/day or acetylcysteine 60 mg twice a day; [d] Fish oil contains 1800-2700 mg of EPA and DHA per day; [e] Malignancy, haematological events, gastrointestinal events, and infection; AE = Adverse event; CV = Cardiovascular; CVD = Cardiovascular disease; GI = Gastrointestinal; KT = Kidney transplant; n = Number of the population; RR = Risk ratio; vs. = versus

The three RCTs, which measured improvement of kidney function and reduction of proteinuria in glomerular diseases, found that *Abelmoschus manihot* significantly decreased proteinuria, compared with losartan (Zhang et al., 2014), whilst a mix of four types of CHM significantly improved kidney function and significantly decreased proteinuria, compared with benazepril (Wang et al., 2012). Ten mixed CHM together with prednisolone for treating idiopathic nephrotic syndrome which resulted in a lower recurrence rate (13%) compared to prednisone therapy (40%) (Qing et al., 2001).

One RCT examined the immunosuppressive effect of Cordyceps as an adjuvant therapy (with cyclosporine), or cyclosporine alone (usual care) in participants who had received a kidney transplant (Li et al., 2009). The results of this RCT found that participants who received Cordyceps adjuvant therapy had the same graft survival rates, incidence rate of acute renal allograft rejection, and levels of serum creatinine; however, it significantly decreased the risk of cyclosporine related side effects (Table 5).

A Review of Observational Studies

There were two Taiwanese observational studies, including one cohort and one case-control study, which assessed the association between CHMs and CKD. Observational studies provide important evidence for the effectiveness and safety of CHMs when participants cannot be randomised or for when various types of CHMs have been used; or when it is difficult to blind either participants or practitioners. However, there are limited numbers of them available as CHM services are only embedded in the health care systems in a few countries. In addition, the effectiveness of CHMs derived from observational studies still need to be confirmed by RCTs.

Cohort Study

Lin et al. (2015) conducted a large retrospective cohort study (n = 24,971) assessing the risk of end-stage renal disease (ESRD) associated with prescribed CHMs in Taiwanese patients with stages 3-5 CKD. Newly diagnosed CKD patients were prescribed one of the 25 different formulas of the CHMs for kidney diseases (n = 11,351; median duration of CHM use was 22 days), compared with those who were not prescribed CHM (n = 13,620). They were followed up to death or dialysis initiation. The hazard ratio of ESRD was adjusted by age, sex, comorbidities, diabetic and hypertensive, nonsteroidal anti-inflammatory, or analgesic drugs to derive the adjusted cause-specific hazard ration (aCSHR). Results showed that herbal medicine users had a lower risk of ESRD, compared with non-users (aCSHR: 0.41; 95%CI: 0.37, 0.46) (Lin et al., 2015). Subgroup analyses were also conducted comparing different CHM formulas. Two formulas of CHM (active ingredients in Table 6), i.e. the wind dampness-dispelling formulas (aCSHR: 0.63; 95%CI: 0.51,

Table 5. CHMs for glomerular diseases and kidney transplant

Authors	Study design and country	Population	Intervention	Finding
Zhang et al. (2014b)	Open label RCT (n = 417) China	Patients had primary glomerular disease and stages 1-2 CKD	(1) A huangkui capsule[a] 2.5 g 3 times a day for 6 months (2) Losartan 50 mg/d (3) CHM + Losartan 50 mg/d	**Mean difference in reduction of 24 hr proteinuria** CHM vs. losartan: -508±457 mg/day (p < 0.01) Combination vs. losartan: -529±509 mg/day (p < 0.01) Combination vs. CHM: -708±588 mg/day (p = 0.4) **A/E of CHM**: GI discomfort and liver injury (n = 3)
Y.J. Wang et al. (2012)	Double-blinded RCT (n = 578) China	Patients had primary glomerulonephritis and stage 3 CKD	(1) 4 types of CHM[b] for 6 months based on traditional Chinese medicine syndrome (2) CHM + Benazepril 10 mg/d (3) Benazepril 10 mg/d	**eGFR in each arm comparing with baseline** CHM: 48±16 ml/min vs.45±10 ml/min (p< 0.01) Benazepril: 43±12 ml/min vs. 45±9 ml/min (p> 0.05) Combination 48+18 ml/min vs. 45±10 ml/min (p< 0.05) **Median reduction rate of UP comparing with baseline** CHM (-24.8%) decreased 24 hr proteinuria similar to combination (-8.8%) and Benazepril (0%) (p<0.05) **A/E of CHM**: hyperkalemia and liver injury; no difference between CHM and ACEI groups
Li et al. (2009)	RCT did not report blinding procedure (n = 202) China	Kidney transplant recipients	Cordyceps 1 g 3 times a day for one year + CsA 0.2-0.4 mg/kg/d lower dose than treatment gr. vs. CsA	No significant difference in graft survival rates, incidences of acute renal allograft rejection, and Scr between the treatment (Cordyceps adjuvant to CsA) and control groups (standard dose of CsA) Incidences of nephrotoxicity (19% vs. 34%) and hepatotoxicity (13% vs. 25%) were lower in Cordyceps adjuvant group (p< 0.05)
Qing et al. (2001)	RCT did not report blinding procedure (n = 120) China	Patients with remitted idiopathic nephrotic syndrome	CHM[c] twice a day for 6 months during reduced dose of prednisone vs. Prednisone 1 mg/kg/day for 10 weeks	Recurrence rate of nephrotic syndrome was lower in CHM group (13% vs. 40%) A/E of prednisone was lower in the CHM group.

[a]*Abelmoschus manihot;*[b] 1) Treatment of Qi Yin/Xue deficiency: *Astragalus membranaceus, Radix Pesudostellariae, Radix angelicae sinensis*, and *Ligustrum lucidum*; 2) treatment of blood stasis: *Radix Salviae Miltiorrhizae, Semen persicae, Herba centellae*, and Radix et rhizome rhei; 3) treatment of wind-dampness: *Tripterygium wilfordii, Radix Stephaniae Tetrandrae, Euonymus alatus*; 4) treatment of damp heat: *Rhizoma polygoni cuspidate, Rhizoma coptidis, Rhizoma smilacis glabrae*, and *Serissa serissoides;*[c] Concoction contains *Radix Astragali* 30 g, *Radix Angelicae Sinensis* 15 g, *Radix Saposhnikoviae* 15 g, *Rhizoma Atractylodis alba* 15 g, *Herba Leonuri* 15 g, *Radix Salviae Miltiorrhizae* 15 g, *Fructus Pyrrosia Sheareri* 15 g, *Radix Rehmanniae* 15 g, *Rhizoma Anemarrhenae* 15 g, and *Radix Glycyrrhizae* 9 g.; ACEI = Angiotensin-converting enzyme inhibitor; A/E = Adverse events; CsA = Cyclosporine; GI = Gastrointestinal; Scr = Serum creatinine; UP = Urine protein; vs. = versus

0.77), and harmonizing formulas (aCSHR: 0.59; 95%CI: 0.46, 0.74) were associated with the lower risk of ESRD. In contrast, the dampness-dispelling (aCSHR: 1.47; 95%CI: 1.20, 1.79), and purgative formulas (aCSHR: 1.58; 95%CI: 1.22, 2.05) were associated with a higher risk of ESRD, this may be due to them containing aristolochic acid known as a nephrotoxicity (Lin, et al., 2015), and both having a diuretic effect which may induce dehydration, therefore increasing the risk of AKI.

Case-Control Study

Hsu et al. (2014) conducted a case-control study to compare CHM as an adjuvant therapy to anti-diabetic drugs in patients with type 2 diabetes mellitus (DM) who had either developed CKD (n = 1,346) or who did not (n = 14,059). 'Liu-Wei-Di-Huang-Wan' - a traditional CHM formula consisting of six herbal medicines, i.e. *Rehmannia glutinosa*, *Cornus officinalis*, *Dioscorea oppositifolia*, *Alisma plantago-aquatica*, *Paeonia suffruticosa*, and *Poria cocos* was the targeted exposure, as its pharmacological effect of decreasing proteinuria may slow the progression of CKD (Sun et al., 2016). The results found that DM patients who took CHM were less likely to develop CKD (OR: 0.69; 95%CI: 0.61,0.77) (Hsu et al., 2014). However, they did not find a linear association between dose-response and the prevention of developing CKD.

EFFICACY OF OTHER CAM FOR COMPLICATIONS OF END-STAGE RENAL DISEASE

This section summarises evidence from clinical trials assessing the efficacy of CAM for managing complications and symptoms of ESRD as well as CAM's impacts on biomarkers in patients with ESRD. Current evidence emerged from 12 clinical trials which were published 2000 to 2015. They indicated that CAM may relieve complications of ESRD, i.e. pain, anxiety, depression, uraemic pruritus, and uremia. However, the quality of these trials was generally poor due to small sample sizes, and lack of randomisation and blinding. Therefore, the results have to be interpreted with caution.

Table 6. CHM formulas relating to the slow progression of CKD and risk of ESRD

Formulas	Active Ingredients
Benefit of CKD	
Wind dampness-dispelling formula (containing 46 herbal products)	Dwu Hwo Jih Sheng Tang; Mu Gua/Chaenomelis Fructus;Dang Guei Nian Tong Tang; Fang Feng/Saposhnikoviae Radix; Di Long/Lumbricus; Wei Ling Xian/ Clematidis Raix; Cang Er Sang; Tian Ma Kou Ten Yin; Xiao Feng San; Sang Zhi/ Mori Ramulus; Sang Ji Sheng/Taxillus Ramulis; Shang Zhong Xia Tong Yong Tong Feng Wan; Gou Ji/Cibotii Rhizoma; Kuei Chih Shao Yao Chih Mu Tang; Qin Jiao/Gentiana Macrophyllae Radix; Xiao Huo Luo Dan; Juan Bi Tang; Kou Ten San; Lu Lu Tong /Liquidambaris Fructus; Jiang Can/Bombyx Batryticatus ; Ching Shang JiuanTong Tang; Fang Ji/Stephaniae Tetrandrae Radix; Du Huo/ Angelicae Pubescentis Radix; Ching Kong Gau; Wu Chia Pee/Acanthopanacis Cortex; San Bi Tang; Jih Sheng San; Hsiao Hsu Ming Tang; Qian Nian Jian/Homalomena Rhizoma; Chuan Xiong Cha Tiao Sang; Di Wu Gong /Heliminthostachydis Rhizoma; Ba Xian Tang; Xi Xian Cao/Siegesbeckiae Herba; San Bih Tang; Chuan Shan Long/Rhizoma Dioscoreae Nipponicae; Da Qin Jiao Tang; Niao Bu Xiu/Zanthoxylum Nitidum (Roxb.) DC; Da Ding Cao/Leibnitzia anandria; Han Fang Ji/Sinomenium acutum; Dwu Hwo Jih Sheng Wan; Song Jie/Pinus tabulaeformis Carr; Bai Hualien/Chinese Lizarbtail Herba; Da Fang Feng Tang; Jiow Fei Ba Xian Tang; Hsu Ming Tang; Yi Yi Ren Tang
Harmonizing formula (containing 16 herbal products)	Jia Wei Xiao Yao San; Shao Yao Gan Cao Tang; Xiao Chai Hu Tang; Chai Hu Shu Gan Tang; Si Ni Sang; Chai Hu Gui Zhi Tang; Xiao Yao San; Chair ShiannTang; Huang Lian Tang; Chai Hu Gui Zhi Gan Jiang Tang; Xiao Chai Hu Tang; Jia Wei Xiao Yao Wan; Xiao Chai Hu Tang Qu Ngin Sam; Sheng Jiang Xie Xin Tang; Gan Cao Xie Xin Tang; Chai Hu Jia Long Gu Mu Li Tang; Huang Lian E Jiao Tang
Risk of ESRD	
Dampness-dispelling formula (containing 70 herbal products)	Che Qian Zi /Plantaginis Semen; Fu Ling/Poriae; Huang Bo/Phellodendri Cortex; Wu Ling Sang; Zhu Ling Tang; Yi Yi Ren/Coix Seed; Huang Lian/ Coptidis Rhizoma; Huo Xiang Zheng Qi San; Ling Gui Zhu Gan Tang; Cang Zhu/ Atractylodis Rhizoma; Ze Xie/Alismatis Rhizoma; Qiang Huo Sheng Shi Tang; Yin Chen Wu Ling San; Huo Xiang/AgastachesHerba; Bi Xie Fuen Ching Yin; Ba Zheng San; Yin Chen Hao/Artemisia capillaries Herba; Bi Xie /Dioscoreae Septemlobae Rhizoma; Fang Ji Huang Qi Tang; Hua Shi, Talcum; Hu Zhang/ Polygoni Cuspidati Rhizoma; Yi Yi Ren Tang; Bai Xian Pi/Dictamni Cortex; Erh Chu Tang; Wu Lin San; Zhu Ling/Polyporus; Di Fu Zi/ Kochiae Fructus; Dong Gua Zi/Benincasae Seed; Tao Shui Fu Lien Tang; Yueh Bih Jia Jwu Tang; Hua Shi Cao/ Orthosiphon Herba; Yin Chen/Artemisiae Capillaris Herba; Wu Pi Yin; Long Dan/ Gentianae Radix; Ding Shu Xiu/Elephantopus Herba; Suo Sha Ren/Amomi Fructus; Chi Xiao Dou/Phaseoli Seed; Mu Tong/Clematidis Armandi Caulis; Yu Mi Xu/ Maydis Stigma; Dong Kui Zi/Abutili Semen; Liu Ho Tong; Bai Dou Kou/Amomi Rotundus Fructus; Che Gian Cao/Plantaginis Herba; Pei Lan/Eupatorii Herba; Yin Chen Hao Tang; Ku Shen/Sophorae Flavescentis Radix; Qu mai/Dianthi Herba; Mu Fang Ji Tang; Chong Wei Zi/Leonuri Herba; Shen Jue Tang; Tong Cao/Medulla Tetrapanacis Papyriferi; Fen Hsiao Tang; Shi Wei/ Pyrrosiae Folium; Xiao Ban Xia Jia Fu Ling; Be Yin Chen/Origanum vulgare L.; Chun Gen Pi/Ailanthi Cortex; Deng Xin Cao/Junci Medulla; Bian Xu/Polygoni avicularis Herba; Ma Ti Jin/Dichondrae Herba; Hai Jin Sha/Lygodii Spora; Chai Ling Tang; Cao Guo/Tsaoko Fructus; Fu Ling/Poria; Ji Ming San; Zhi Ju Zi/Hoveniae Semen; Ping Wei Sang; Yue Bi Tang; Ze Qi/Sun Euphorbia; Guang Jin Qian Cao/Herba Desmodii Styracifolii; Jiang Hwo Shenq Shy Tang
Purgative formula (containing 10 herbal products)	Da Huang/Rhubarb; Gua Lou Ren/Trichosanthis Semen; Tiao Wei Cheng Qi Tang; Tao Ren Cheng Qi Tang; Hsiao Cheng Qi Tang; Da Cheng Qi Tang; Fan Xie Ye/ Sennae Folium; Fu Ma Ren/Sesami Nigrum Semen; Shu Zao Yin Zi; Qian Niu Zi/ Pharbitidis Semen

Pain, Anxiety and Depression

Five clinical trials assessed the efficacy of CAMs for managing the complications of ESRD compared with placebo, active control, or standard treatment (Table 7). The primary outcomes include symptoms of anxiety, depression, sleep, fatigue, and pain which were measured by validated self-reports. Four trials were conducted in haemodialysis patients to assess the efficacy of acupressure, Yoga, or aromatherapy on ESRD symptoms (Hmwe et al., 2015; Itai et al., 2000; Kim et al., 2011; Yurtkuran et al., 2007). One open-label RCT was conducted in kidney transplant recipients to assess the efficacy of mindfulness-based stress reduction (MBSR) on symptoms of anxiety, depression, and sleep quality (Gross et al., 2010).

Acupuncture relieved pain and improved quality of sleep (Kim et al., 2011) and depression (Hmwe et al., 2015). The potential mechanism of action of acupuncture for analgesic effects may be mediated by the release of the endogenous opiate β-endorphin and acetylcholine (Garcia et al., 2005). Acupoint massage seems to alleviate sleep disturbance in patients with ESRD due to stimulating the secretion of serotonin (Tsay, et al., 2003). Aromatherapy improved symptoms of anxiety and depression in haemodialysis patients as fragrance is likely to have sedative effects (Itai et al., 2000). Yoga relieved pain, fatigue, and sleep disturbance (Yurtkuran et al., 2007). Regarding yoga, Kashinath et al. (2014) suggested that patients with CKD should practice yoga under medical supervision and avoid some positions, such as complete inverted poses, and fast breathing practices. The MBSR decreased anxiety and sleep symptoms; but its mechanism is still unknown (Gross et al., 2010). However, the quality of these trials was poor due to limited sample sizes, unblinding (four trials), non-randomisation (two trials), and measuring subjective outcomes. These biases may contribute to the positive effects of CAM reported by participants. Reports of adverse effects of CAM are also lacking.

Uraemic Pruritus

Uraemic pruritus may be associated with neuropathy and neurologic changes, so acupuncture and acupressure may have an impact on relieving symptoms (Garcia et al., 2005). Currently, there are six studies which assessed the efficacy of CAM (aromatherapy with massage, turmeric, acupuncture, acupressure, and thermal therapy) compared to placebo or usual care for managing uraemic pruritus in patients who have received haemodialysis (Table 8), including a

Table 7. Clinical trials assessing the efficacy of CAM for managing pain, anxiety and depression in patients with ESRD and kidney transplants

Authors	Study Design	Population	Intervention	Outcome And Finding
Hmwe et al. (2015) in Malaysia	Open-label RCT (n = 108)	HD patients	Acupressure 3 times a week for 4 weeks for depression vs. a standard therapy	Measure depression scores using DASS-21 Significantly decreased DASS scores, compared with the control group. S/E: intra-dialytic hypotension
Kim et al. (2011) in Korea	Before and after study (n = 24) Non-randomisation Unblinding	HD patients	Acupuncture twice a week for 6 weeks	Assess symptoms using MYMOP2 Significantly improved symptoms[a], compared with participants' baseline
Gross et al. (2010) in the U.S.	Open-label RCT (n = 72)	Kidney, liver, heart or lung transplant	MBSR 2.5 hr classes weekly for 2 months vs. an active control (practising non-specific elements of MBSR)	Assess anxiety, depression and sleep quality using self-report for one year Significantly decreases anxiety and sleep symptoms, compared with the group of active control
Yurtkuran et al. (2007) in Turkey	Single blinded RCT (n = 37)	HD patients (almost all women)	Yoga-based exercise 30 minutes twice a week for 3 months vs. a standard therapy	Assess symptoms using VAS Significantly improved symptoms[a], compared with the control group No S/E
Itai et al. (2000) in Japan	Controlled trial (n = 14) Non-randomisation Unblinding	Female HD patients	Aromatherapy for 1 week (lavender and hiba oil) vs. control group (natural smell)	Assess anxiety and depression using self-report Significantly improved anxiety and depression, compared with the control group

[a]Pain, fatigue and sleep disturbance; DASS = The Depression, Anxiety, Stress Scales; ESRD = End-stage renal disease; HD = Haemodialysis; MBSR = Mindfulness-Based Stress Reduction; MYMOP2 = The Measure Your Medical Outcome Profiles 2 questionnaire; RCT = Randomised controlled trial; S/E = Side effects; vs. = versus

systematic review (Kim et al., 2010), two double-blinded RCTs (Hsu et al., 2009; Pakfetrat et al., 2014), and three non-randomised and unblind trials (Cürcani & Tan, 2014; Kiliç et al., 2013; Shahgholian et al., 2009). The primary outcome (pruritus symptoms) was measured by a self-reported visual analogue scale or pruritus score (Table 8).

Most studies reported that CAM significantly relieved uraemic pruritus, except for a double-blinded RCT which found no significant benefits of thermal therapy compared to placebo (Hsu, et al., 2009). This negative finding may be due to an ineffective intervention, small sample size, or insufficient time to detect a change. Aromatherapy with massage significantly relieved the symptoms of uraemic pruritus in dialysis patients (Cürcani & Tan, 2014; Shahgholian et al., 2009). It is likely that massage attributed to relieving pruritus rather than the aromatherapy. Turmeric significantly relieved uraemic

Table 8. Research for the efficacy of CAM for uraemic pruritus in haemodialysis patients

Authors	Study Design	Intervention	Outcome and Finding
Cürcani and Tan (2014) in Turkey	Quasi-experimental clinical trial (n = 134) Non-randomisation Unblinding	Aromatherapy (lavender, tea tree, almond and jojoba oils) massage the oils into skin 3 times a week for 6 weeks vs. control group received routine care	Assess uraemic pruritus using VAS and a pruritus score Mean pruritus scores (7.2±3.14), compared with the control group (10.0±2.47), $p < 0.01$ A/E: not reported
Pakfetrat et al. (2014) in Iran	Double- blinded RCT (n = 100) No report of blinding procedure	Turmeric 500 mg 3 times a day for 8 weeks vs. placebo	Assess uraemic pruritus using the Detailed Pruritus Score Reduced pruritus scores (-13.6±2.6), compared with the placebo group (-7.2±2.6), $p < 0.01$ Observing no A/E
Kiliç Akça et al. (2013) in Turkey	Open-label controlled trial (n = 78) Non-randomisation	Acupressure 3 times weekly for 6 weeks vs. control group received routine care	Assess uraemic pruritus using VAS and a pruritus score Significant decreases mean VAS and mean pruritus scores, compared with the control group A/E: not reported
Kim et al. (2010)	Systematic review of RCT (n = 3) and uncontrolled trials (n = 3)	(1) Acupuncture (2) Sham acupuncture (3) Conventional medicine, i.e. oral anti-histamine or oral calcitriol	Assess uraemic pruritus using self-report 5 out of 6 studies reported significantly alleviated uraemic pruritus, compared with Sham acupuncture or oral anti-histamine No difference in relieved pruritus between acupuncture and calcitonin High risk of bias in most of studies A/E: elbow soreness
Shahgholian et al. (2009) in Iran	Before and after study (n = 24) Non-randomisation	Aromatherapy (lavender, tea tree mint and almond oil) massage the oils into skin for 2 weeks	Assess uraemic pruritus using self-report Significant relieved uraemic pruritus Three patients left the study due to complaining the oil odor and greasy sensation
Hsu et al. (2009) in Taiwan	Double- blinded RCT (n = 41)	40°C thermal therapy with far-infrared rays at the Sanyinjiao acupoint for 15 minutes twice a week for 9 weeks vs. placebo	Assess uraemic pruritus using VAS and a pruritus score No difference in relieved pruritus between two groups Observing no A/E

A/E = Adverse effects; MBSR = Mindfulness-Based Stress Reduction; RCT = Randomised controlled trial; VAS = the Visual Analogue Scale; vs. = versus pruritus due to its anti-inflammatory effect (Pakfetrat et al., 2014). However, the limitations of these studies are similar to the previous ones. Most CAM studies are small, open-label, and non-RCT, and do not report adverse effects. Although the pruritus outcome was measured by using a validated, self-reported scale, it may still lead to measurement bias.

Uraemia

Nizhi et al. (2000) conducted an open-label, non-randomised controlled trial to assess the efficacy of adjuvant CHM with haemodialysis therapy compared with haemodialysis only for alleviating uremia in haemodialysis patients (n = 60). The intervention was 'Tongmai' solution (10 ml/ampule) containing Astragalus root 5 grams, notoginseng 1.5 grams, and 0.5 gram of Rhubarb. The treatment group received haemodialysis therapy combined with Tongmai 20 ml 3 times a day and rhubarb 2 pills 3 times a day for 3 months. The Kt/V is a fundamental parameter for measuring dialysis clearance. The end point was the Kt/V value at 1 and 3 months. The Kt/V target should be 1.2-1.4 ml/min. The authors found that the adjuvant CHM with haemodialysis significantly achieved the Kt/V target (1.18±0.35 ml/min) compared to the control group (Kt/V 0.98±0.28 ml/min, $p < 0.05$). This study did not report adverse effects. However, notoginseng and rhubarb have been reported as a cause of AKI (Albersmeyer et al., 2012; Lin, et al., 2011). The quality of Nizhi's study is limited and the confounding factors related to the outcome, such as fluid and protein intake were not mentioned.

Evidence for the Effects of CAM on Biomarkers

There are two clinical trials assessing the efficacy of CAM in decreasing oxidative stress in haemodialysis patients (Table 9) (Gordon, et al., 2013; Yeung et al., 2015). Oxidative stress is one factor associated with accelerated atherosclerosis in haemodialysis patients. Plasma levels of isofuran and plasma F_2-isoprostane are standard indicators for measuring oxidative stress. One open-label trial evaluated the efficacy and safety of varying doses of Coenzyme Q_{10} (300, 600, 1,200, and 1,800 mg/day) in 15 haemodialysis patients. They found increased doses of CoQ_{10} were associated with greater reduction in oxidative stress. Although most participants could tolerate the higher dose of CoQ_{10}, some patients suffered from abdominal pain and nausea (Yeung, et al., 2015). Another unblind RCT examined the effects of Hatka

Table 9. Clinical trials of CAM's influence on biomarker measure in haemodialysis patients

Authors	Study design	Population	Intervention	Outcome and finding
Yeung et al. (2015) in the U.S.	Open label trial (n = 15)	HD patients	CoQ_{10} 300,600,1,200, and 1,800 mg/day	Measure oxidative stress biomarkers in plasma Significantly decreased oxidative stress, compared with the participants' baseline Adverse effects: nausea (n = 3)
Gordon et al. (2013) in Jamaica	UnblindRCT (n = 68)	HD patients	Hatha Yoga 30 minutes daily for 4 months vs. Regular lifestyle practice	Measure oxidative stress biomarkers in plasma Significantly decreased oxidative stress, compared with the participants' baseline

vs. = versus

yoga in haemodialysis patients and found that yoga significantly decreased oxidative stress (Nguyen-Khoa et al., 2001). Currently, there is a limited number of RCTs studying the effects of CAM on biomarkers. Further RCTs are needed to link the clinical outcomes of oxidative stress with CAM such as incidence of cardiovascular disease.

NEPHROPATHY OF HERBAL MEDICINES AND DIETARY SUPPLEMENTS

Herbal medicine is more likely to cause AKI than other CAMs. Aristolochic acid contained in slimming pills was the first herbal medicine reported to be associated with nephropathy. This situation alerted conventional practitioners worldwide since 1992 (Debelle et al., 2008; Vanherweghem et al., 1993). Herbal medicines are likely to cause AKI rather than chronic kidney disease (Luyckx, 2012; Tangkiatkumjai et al., 2015). They also worsen electrolyte imbalance in patients with advanced CKD, particularly hyperkalemia and hyperphosphatemia. Adulterants in the products can also cause nephropathy, such as conventional medicines or heavy metals. Patients with renal insufficiency are more vulnerable to AKI related nephrotoxicity, compared with general populations. The manifestation of toxicity depends on the susceptible individual as well as dose, duration, and type of substance administered (The Indian Society of Nephrology, 2005). However, current epidemiological evidence for HDS related nephropathy is limited and most

Figure 1. Eosinophiluria in patients with acute interstitial nephritis; Eosinophiluria (Wright's stain, magnification: 1000x) (black arrow) from urine sample from patient with acute interstitial nephritis taking HDS and other medication. (Courtesy of Department of pathology, HRH Princess Maha Chakri Sirindhorn Medical Center, Faculty of Medicine, Srinakharinwirot University, Nakorn Nayok, Thailand)

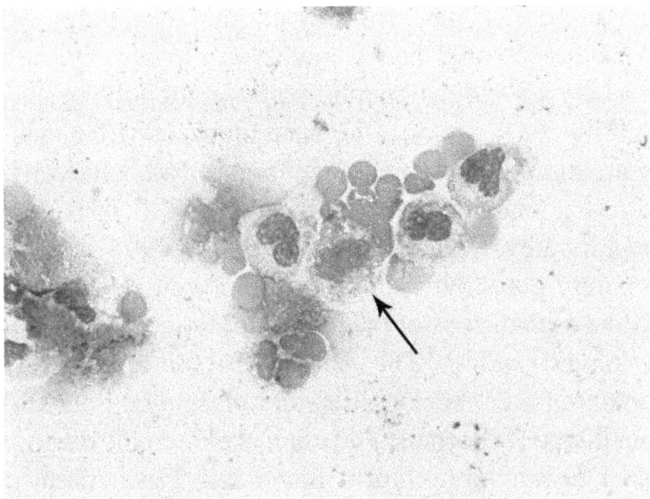

of the adverse event information are acquired from anecdotes (case reports or case series).

Pathology of Nephropathy Related to HDS

Kidneys are the one of most susceptible organs to toxic insult due to (1) approximately one-fourth of the cardiac output supplies the kidney hence prompt delivery of the toxic substance; (2) large surface area of the tubular epithelium provide sites for toxin exposure; (3) concentability of urine solutes also increase the concentration of toxin in renal medulla, further enhancing its toxic effect; and (4) changes of urine pH may affect the solubility of certain excreted substance, active toxic metabolites and precipitating formation causing damage renal tubules (Bennett, 1997; The Indian Society of Nephrology, 2005). Nephrotoxicity is classified as direct or indirect. The direct effect is an injury of the tubular system or renal parenchyma from the toxic substance itself, such as intratubular oxalate crystal precipitation from star fruit (Jang, 2012). Meanwhile, the indirect effect is an injury mediated by immunologic response to the toxic substance such as acute interstitial nephritis as a result of reduction of prostaglandin from nonsteroidal anti-inflammatory drugs (NSAIDs). It should be noted that a substance may induce nephrotoxicity by more than one pathogenic mechanism. For example, NSAIDs are known to cause four different AKI phenotypes, i.e. reduced renal perfusion, ischemic ATN, drug-induced acute interstitial nephritis (AIN), and minimal change disease which present as nephrotic syndrome (Naughton, 2008). HDS, conventional medicines, and heavy metals can cause diverse phenotypes of AKI such as crystal-induced nephropathy, acute tubular necrosis, acute interstitial nephritis, etc (Luyckx, 2012; Naughton, 2008). Patients with kidney insufficiency are more vulnerable to nephropathy associated with HDS.

Aistolochia is a main toxic substance in CHM, causing progressive interstitial nephropathy (Vanherweghem, et al., 1993). In general, cell-mediated immunity plays the major pathogenic role in drug-induced AIN. Interstitial edema with diffuse or patchy infiltration of inflammatory cells is the typical histologic findings. The infiltrative cells are mainly lymphocytes, monocytes, macrophages, eosinophils, and plasma cells, whilst glomeruli and vessels are distinctly normal. The clinical clue to the diagnosis is sterile pyuria, declined GFR in non-oliguric individuals. Eosinophiluria is a strong indicator for AIN but found in around 23% of cases (Figure 1) (Baker & Pusey, 2004; Choudhury & Ahmed, 2006; Kodner & Kudrimoti, 2003; Naughton, 2008; Rossert, 2001).

Nevertheless, CHM might cause a form of chronic interstitial nephritis called 'Chinese Herbal Nephropathy' caused by *Aristolochia.* It presents as progressive renal function impairment, increased blood pressure, and increased proteinuria (usually less than 1500 mg/day) with absence of *urinary sediment and esionophiluria.* The rate of progression is influenced by the dose and duration of intake of the herbs (Jha & Chugh, 2003). The pathogenesis of Aristolochia-induced Nephropathy is not fully understood. Many studies report that *Aristolochia* injections could promote progressive renal failure along with a 'hypocellular interstitial nephritis' which differed from typical drug-induced AIN (Cosyns et al., 2001; Depierreux et al., 1994; Jha & Chugh, 2003; Kanaan et al., 2003). The renal histology of Aristolochia-Induced Nephropathy shows scanty inflammatory cells within the interstitial space and endothelial cell swelling, which leads to thickening of the walls of arterioles (Figure 2). The glomeruli are relatively spared, and no immune deposits are observed.

Several reports also have suggested that *Aristolochia* might be associated with a gene mutation involved in the development of urothelial cancer. A series of case reports have suggested that long-term use of CHM is associated

Figure 2. Comparison of renal histological findings; normal, conventional, and hypocellular interstitial nephritis; Figure 2. A. Normal renal histology (Hematoxylin and Eosin stain (H&E), magnification 200x): Normal glomeruli appears as thin capillaries with normocellularity and matrix of mesangium. In renal cortex, the tubules are almost back to back and there is very little interstitial space and fewer cells between the tubules; Figure 2. B. Conventional interstial nephritis (H&E, magnification 200x): Renal pathology in patient with drug-induced interstitial nephritis. There is widening of interstial space which indicates interstitial edema and fibrosis. The diffuse infiltration by lymphocytes, macrophages (black arrow) and focal dense eosinophils (Torquoise blue arrow) are also seen; Figure 2. C. Hypocellular interstial nephritis (H&E, magnification 200x): Showing a renal pathology in patient taking CHM or Helicteres isora. There is markedly widening interstitial space and fibrosis with diffuse tubular atrophy. The cellular infiltration is markedly decreased when compare to the findings in conventional interstitial nephritis, mostly are mononuclear cells, plasma cells and eosinophils. The dilatation of Bowman's space with wrinkling and thickening of glomerular basement membrane is seen in glomeruli; Abbrevations: G = Glomerulus, I = Interstitial, T = Tubule, Eo = Eosinophil; [Courtesy of Dr. Vijitr Boonpucknavig, Bangkok, Thailand (Figure 2-A and 2-B) and Dr. Worapon Buranachokpaisan, Phitsanulok, Thailand (Figure 2-C)]

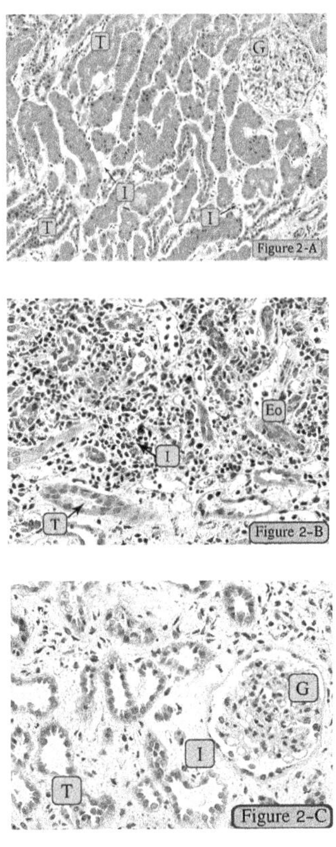

Figure 3. The Helicteres isora tree. (The Indian screw tree); Figure 3. Helicteres isora (Indian screw tree): The trees are known in Thailand as "Por Bid". Figure A-B show its stem and leaves. Figure C-D indicate its fruits which has been used as a medicinal agent for treating diabetes and hyperlipidaemia (Gupta et al., 2009; Kumar & Singh, 2014)

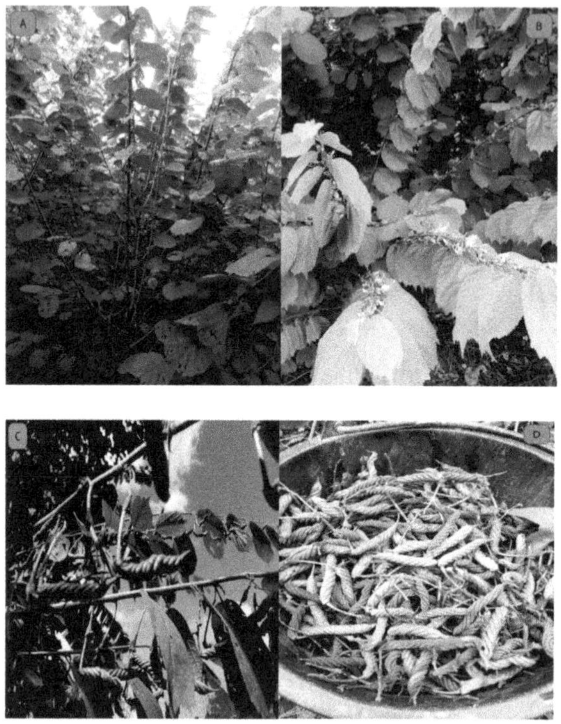

with a high incidence of urothelial dysplasia of the genitourinary tract, and urothelial cancer (Arlt et al., 2002; Cosyns et al., 1999; Jha & Chugh, 2003; Nortier et al., 2000). In addition, a case report from Thailand has indicated that *Helicteres isora,* can cause renal pathology similar to CHM (Figure 3) (Gupta et al., 2009; Kumar & Singh, 2014). To specify a nephrotoxic substance in this plant, further animal toxicity studies are needed. Figure 4 demonstrates oxalate crystals related to star fruit or vitamin C.

Figure 4. Calcium oxalate crystals (Fresh urine sample, magnification: 400x): seen as envelop-shaped crystal (red arrow) from fresh urine sample from patient with oxalate nephropathy taking star fruits or high dose of vitamin C.

Figure 4. Urine calcium oxalate crystals in patient taking star fruits or vitamin C; (Courtesy of Department of pathology, HRH Princess Maha Chakri Sirindhorn Medical Center, Faculty of Medicine, Srinakharinwirot University, Nakorn Nayok, Thailand)

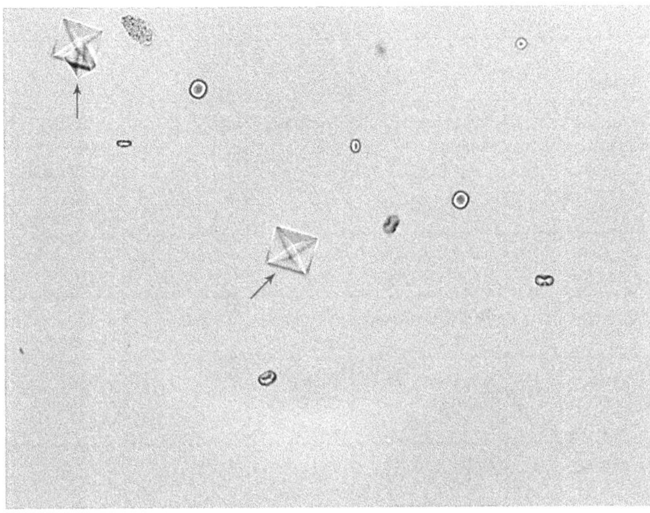

Acute Kidney Injury

AKI is an abrupt reduction in kidney function within a period ranging from minutes to days that results in volume overload and electrolyte imbalance. The potential mechanisms of AKI related to HDS include renal tubular injury, acute interstitial nephritis or obstructive nephropathy. These mechanisms are similar to nephrotoxicity due to conventional medicines. Approximately 35% of AKI may be related to herbal medicine in the developing countries (Luyckx, 2012), whilst 20% of AKI results from conventional medicines (Li, et al., 2013). Due to limited RCTs reporting adverse events of HDS, case reports are likely to be the main evidence source for suggesting which HDS should be avoided. Luyckx (2012) gathered many case reports on HDS related to AKI worldwide and reported that *Tripterygium wilfordii* caused AKI. In contrast, some meta-analyses show the efficacy of *Tripterygium wilfordii* for treating kidney diseases. Hence contrasting information suggests that some herbal medicines may have both the beneficial and adverse effects on the kidneys. Overall, there were 32 anecdotes of reported HDS associated with AKI in both general populations and patients with CKD (Table 10). Of

Table 10. Case reports on HDS or traditional medicine associated with acute kidney injury

Common Name	Scientific Name	Mechanism of AKI	Kidney Function at Baseline	Time Exposure/ Onset of AKI	Dosage Regimen	Reference
African Mango	*Irvingia gabonensis*	Unknown	Stage 3a	3 mo	1 g/d	(Özkan & Ulusoy, 2015)
Anatolian Hawthorn	*Crataegus orientalis*	Acute interstitial nephritis	Normal	3 d	½ kg of fresh weight and 5 cups of tea (leaves)	(Horoz et al., 2008)
Autumn crocus	*Colchicum autumnale*	Kidney necrosis Rhabdomyolysis	Renal insuff.	within 12 hr	2 whole plants	(Brvar et al., 2004)
Bee pollen		Acute interstitial nephritis	Normal	5 mo	Not reported	(Akiyasu et al., 2010)
Bindii	*Tribulus terrestris*	Acute tubular necrosis	History of kidney stones	2 d	2 L/d	(Talasaz, Abbasi, Abkhiz et al., 2010)
Black cumin	*Nigella sativa*	Unknown	Unknown	6 d	2-2.5 g/d	(Arslan et al., 2013)
Cape Aloe	*Aloe capensis*	Acute tubular necrosis	Unknown	1 mo	Not reported	(Luyckx et al., 2002)
Cat's claw	*Uncaria tomentosa*	Acute interstitial nephritis	Stage 3b	Not reported	1 cap 4 times/d	(Hilepo, Bellucci, & Mossey, 1997)
Cherry concentrate	*Prunus cerasus*	Prerenal azotemia	Stage 3b	1 mo	2-4 ounces/d	(Luciano, 2014)
CKLS*	*Aloe vera, Cascara sagrada*	Acute tubulointerstitial nephritis	Normal	5 d	3 capsules/d	(Adesunloye, 2003)
	Uva ursi	Albuminuria				
Creatine		Acute focal interstitial nephritis	Normal	1 mo	5 g/d	(Koshy, Griswold, & Schneeberger, 1999)
Djenkol beans	*Pithecellobium jeringa*	Obstructive nephropathy	Unknown	1 d	Not reported	(Wong, Ong, Chua et al., 2007)
Mourning Cypress	*Cupressus funebris*	Acute tubular necrosis and Acute interstitial nephritis	Normal	1 d	Not reported	(Lee & Chen, 2006)
Glucosamine		Acute interstitial nephritis	Unknown	2-3 mo	Not reported	(Audimoolam & Bhandari, 2006)

continued on following page

Table 10. Continued

Common Name	Scientific Name	Mechanism of AKI	Kidney Function at Baseline	Time Exposure/ Onset of AKI	Dosage Regimen	Reference
Gongjin-dan	*Moschus mschiferus* Linne *Cervus elaphus* sibiricus	Focal tubulointerstitial nephritis	Normal	20 d	4 g/d	(Lee, Jeong, & Rhee, 2014)
Hemlock	*Conium maculatum*	Acute tubular necrosis Rhabdomyolysis	Unknown	Within 24 hr	Accidental taking	(Rizzi et al., 1991)
Kariyat	*Andrographis paniculata*	Acute tubular necrosis	Normal	6-48 hr	100-750 mg iv	(Zhang, Zhang, Zhang et al., 2014)
Khat	*Catha edulis*	AKI caused by rhabdomyolysis	Unknown	14 d	Chewing 2-3 g/d of fresh leaves	(Tratenberg, Mehta, Kleinman et al., 2015)
Licorice	*Glycyrrhiza glabra*	AKI caused by hypokalaemic rhabdomyolysis	Stage 3a	9 mo	150 mg/d	(Chubachi, et al., 1992)
L-lysine		Proximal tubular necrosis Fanconi's syndrome	Normal	5 yr	3 g/d	(Lo, Chertow, Rennke et al., 1996)
Pro-Lift®	6% ephedrine/ tablet	Kidney stones	Single kidney with history of kidney stones	10 mo	4-12 tablets/d	(Powell, Hsu, Turk et al., 1998)
Wild mushroom	*Cortinarius orellanus*	Acute interstitial nephritis	Unknow	10 d	Eating in a soup	(Kilner et al., 1999)
Notoginseng	*Panax notoginseng*	Prerenal azotemia	Normal	1 wk	10-400 mg/kg/d	(Lin, et al., 2011)
Propolis		Acute interstitial nephritis	Normal	2 wk	5 ml 3 times/d	(Li, Lin, Yang et al., 2005)
Energy drink	Caffeine, vitamins B3, B5, B6, B12, sucrose, glucose, taurine, and glucuronolactone	Acute tubular necrosis	Normal	Several wk	6 bottles/d (20 oz)	(Greene, Oman, & Lefler, 2014)
Rhubarb	*Rheum officinale*	Oxalate nephropathy	Normal	1 mo	500 mg/d (fresh weight)	(Albersmeyer, et al., 2012)
Sea spurge	*Euphorbia paralias*	Acute tubular necrosis Acute interstitial nephritis	History of nephrotic syndrome	10 d	Taking boiled spurge once	(Boubaker et al., 2013)

continued on following page

Table 10. Continued

Common Name	Scientific Name	Mechanism of AKI	Kidney Function at Baseline	Time Exposure/ Onset of AKI	Dosage Regimen	Reference
Senna	*Sennae fructus angustifoliae*	Renal tubular acidosis	Unknown	> 3 yr	1 L of 70 g of dry senna	(Vanderperren et al., 2005)
Spanish fly	*Cantharis vesicatoria*	tubular Acute necrosis	Normal	10 hr	Drinking as a beverage	(Karras, Farrell, Harrigan et al., 1996)
Star fruit	*Averrhoa carabola*	Oxalate nephropathy Acute tubulointerstitial disease	Normal (n = 1) and renal insuff. (n = 1)	4-12 days	4-6 star fruits	(Abeysekera et al., 2015)
Vitamin C		Oxalate nephropathy Acute tubular injury	Stage 3a	2-6 mo	500-1,000 mg/d	(Lamarche, Nair, Peguero, & Courville, 2011)
Wormwood oil	*Artemisia absinthium*	AKI caused by rhabdomyolysis	Unknown	≤ 6 hr	10 ml once	(Weisbord, et al., 1997)

* CKLS = Colon, Kidney, Liver, Spleen

which, 16 reports were included in Luyckx' review (2012) and the remaining reports emerged from a systematic search by the authors of this chapter. The case reports indicate that risk factors related to AKI; are pre-existing CKD, advanced age, taking high doses and/or long-term use of HDS. A seizure may provoke rhabdomyolysis induced AKI (Chubachi et al., 1992; Weisbord et al., 1997). Most patients from those case reports recovered from AKI after stopping HDS, although a small number of the patients suffered from ESRD and died.

Bee pollen is able to induce AKI related to both short-term (within 24 hour) and long-term periods (> 3 months) (Akiyasu, et al., 2010). Cherry concentrate for gout may cause AKI due to its effect as a cyclooxygenase inhibitor (Luciano, 2014). Herbal medicines containing a high amount of flavonoids are likely to damage the kidneys via acute interstitial nephritis, such as Mourning Cypress and Anatolian Hawthorn (Horoz et al., 2008; Lee & Chen, 2006). Gongjin-dan contains four ingredients that are associated with nephropathy (Lee et al., 2014). Case series have reported that kariyat infusion and Hemlock are related to AKI (Rizzi et al., 1991; Zhang, et al., 2014). Some patients have AKI from accidentally taking plants, such as

Hemlock and Autumn crocus (Brvar et al., 2004; Rizzi et al., 1991). Some bird meats eaten by the patients have been contaminated by Hemlock as the birds consume the buds. Additionally, one patient mistakenly took Autumn crocus (nephrotoxicity) rather than wild garlic because these two plants are quite similar. Likewise, toxic mushrooms were mistakenly took by two patients, who then developed AKI (Kilner et al., 1999). Khat has been used for stimulation and euphoria, and may cause AKI (Tratenberg et al., 2015).

Some patients suffer from AKI due to taking a high amount of HDS, such as an energy drink (Greene et al., 2014), licorice, or *Nigella sativa*. Chubachi et al. (1992) reported that a patient with stage 3 CKD took licorice for a long-term period, and then developed chronic hypokalaemia, which might lead to tubulointerstitial nephritis and AKI. Dehydration is another risk factor of licorice induced AKI. *Nigella sativa* has an effect on preventing kidney damage in rats (Bayrak et al., 2008; Havakhah et al., 2014). However, one case report indicates that a high dose of *Nigella sativa* may cause AKI within 6 days in humans (Arslan et al., 2013). Therefore, people should not take a higher than recommended dose of HDS.

Several HDS result in AKI associated with nephrolithiasis. An energy supplement containing ephedrine (Ma-Huang) may induce nephrolithiasis, particularly in patients with high risk of kidney stones (Powell et al., 1998). Abeysekera et al. (2015) have reported that patients with both normal kidney function or diabetic nephropathy might develop AKI from taking star fruit, which causes oxalate nephropathy. Whilst vitamin C (500-1,000 mg/day) is likely to induce oxalate nephropathy in patients with renal insufficiency. People with normal kidney function may develop oxalate nephropathy when they take more than 2 g/day of vitamin C (Lamarche et al., 2011). Diuretic effects of Notoginseng may cause AKI related to dehydration (Lin et al., 2011). A case report reveals that alfalfa combined with black cohosh may cause acute graft rejection with vasculitis in a kidney transplant recipient (Light & Light, 2003).

Electrolyte Imbalance

Of the HDS related to electrolyte imbalance, HDS users with advanced CKD may frequently suffer from uncontrolled hyperkalemia and hyperphosphatemia. Severe hyperkalemia is life-threatening as it may lead to ventricular arrhythmias and respiratory failure whilst hyperphosphatemia may increase cardiovascular calcification in patients with CKD. Evidence from animal studies has demonstrated that some herbal diuretics are likely to induce AKI and uncontrolled hyperkalemia in patients with renal insufficiency (Wright et al., 2007). For example, one HDS known as Noni juice may lead to hyperkalemia in CKD patients (Mueller et al., 2000). A cohort study with a one year follow-up recruited 357 patients with stages 3-5 CKD and found that patients who took dietary supplements containing phosphate and/or vitamin D (i.e. bee pollen, cod liver oil, multivitamins, protein supplements, rice bran oil, and wheatgrass) were more likely to have worsening hyperphosphatemia (Tangkiatkumjai et al., 2015).

Adulteration and Contamination

Asian traditional medicine can be contaminated or adulterated by conventional medicine, heavy metals, or microorganisms. Posadzki et al. (2013) reviewed 26 systematic reviews of the contaminations of herbal medicine and reported that Indian and Chinese herbal medicines were the most frequently adulterated and contaminated. NSAIDs, indomethacin, and prednisolone are common adulterations in herbal products, and could cause AKI (Posadzki et al., 2013). In terms of heavy metals (i.e. cadmium and mercury) related to AKI, Kim et al. (2014) reviewed 10 studies of the contaminations of Traditional Chinese Medicines (TCM) and found contamination by cadmium which led to Faconi's syndrome and AKI (Kim et al., 2014). An older patient received chronic inhalation of cinnabar (containing mercury sulfide) and calomel, and then developed nephrotoxicity (Liu et al., 2008).

Recommendations for Preventing Acute Kidney Injury From Using Herbal and Dietary Supplements

Based on the current anecdotal evidence and knowledge of potential mechanisms leading to nephropathy, it is important that the health care professionals should be mindful of the risks in routine practices, particularly in Asian and African countries, where the use of HDS is highly prevalent. To prevent nephopathy from using HDS, conventional practitioners, should regularly ask CKD patients about HDS use, and recommend to patients which HDS should be avoided. The common rule of thumb to prevent HDS related nephropathy is to avoid using unregistered HDS, HDS which are associated with dehydration, AKI or nephrotoxicity. Also, high doses or long-term use. In particular, herbal diuretics, laxatives, and herbal medicines with the risk of over diuresis, diarrhea, or vomiting which may cause dehydration. Hemlock, Autumn crocus, and toxic mushrooms are notoriously related to nephropathy. High doses of vitamin C, rhubarb and Nigella sativa should also be avoided. It is noteworthy that the recommended dose for general populations may cause AKI in patients with renal insufficiency; therefore, these patients should consult their doctor before taking any HDS.

ADVERSE EFFECTS OF OTHER COMPLEMENTARY AND ALTERNATIVE MEDICINE

Acupuncture and massage are likely to be safe in patients with CKD as shown in several systematic reviews (MacPherson et al., 2001; Wu et al., 2015; Xu et al., 2013; Yin et al., 2014). However, acupuncture may cause infection, such as hepatitis, or minor adverse events, i.e. bruising, pain and bleeding. Serious adverse events of acupuncture and massage are rare. Acupuncture may cause pneumothorax and central nervous system injury (Wu et al., 2015). Massage may result in hemiparesis, spinal epidural hematoma, and atlantoaxial dislocation (Yin et al., 2014). Thus, people should keep in mind that these CAMs are not totally safe.

CONCLUSION

Herbal medicine could be an option for treating kidney diseases when conventional medicines fail to achieve the satisfactory effect. Chinese herbal medicine, i.e. Astragalus, Cordyceps, and Tripterygium, as an adjuvant therapy to conventional medicine may improve CKD, proteinuria, and glomerular diseases. The pharmacological effects of CHMs in treating CKD, may be associated with the stimulation of immune system, antioxidants and anti-inflammation. Regarding evaluation of the efficacy of the CHM combined with usual treatment for managing CKD, there is evidence for Astragalus and Tripterygium. The RCTs included in the meta-analyses for these CHMs had same methodological issues, i.e. small sample sizes, unclear randomisation, unclear blinding, short-term follow-up, and lack of reported adverse effects. However, these issues may due to the fact that double-blinded clinical trials of CHM are difficult to conduct. Current systematic reviews revealed convincing benefits for a combination of Astragalus, Tripterygium, and Cordyceps together with conventional medicine for treating CKD. There is a lack of studies to prove benefits of *Rheum officinale*. Acupuncture, yoga and aromatherapy with massage may reduce symptoms in patients with ESRD, such as muscle pain, anxiety, and pruritus. However, further studies are required to confirm their efficacy and safety.

To ensure the safe use of HDS, patients with renal insufficiency should avoid using unregistered herbal products or those that may lead to AKI, such as CHM containing Aristolochic acids, Cape aloe, creatine, Mourning cypress, Gongjin-dan, licorice, rhubarb, vitamin C, or star fruit. In addition, patients with advanced CKD should not take dietary supplements containing a high amount of phosphate and/or vitamin D. Further research is needed to examine whether *Tripterygium wilfordii*, Black cumin and herbal medicines which contain a high amount of flavonoids have either beneficial effects on CKD or risk of AKI. Chapter 10 will propose further research on CAM for kidney diseases.

REFERENCES

Abeysekera, R. A., Wijetunge, S., Nanayakkara, N., Wazil, A. W., Ratnatunga, N. V., Jayalath, T., & Medagama, A. (2015). Star fruit toxicity: a cause of both acute kidney injury and chronic kidney disease: a report of two cases. *BMC Research Notes*, *8*(1), 796. doi:10.1186/s13104-015-1640-8 PMID:26680759

Adesunloye, B. A. (2003). Acute renal failure due to the herbal remedy CKLS. *The American Journal of Medicine*, *115*(6), 506–507. doi:10.1016/S0002-9343(03)00427-3 PMID:14563511

Akiyasu, T., Paudyal, B., Paudyal, P., Kumiko, M., Kazue, U., Takuji, N., & Minoru, K. et al. (2010). A case report of acute renal failure associated with bee pollen contained in nutritional supplements. *Therapeutic Apheresis and Dialysis*, *14*(1), 93–97. doi:10.1111/j.1744-9987.2009.00707.x PMID:20438524

Albersmeyer, M., Hilge, R., Schrottle, A., Weiss, M., Sitter, T., & Vielhauer, V. (2012). Acute kidney injury after ingestion of rhubarb: Secondary oxalate nephropathy in a patient with type 1 diabetes. *BMC Nephrology*, *13*(1), 141. doi:10.1186/1471-2369-13-141 PMID:23110375

Arlt, V. M., Stiborova, M., & Schmeiser, H. H. (2002). Aristolochic acid as a probable human cancer hazard in herbal remedies: A review. *Mutagenesis*, *17*(4), 265–277. doi:10.1093/mutage/17.4.265 PMID:12110620

Arslan, E., Sayın, S., Demirbaş, Ş., Çakar, M., Somak, N. G., Yeşilkaya, Ş., & Sağlam, K. (2013). A case study report of acute renal failure associiaed with *Nigella sativa* in a diabetic patient. *Journal of Internal Medicine*, *11*(1), 64–66. PMID:23464648

Audimoolam, V. K., & Bhandari, S. (2006). Acute interstitial nephritis induced by glucosamine. *Nephrology, Dialysis, Transplantation*, *21*(7), 2031. doi:10.1093/ndt/gfl025 PMID:16504980

Baker, R. J., & Pusey, C. D. (2004). The changing profile of acute tubulointerstitial nephritis. *Nephrology, Dialysis, Transplantation*, *19*(1), 8–11. doi:10.1093/ndt/gfg464 PMID:14671029

Bakris, G. L. (2008). Slowing nephropathy progression: Focus on proteinuria reduction. *Clinical Journal of the American Society of Nephrology; CJASN*, *3*(Suppl 1), S3–S10. doi:10.2215/CJN.03250807 PMID:18178794

Bayrak, O., Bavbek, N., Karatas, O. F., Bayrak, R., Catal, F., Cimentepe, E., & Akcay, A. et al. (2008). *Nigella sativa* protects against ischaemia/reperfusion injury in rat kidneys. *Nephrology, Dialysis, Transplantation*, *23*(7), 2206–2212. doi:10.1093/ndt/gfm953 PMID:18211980

Bennett, W. M. (1997). Drug nephrotoxicity: An overview. *Renal Failure*, *19*(2), 221–224. doi:10.3109/08860229709026280 PMID:9101595

Boubaker, K., Ounissi, M., Brahmi, N., Goucha, R., Hedri, H., Abdellah, T. B., & Kheder, A. et al. (2013). Acute renal failure by ingestion of *Euphorbia paralis*. *Saudi Journal of Kidney Diseases and Transplantation*, *24*(3), 571–575. doi:10.4103/1319-2442.111069 PMID:23640634

Brvar, M., Ploj, T., Kozelj, G., Mozina, M., Noc, M., & Bunc, M. (2004). Case report: Fatal poisoning with *Colchicum autumnale*. *Critical Care (London, England)*, *8*(1), R56–R59. doi:10.1186/cc2427 PMID:14975056

Chen, Y., Gong, Z., Chen, X., Tang, L., Zhao, X., Yuan, Q., & Cai, G. (2013). *Tripterygium wilfordii* Hook F (a traditional Chinese medicine) for primary nephrotic syndrome. *Cochrane Database of Systematic Reviews*, *11*(8), CD008568. PMID:23934958

Cheung, A. K., Sarnak, M. J., Yan, G., Berkoben, M., Heyka, R., Kaufman, A., & Levey, A. S et al.. (2004). Cardiac diseases in maintenance hemodialysis patients: Results of the HEMO Study. *Kidney International*, *65*(6), 2380–2389. doi:10.1111/j.1523-1755.2004.00657.x PMID:15149351

Chou, W. C., Wu, C. C., Yang, P. C., & Lee, Y. T. (1995). Hypovolemic shock and mortality after ingestion of *Tripterygium wilfordii* hook F.: A case report. *International Journal of Cardiology*, *49*(2), 173–177. doi:10.1016/0167-5273(95)02282-2 PMID:7628889

Choudhury, D., & Ahmed, Z. (2006). Drug-associated renal dysfunction and injury. *Nature Clinical Practice. Nephrology*, *2*(2), 80–91. doi:10.1038/ncpneph0076 PMID:16932399

Chubachi, A., Wakui, H., Asakura, K. I., Nishimura, S., Nakamoto, Y., & Miura, A. B. (1992). Acute renal failure following hypokalemic rhabdomyolysis due to chronic glycyrrhizic acid administration. *Internal Medicine (Tokyo, Japan)*, *31*(5), 708–711. doi:10.2169/internalmedicine.31.708 PMID:1504440

Cosyns, J. P., Dehoux, J. P., Guiot, Y., Goebbels, R. M., Robert, A., Bernard, A. M., & van Ypersele de Strihou, C. (2001). Chronic aristolochic acid toxicity in rabbits: A model of Chinese herbs nephropathy? *Kidney International*, *59*(6), 164–173. doi:10.1046/j.1523-1755.2001.00731.x PMID:11380818

Cosyns, J. P., Jadoul, M., Squifflet, J. P., Wese, F. X., & van Ypersele de Strihou, C. (1999). Urothelial lesions in Chinese-herb nephropathy. *American Journal of Kidney Diseases*, *33*(6), 1011–1017. doi:10.1016/S0272-6386(99)70136-8 PMID:10352187

Cürcani, M., & Tan, M. (2014). The effect of aromatherapy on haemodialysis patients pruritus. *Journal of Clinical Nursing*, *23*(23-24), 3356–3365. doi:10.1111/jocn.12579 PMID:24646128

Debelle, F. D., Vanherweghem, J. L., & Nortier, J. L. (2008). Aristolochic Acid Nephropathy: A Worldwide Problem. *Kidney International*, *74*(2), 158–169. doi:10.1038/ki.2008.129 PMID:18418355

Depierreux, M., Van Damme, B., Vanden Houte, K., & Vanherweghem, J. L. (1994). Pathologic aspects of a newly described nephropathy related to the prolonged use of Chinese herbs. *American Journal of Kidney Diseases*, *24*(2), 172–180. doi:10.1016/S0272-6386(12)80178-8 PMID:8048421

Garcia, G. E., Ma, S. X., & Feng, L. (2005). Acupuncture and kidney disease. *Advances in Chronic Kidney Disease*, *12*(3), 282–291. doi:10.1016/j.ackd.2005.04.002 PMID:16010643

Gordon, L., McGrowder, D. A., Pena, Y. T., Cabrera, E., & Lawrence-Wright, M. B. (2013). Effect of yoga exercise therapy on oxidative stress indicators with end-stage renal disease on hemodialysis. *Int J Yoga*, *6*(1), 31–38. doi:10.4103/0973-6131.105944 PMID:23440311

Greene, E., Oman, K., & Lefler, M. (2014). Energy drink-induced acute kidney injury. *The Annals of Pharmacotherapy*, *48*(10), 1366–1370. doi:10.1177/1060028014541997 PMID:24986632

Gross, C. R., Kreitzer, M. J., Thomas, W., Reilly-Spong, M., Cramer-Bornemann, M., Nyman, J. A., & Ibrahim, H. N. et al. (2010). Mindfulness-based stress reduction for solid organ transplant recipients: A randomized controlled trial. *Alternative Therapies in Health and Medicine*, *16*(5), 30–38. PMID:20882729

Gupta, R. N., Pareek, A., Suthar, M., Rathore, G. S., Basniwal, P. K., & Jain, D. (2009). Study of glucose uptake activity of Helicteres isora Linn. fruits in L-6 cell lines. *Int J Diabetes Dev Ctries*, *29*(4), 170–173. doi:10.4103/0973-3930.57349 PMID:20336200

Havakhah, S., Sadeghnia, H. R., Hajzadeh, M. A. R., Roshan, N. M., Shafiee, S., Hosseinzadeh, H., & Rad, A. K. et al. (2014). Effect of *Nigella sativa* on ischemia-reperfusion induced rat kidney damage. *Iranian Journal of Basic Medical Sciences.*, *17*(12), 986–992. PMID:25859302

Hilepo, J. N., Bellucci, A. G., & Mossey, R. T. (1997). Acute renal failure caused by Cats Claw herbal remedy in a patient with systemic lupus erythematosus. *Nephron*, *77*(3), 361. doi:10.1159/000190304 PMID:9375835

Hmwe, N. T. T., Subramanian, P., Tan, L. P., & Chong, W. K. (2015). The effects of acupressure on depression, anxiety and stress in patients with hemodialysis: A randomized controlled trial. *International Journal of Nursing Studies*, *52*(2), 509–518. doi:10.1016/j.ijnurstu.2014.11.002 PMID:25468282

Horoz, M., Gok, E., Genctoy, G., Ozcan, T., Olmaz, R., Akca, M., & Gurses, I. et al. (2008). Crataegus Orientalis associated multiorgan hypersensitivity reaction and acute renal failure. *Internal Medicine (Tokyo, Japan)*, *47*(23), 2039–2042. doi:10.2169/internalmedicine.47.1502 PMID:19043257

Hsu, M. C., Chen, H. W., Hwu, Y. J., Chanc, C. M., & Liu, C. F. (2009). Effects of thermal therapy on uremic pruritus and biochemical parameters in patients having haemodialysis. *Journal of Advanced Nursing*, *65*(11), 2397–2408. doi:10.1111/j.1365-2648.2009.05100.x PMID:19737321

Hsu, P. C., Tsai, Y. T., Lai, J. N., Wu, C. T., Lin, S. K., & Huang, C. Y. (2014). Integrating traditional Chinese medicine healthcare into diabetes care by reducing the risk of developing kidney failure among type 2 diabetic patients: A population-based case control study. *Journal of Ethnopharmacology*, *156*, 358–364. doi:10.1016/j.jep.2014.08.029 PMID:25178949

Itai, T., Amayasu, H., Kuribayashi, M., Kawamura, N., Okada, M., Momose, A., & Kaneko, S. et al. (2000). Psychological effects of aromatherapy on chronic hemodialysis patients. *Psychiatry and Clinical Neurosciences*, *54*(4), 393–397. doi:10.1046/j.1440-1819.2000.00727.x PMID:10997854

Jang, J. L. (2012). Intrinsic causes of acute kidney injury. In S. Cheng & A. Vijayan (Eds.), *The Washington Manual of Nephrology Subspecialty Consult* (pp. 133–162). Philadelphia: Lippincott Williams & Wilkins.

Jha, V., & Chugh, K. S. (2003). Nephropathy associated with animal, plant, and chemical toxins in the tropics. *Seminars in Nephrology*, *23*(1), 49–65. doi:10.1053/snep.2003.50003 PMID:12563601

Jun, M., Venkataraman, V., Razavian, M., Cooper, B., Zoungas, S., & Ninomiya, T. et al.. (2012). Antioxidants for chronic kidney disease. *Cochrane Database of Systematic Reviews*, *17*(10), CD008176. PMID:23076940

Kanaan, N., Cosyns, J. P., Jadoul, M., & Goffin, E. (2003). The importance of a histology-based diagnosis of interstitial nephropathy in two patients with renal insufficiency. *Nephrology, Dialysis, Transplantation*, *18*(2), 440–442. doi:10.1093/ndt/18.2.440 PMID:12543907

Karras, D. J., Farrell, S. E., Harrigan, R. A., Henretig, F., & Gealt, L. (1996). Poisoning from Spanish Fly (Cantharidin). *The American Journal of Emergency Medicine*, *14*(5), 478–483. doi:10.1016/S0735-6757(96)90158-8 PMID:8765116

Kashinath, G. M., Hemant, B., Praerna, C., Nagarathna, R., & Nagendra, H. R. (2014). Role of Yoga in chronic kidney disease: A hypothetical review. *J Nephrol Ther*, *4*(3).

Kiliç Akça, N., Taşçi, S., & Karataş, N. (2013). Effect of acupressure on patients in Turkey receiving hemodialysis treatment for uremic pruritus. *Alternative Therapies in Health and Medicine*, *19*(5), 12–18. PMID:23981400

Kilner, R. G., DSouza, R. J., Oliveira, D. B., MacPhee, I. A., Turner, D. R., & Eastwood, J. B. (1999). Acute renal failure from intoxication by Cortinarius orellanus: Recovery using anti-oxidant therapy and steroids. *Nephrology, Dialysis, Transplantation*, *14*(11), 2779–2780. doi:10.1093/ndt/14.11.2779-a PMID:10534536

Kim, H., Hughes, P., & Hawes, E. M. (2014). Adverse events associated with metal contamination of traditional Chinese medicines in Korea: A clinical review. *Yonsei Medical Journal*, *55*(5), 1177–1186. doi:10.3349/ymj.2014.55.5.1177 PMID:25048473

Kim, K. H., Kim, T. H., Kang, J. W., Sul, J. U., Lee, M. S., Kim, J. I., & Choi, S. M. et al. (2011). Acupuncture for symptom management in hemodialysis patients: A prospective, observational pilot study. *Journal of Alternative and Complementary Medicine (New York, N.Y.)*, *17*(8), 741–748. doi:10.1089/acm.2010.0206 PMID:21721925

Kim, K. H., Lee, M. S., Choi, S. M., & Ernst, E. (2010). Acupuncture for treating uremic pruritus in patients with end-stage renal disease: A systematic review. *Journal of Pain and Symptom Management*, *40*(1), 117–125. doi:10.1016/j.jpainsymman.2009.11.325 PMID:21796811

Kodner, C. M., & Kudrimoti, A. (2003). Diagnosis and management of acute interstitial nephritis. *American Family Physician*, *67*(12), 2527–2534. PMID:12825841

Koshy, K. M., Griswold, E., & Schneeberger, E. E. (1999). Interstitial nephritis in a patient taking creatine. *The New England Journal of Medicine*, *340*(10), 814–815. doi:10.1056/NEJM199903113401017 PMID:10075534

Kumar, N., & Singh, A. K. (2014). Plant profile, phytochemistry and pharmacology of Avartani (Helicteres isora Linn.): A review. *Asian Pac J Trop Biomed*, *4*(Suppl 1), S22–S26. doi:10.12980/APJTB.4.2014C872 PMID:25183085

Lamarche, J., Nair, R., Peguero, A., & Courville, C. (2011). Vitamin C-induced oxalate nephropathy. *International Journal of Nephrology*, *146927*. doi:10.4061/2011/146927 PMID:21603151

Lee, J. J., & Chen, H. C. (2006). Flavonoid-induced acute nephropathy by *Cupressus funebris* Endl (Mourning Cypress). *American Journal of Kidney Diseases*, *48*(5), E81–E85. doi:10.1053/j.ajkd.2006.08.011 PMID:17059987

Lee, K. H., Jeong, H. S., & Rhee, H. (2014). A patient with minimal change disease and acute focal tubulointerstitial nephritis due to traditional medicine: A case report and small literature review. *Explore (New York, N.Y.)*, *10*(5), 319–323. doi:10.1016/j.explore.2014.06.001 PMID:25037506

Li, M., Wang, W., Xue, J., Gu, Y., & Lin, S. (2011). Meta-analysis of the clinical value of *Astragalus membranaceus* in diabetic nephropathy. *Journal of Ethnopharmacology*, *133*(2), 412–419. doi:10.1016/j.jep.2010.10.012 PMID:20951192

Li, P. K., Burdmann, E. A., & Mehta, R. L. (2013). World kidney day 2013: Acue kidney injury-global halth alert. *American Journal of Kidney Diseases*, *61*(3), 359–363. doi:10.1053/j.ajkd.2013.01.002 PMID:23414727

Li, Y., Xue, W. J., Tian, P. X., Ding, X. M., Yan, H., Pan, X. M., & Feng, X. S. (2009). Clinical application of *Cordyceps sinensis* on immunosuppresive therapy in renal transplantation. *Transplantation Proceedings*, *41*(5), 1565–1569. doi:10.1016/j.transproceed.2009.02.085 PMID:19545680

Li, Y. J., Lin, J. L., Yang, C. W., & Yu, C. C. (2005). Acute renal failure induced by a Brazilian variety of propolis. *American Journal of Kidney Diseases*, *46*(6), E125–E129. doi:10.1053/j.ajkd.2005.08.028 PMID:16310564

Light, T. D., & Light, J. A. (2003). Acute renal transplant rejection possibly related to herbal medications. *American Journal of Transplantation*, *3*(12), 1608–1609. doi:10.1046/j.1600-6135.2003.00270.x PMID:14629295

Lim, A. K. H., Manley, K. J., Roberts, M. A., & Fraenkel, M. B. (2016). Fish oil for kidney transplant recipients. *Cochrane Database of Systematic Reviews*, *8*, CD005282. PMID:27535773

Lin, M. Y., Chiu, Y. W., Chang, J. S., Lin, H. L., Lee, C. T. C., & Chiu, G. F. (2015). Association of prescribed Chinese herbal medicine use with risk of end-stage renal disease in patients with chronic kidney disease. *Kidney International*, 5. PMID:26244923

Lin, Y. C., Chen, Y. C., Chen, T. H., Chen, H. H., & Tsai, W. J. (2011). Acute kidney injury associated with hepato-protective Chinese herb - Pien Tze Huang. *J Exp Clin Med*, *3*(4), 184–186. doi:10.1016/j.jecm.2011.07.005

Liu, J., Zheng, S. J., Yu, L. M., Goyer, R. A., & Waalkes, M. P. (2008). Mercury in traditional medicines: Is cinnabar toxicologically similar to common mercurials. *Experimental Biology and Medicine (Maywood, N.J.)*, *233*(7), 810–817. doi:10.3181/0712-MR-336 PMID:18445765

Lo, J. C., Chertow, G. M., Rennke, H., & Seifter, J. L. (1996). Fanconis syndrome and tubulointerstitial nephritis in association with L-lysine ingestion. *American Journal of Kidney Diseases*, *28*(4), 614–617. doi:10.1016/S0272-6386(96)90476-X PMID:8840955

Luciano, R. L. (2014). Acute kidney injury from cherry concentrate in a patient with CKD. *American Journal of Kidney Diseases*, *63*(3), 503–505. doi:10.1053/j.ajkd.2013.09.021 PMID:24290246

Luyckx, V. A. (2012). Nephrotoxicity of alternative medicine practice. *Advances in Chronic Kidney Disease*, *19*(3), 129–141. doi:10.1053/j.ackd.2012.04.005 PMID:22578672

Luyckx, V. A., Ballantine, R., Claeys, M., Cuyckens, F., Van den Heuvel, H., Cimanga, R. K., & Katz, I. J. et al. (2002). Herbal Remedy-Associated Acute Renal Failure Secondary to *Cape aloes*. *American Journal of Kidney Diseases*, *39*(3), E13–E17. doi:10.1053/ajkd.2002.31424 PMID:11877593

MacPherson, H., Thomas, K., Walters, S., & Fitter, M. (2001). A prospective survey of adverse events and treatment reactions following 34,000 consultations with professional acupuncturists. *Acupuncture in Medicine*, *19*(2), 93–102. doi:10.1136/aim.19.2.93 PMID:11829165

Mueller, B. A., Scott, M. K., Sowinski, K. M., & Prag, K. A. (2000). Noni juice (*Morinda citrifolia*): Hidden potential for hyperkalemia? *American Journal of Kidney Diseases*, *35*(2), 310–312. doi:10.1016/S0272-6386(00)70342-8 PMID:10676732

Naughton, C. A. (2008). Drug-induced nephrotoxicity. *American Family Physician*, *78*(6), 743–750. PMID:18819242

Nguyen-Khoa, T., Massy, Z. A., de Bandt, J. P., Kebede, M., Salama, L., & Lambrey, G. et al.. (2001). Oxidative stress and haemodialysis: Role of inflammation and duration of dialysis treatment. *Nephrology, Dialysis, Transplantation*, *16*(2), 335–340. doi:10.1093/ndt/16.2.335 PMID:11158409

Nizhi, Y., Xusheng, L., Qizhan, L., Daji, X., Lixin, W., & Lili, D. et al.. (2000). Clinical study on effect of Chinese herbal medicine combined with hemodialysis in treating uremia. *CJIM*, *6*(1), 18–21.

Nortier, J. L., Martinez, M. C., Schmeiser, H. H., Arlt, V. M., Bieler, C. A., Petein, M., & Vanherweghem, J.-L. et al. (2000). Urothelial carcinoma associated with the use of a Chinese herb (Aristolochia fangchi). *The New England Journal of Medicine*, *342*(23), 1686–1692. doi:10.1056/NEJM200006083422301 PMID:10841870

Okuda, M., Horikoshi, S., Matsumoto, M., Tanimoto, M., Yasui, H., & Tomino, Y. (2012). Beneficial effect of *Astragalus membranaceus* on estimated glomerular filtration rate in patients with progressive chronic kidney disease. *Hong Kong J Nephrol*, *14*(1), 17–23. doi:10.1016/j.hkjn.2012.01.001

Özkan, G., & Ulusoy, Ş. (2015). A case of renal failure developing in association with African mango consumption. *Int J Clin Exp Med*, *8*(4), 6374–6378. PMID:26131261

Pakfetrat, M., Basiri, F., Malekmakan, L., & Roozbeh, J. (2014). Effects of turmeric on uremic pruritus in end stage renal disease patients: A double-blind randomized clinical trial. *Journal of Nephrology*, *27*(2), 203–207. doi:10.1007/s40620-014-0039-2 PMID:24482090

Posadzki, P., Watson, L., & Ernst, E. (2013). Contamination and adulteration of herbal medicinal products (HMPs): An overview of systematic reviews. *European Journal of Clinical Pharmacology*, *69*(3), 295–307. doi:10.1007/s00228-012-1353-z PMID:22843016

Powell, T., Hsu, F. F., Turk, J., & Hruska, K. (1998). Ma-Huang strikes again: Ephedrine nephrolithiasis. *American Journal of Kidney Diseases*, *32*(1), 153–159. doi:10.1053/ajkd.1998.v32.pm9669437 PMID:9669437

Qing, X., Xue-lan, Z., Min, G., & Yao, Z. (2001). Assessment on application of Chinese herbal medicine in the process of corticosterone reduction in nephrotic syndrome. *Chinese Journal of Integrative Medicine*, *7*(3), 180–182.

Rizzi, D., Basile, C., Di Maggio, A., Sebastio, A., Introna, F. J., Rizzi, R., & Smialek, J. E. et al. (1991). Clinical spectrum of accidental hemlock poisoning: Neurotoxic manifestations, rhabdomyolysis and acute tubular necrosis. *Nephrology, Dialysis, Transplantation*, *6*(12), 939–943. doi:10.1093/ndt/6.12.939 PMID:1798593

Rossert, J. (2001). Drug-induced acute interstitial nephritis. *Kidney International*, *60*(2), 804–817. doi:10.1046/j.1523-1755.2001.060002804.x PMID:11473672

Shahgholian, N., Dehghan, M., Mortazavi, M., Gholami, F., & Valiani, M. (2009). Effect of aromatherapy on pruritus relief in hemodialysis patients. *Iran J Nurs Midwifery Res*, *15*(4), 240–244. PMID:22049288

Sun, G. D., Li, C. Y., Cui, W. P., Guo, Q. Y., Dong, C. Q., Zou, H. B., & Miao, L. et al. (2016). Review of herbal traditional Chinese medicine for the treatment of diabetic nephropathy. *J Diabetes Res*, *2016*, 5749857. doi:10.1155/2016/5749857 PMID:26649322

Talasaz, A. H., Abbasi, M. R., Abkhiz, S., & Dashti-Khavidaki, S. (2010). *Tribulus terrestris*-induced severe nephrotoxicity in a young healthy male. *Nephrology, Dialysis, Transplantation*, *25*(11), 3792–3793. doi:10.1093/ndt/gfq457 PMID:20667992

Tangkiatkumjai, M., Boardman, H., Praditpornsilpa, K., & Walker, D.-M. (2015). Association of herbal and dietary supplements with progression and complications of chronic kidney disease: A prospective cohort study. *Nephrology (Carlton, Vic.)*, *20*(10), 679–687. doi:10.1111/nep.12531 PMID:26040915

The Indian Society of Nephrology. (2005). Drugs and the kidney. *Indian J Nephrol*, *15*(Suppl 1), S75–S79.

Tratenberg, M., Mehta, S., Kleinman, G., Gazivoda, V., & Tassiulas, I. (2015). Severe rhabdomyolysis associated with catha edulis (khat) use. *Case Reports in Clinical Pathology*, *2*(1), 87–90.

Tsay, S. L., Rong, J. R., & Lin, P. F. (2003). Acupoints massage in improving the quality of sleep and quality of life in patients with end-stage renal disease. *Journal of Advanced Nursing*, *42*(2), 134–142. doi:10.1046/j.1365-2648.2003.02596.x PMID:12670382

Vanderperren, B., Rizzo, M., Angenot, L., Haufroid, V., Jadoul, M., & Hantson, P. (2005). Acute liver failure with renal impairment related to the abuse of senna anthraquinone glycosides. *The Annals of Pharmacotherapy*, *39*(7-8), 1353–1357. doi:10.1345/aph.1E670 PMID:15956233

Vanherweghem, J. L., Depierreux, M., Tielemans, C., Abramowicz, D., Dratwa, M., & Jadoul, M. et al.. (1993). Rapidly progressive interstitial renal fibrosis in young women: Association with slimming regimen including Chinese herbs. *Lancet*, *341*(8842), 387–391. doi:10.1016/0140-6736(93)92984-2 PMID:8094166

Wang, H., Song, H., Yue, J., Li, J., Hou, Y. B., & Deng, J. L. (2012). Rheum officinale (a traditional Chinese medicine) for chronic kidney disease. *Cochrane Database of Systematic Reviews*, *7*, CD008000. PMID:22786510

Wang, Y. J., He, L. Q., Sun, W., Lu, Y., Wang, X., Zhang, P., & Liu, X. et al. (2012). Optimized project of traditional Chinese medicine in treating chronic kidney disease stage 3: A multicenter double-blinded randomized controlled trial. *Journal of Ethnopharmacology*, *139*(3), 757–764. doi:10.1016/j.jep.2011.12.009 PMID:22178174

Weisbord, S. D., Soule, J. B., & Kimmel, P. L. (1997). Poison on line - acute renal failure caused by oil of wormwood purchased through the internet. *The New England Journal of Medicine*, *337*(12), 825–827. doi:10.1056/NEJM199709183371205 PMID:9297113

Wong, J. S., Ong, T.-A., Chua, H. H., & Tan, C. (2007). Acute Anuric Renal Failure Following Jering Bean Ingestion. *Asian Journal of Surgery*, *30*(1), 80–81. doi:10.1016/S1015-9584(09)60134-2 PMID:17337378

Wright, C. I., Van-Buren, L., Kroner, C. I., & Koning, M. M. G. (2007). Herbal medicines as diuretics: A review of the scientific evidence. *Journal of Ethnopharmacology*, *114*(1), 1–31. doi:10.1016/j.jep.2007.07.023 PMID:17804183

Wu, J., Hu, Y., Zhu, Y., Yin, P., Litscher, G., & Xu, S. (2015). Systematic review of adverse effects: A further step towards modernization of acupuncture in China. *Evidence-Based Complementary and Alternative Medicine*, *2015*, 432467. doi:10.1155/2015/432467 PMID:26339265

Xu, S., Wang, L., Cooper, E., Zhang, M., Manheimer, E., Berman, B., & Lao, L. et al. (2013). Adverse events of acupuncture: A systematic review of case reports. *Evidence-Based Complementary and Alternative Medicine*, *2013*, 581203. doi:10.1155/2013/581203 PMID:23573135

Yeung, C. K., Billings, F. T. IV, Claessens, A. J., Roshanravan, B., Linke, L., & Sundell, M. B. et al.. (2015). Coenzyme Q_{10} dose-escalation study in hemodialysis patients: Safety, tolerability, and effect on oxidative stress. *BMC Nephrology*, *16*(183). PMID:26531095

Yin, P., Gao, N., Wu, J., Litscher, G., & Xu, S. (2014). Adverse events of massage therapy in pain-related conditions: A systematic review. *Evidence-Based Complementary and Alternative Medicine*, *2014*, 480956. doi:10.1155/2014/480956 PMID:25197310

Yurtkuran, M., Alp, A., Yurtkuran, M., & Dilek, K. (2007). A modified yoga-based exercise program in hemodialysis patients: A randomized controlled study. *Complementary Therapies in Medicine*, *15*(3), 164–171. doi:10.1016/j.ctim.2006.06.008 PMID:17709061

Zhang, H. W., Lin, Z. X., Tung, Y. S., Kwan, T. H., Mok, C. K., Leung, C., & Chan, L. S. (2014). Cordyceps sinensis (a traditional Chinese medicine) for treating chronic kidney disease. *Cochrane Database of Systematic Reviews*, *12*, CD008353. PMID:25519252

Zhang, H. W., Lin, Z. X., Xu, C., Leung, C., & Chan, L. S. (2014). Astragalus (a traditional Chinese medicine) for treating chronic kidney disease. *Cochrane Database of Systematic Reviews*, *10*, CD008369. PMID:25335553

Zhang, L., Li, P., Xing, C. Y., Zhao, J. Y., He, Y. N., Wang, J. Q., & Chen, X. et al. (2014). Efficacy and safety of *Abelmoschus manihot* for primary glomerular disease: A prospective, multicenter randomized controlled clinical trial. *American Journal of Kidney Diseases*, *64*(1), 57–65. doi:10.1053/j.ajkd.2014.01.431 PMID:24631042

Zhang, W. X., Zhang, Z. M., Zhang, Z. Q., Wang, Y., & Zhou, W. (2014). Andrographolide induced acute kidney injury: Analysis of 26 cases reported in Chinese Literature. *Nephrology (Carlton, Vic.)*, *19*(1), 21–26. doi:10.1111/nep.12172 PMID:24148088

Zhong, Y., Deng, Y., Chen, Y., Chuang, P. Y., & He, J. C. (2013). Therapeutic use of traditional Chinese herbal medications for chronic kidney diseases. *Kidney International*, *84*(6), 1108–1118. doi:10.1038/ki.2013.276 PMID:23868014

Zhong, Y., Menon, M. C., Deng, Y., Chen, Y., & Cijiang, J. (2015). Recent advances in traditional Chinese medicine for kidney disease. *American Journal of Kidney Diseases*, *66*(3), 513–522. doi:10.1053/j.ajkd.2015.04.013 PMID:26015275

Zhu, B., Wang, Y., Jardine, M., Jun, M., Lv, J. C., Cass, A., & Perkovic, V. et al. (2013). *Tripterygium* preparation for the treatment of CKD: A systematic review and meta-analysis. *American Journal of Kidney Diseases*, *62*(3), 515–530. doi:10.1053/j.ajkd.2013.02.374 PMID:23664549

KEY TERMS AND DEFINITIONS

Acupuncture: An alternative therapy uses thin needles which are inserted into the body at acupuncture points in order to treat illnesses or relieve symptoms.

Chinese Herbal Medicine: A traditional remedy contains at least one herbal medicine and has been used more than a thousand years in China. Decoction is the most common preparation of this remedy.

Dietary Supplements: A product contains dietary ingredients, e.g. vitamins, minerals, amino acids, and nutrients.

Efficacy: A beneficial effect of the medicine on treating or alleviating illnesses. This effect should be proved by randomised controlled trials.

Herbal Medicine: A plant has a pharmacological effect on treating illnesses or alleviating symptoms.

Nephropathy: A kidney problem commonly includes acute kidney injury, kidney stones, and chronic kidney disease. This problem relates to both conventional or herbal medicines, and diseases.

Safe: A condition of being no harm from a medicine.

Chapter 8
Herbal Drug Interactions

Mymoona Akhter
Jamia Hamdard, India

ABSTRACT

Use of complementary and alternative medicines (CAM) for preventive and therapeutic purposes has increased tremendously in the last two decades internationally. The manufacturers of these products are not required to submit proof of safety or efficacy to the Food and Drug Administration. As a result, the adverse effects and drug interactions associated with them are largely unknown. In this chapter, the author presents interactions of herbal medicines with other medicines (herbal or non-herbal). A large number of herbal drugs, including from single drug to a variety of mixtures have been used to treat kidney disorders. Herb-herb or herb drug interaction has been reported intensively during last decade, therefore it becomes important to keep an eye on the use of combination herbal therapy in order to avoid serious results because of interactions with each other. Due to the growing awareness about the interactions and side effects of herbal drugs/supplements over the past few years, regulatory bodies are working on these issues and pharmacopoeias are being developed for reference.

INTRODUCTION

The herb drug interaction topic is so vast that a full volume of a book could be dedicated to it. Use of herbal products for preventive and therapeutic purposes has increased tremendously over the last two decades.

DOI: 10.4018/978-1-5225-2882-1.ch008

More than 130 distinct chemical substances which are derived from plants are in use as drugs. Production of modern pharmaceutical compounds requires adherence to good manufacturing practice (GMP). Rigorous safety and efficacy studies are essential before getting approval from regulation bodies for human use. The same is not true with herbal drugs and supplements however as this system is based more on traditional knowledge. Herbal medicines, often dispensed in a crude form of their extracts, form the mainstay of health care for a more than 50% of the population in developing countries due to either non-availability of modern medical care, its cost, or lack of health care knowledge (Brandt and Muller, 1995; Roshni et al., 2014). A large portion of the population in sub-Saharan Africa depend on traditional medicine for its primary health care, whilst 50% of the Chinese population use herbal therapy (Chen et al., 2007). The global annual turnover in herbal medicines is estimated at US$ 60 billion, representing approximately 20% of the overall drug market (Gunjan et al., 2015). CAMs are perceived to be innocuous and safe, therefore there is ignorance of side effects or potential risks of interactions with other drug substances. Chemical compounds, present in crude herbs or their extracts, are responsible for their pharmacological actions. For example, Ginseng (*Panax notoginseng*, family: Araliaceae), which is widely used in China for the treatment of various diseases like cardiovascular, neuropathy or blood disorders, is believed to be safe, though some rare side effects such as anxiety, insomnia, or pain have been reported. Also, a large number of herbal-drug interactions have been reported, e.g. ginkgo products causing bleeding or seizures (Kupiec & Raj, 2005).

BACKGROUND

The kidney is an essential organ when it comes to detoxification of the body. A large number of substances are excreted through the kidney making it vulnerable to toxins. A number of therapeutic drugs can adversely affect the kidney resulting in acute kidney injury (AKI), nephritic syndrome and chronic interstitial nephritis. Medicinal plants are used for the treatment of various diseases (also called 'Herbal medicine' or 'phytomedicine'). Although herbalism has a long tradition of use outside conventional medicine, it is becoming more mainstream as improvements quality control, and clinical research, show the value of herbal medicine in treating and preventing disease. In general, four types of herbal medicine exist: Asian, European, Indigenous, and Neo-Western. The Asian and European systems go back thousands of years, appear in pharmacopoeia, and with such a tradition of use, are better understood than those of indigenous origins that are often only orally recorded (Desmet, 1996). Pharmacopoeia is an official book published usually under the jurisdiction of the government and which contains a list of drugs, their formulas, and methods of identification, requirements and tests for their strength and purity, and other related information. The ones which are most established are of Asian origin, particularly from India (Aryuvedic, Unani, Siddha), China (Wu-Hsing), and Japan (Kampo). Regulatory bodies of various countries have become conscious about the various aspects of herbalism and thus prepared official monographs of these medicines regarding their identity, purity, and analysis. In India a well-established ministry (Ministry of Ayurveda, Yoga and Naturopathy, Unani, Siddha and Homeopathy (AYUSH)) looks after these five systems of indigenous medicines that are widely practiced in India. For every system of medicine, there is an official pharmacopoeia, for instance, India has Unani Pharmacopeia, and Aryuvedic pharmacopoeia. America has the American Herbal Pharmacopoeia. In the Pharmacopoeia of the People's Republic of China (PPRC) volume 1 covers the Traditional Chinese Materia Medica, including Traditional Chinese Patent Medicines, while Volume 2 is dedicated to conventional pharmaceuticals.

The concomitant use of herbal medicines and modern medicine is wide spread globally because of the ready availability. The clinical consequence of herb-drug interactions varies, from being well-tolerated to moderate or serious adverse reactions, even possibly life-threatening. Izzo and Ernst have published a review about interactions between herbal medicines and prescribed drugs (2009). They reported the possible interactions between seven popular herbal medicines: ginkgo, ginseng, St John's wort, Echinacea, garlic, saw palmetto, and kava, and conventional drugs. They found that St John's wort (*Hypericum perforatum*), reduces the plasma concentrations (and/or increases the clearance) of alprazolam, amitriptyline, ciclosporin, atorvastatin, chlorzoxazone, debrisoquine, erythromycin, digoxin, fexofenadine, gliclazide, imatinib, indinavir, ivabradine, mephenytoin, methadone, midazolam, omeprazole, oral contraceptives, quazepam, simvastatin, talinolol, verapamil, voriconazole, and warfarin via cytochrome P450 (CYP) and/or P-glycoprotein induction. Ginkgo (*Ginkgo biloba*) was found to decrease the plasma concentrations of omeprazole, ritonavir and tolbutamide. Clinical cases indicate interactions of ginkgo with antiepileptics, aspirin (acetylsalicylic acid), diuretics, ibuprofen, etc. Kava (*Piper methysticum*) increases the clearance of chlorzoxazone (a CYP2E1 substrate) and may interact with levodopa, alprazolam, and paroxetine. Ginseng (*Panax ginseng*) may interact with phenelzine and warfarin. Garlic

(*Allium sativum*) interacts with chlorpropamide, fluindione, ritonavir and warfarin; it also reduces plasma concentrations of chlorzoxazone (a CYP2E1 probe). Since herbal products are not regulated for purity and potency like conventional drugs, it is possible that some of the adverse effects and herb-drug interactions reported could be due to impurities present or product variability.

MECHANISMS INVOLVED IN HERB-DRUG INTERACTIONS

The mechanisms and clinical implications of herb-drug interactions are well-documented (Chen et al., 2011). Pharmacokinetic interactions are caused by alterations in the absorption, distribution, metabolism, or excretion of drugs which results in altered levels of the drug or its metabolites.

Interaction With Efflux Transporters

The efflux transporters play a role in limiting influx of xenobiotics, thus preventing the intracellular accumulation of their own substrates. The activity of the efflux transporters on interaction with herbs may be inhibited by competitive or non-competitive mechanisms, which may potentially lead to toxic blood plasma concentrations of drugs that are normally substrates. Conversely, the induction of efflux transporters by herbs would result in sub-therapeutic plasma drug levels leading to treatment failure. For example P- Glycoprotein (P-gp), a multi-drug resistance protein 1, plays an important role in regulating the absorption/reabsorption, distribution and elimination of many therapeutic agents. P-gp affects oral drug absorption and decreases bioavailability by pumping back the drug molecules into the gastrointestinal tract lumen. In hepatocytes, most of the substances are pumped into the bile by P-gp and this efflux occurs in many other organs including kidney as well (Takano et al., 2006). Phytoconstituents may inhibit or induce P-gp which will in turn, decreases/potentiates the substrate-induced-fit of drugs resulting in even much slower/higher efflux of most P-gp substrates (Chan et al., 2004).

P-glycoprotein confers high levels of resistance to bulky amphipathic natural product type drugs such as paclitaxel, Vinca alkaloids, anthracyclines, camptothecins, and epipodophyllotoxins. Alisol B23-acetate from *Alisma orientalis* enhances anticancer activity of vinblastine, doxorubicin, rhodamine-123 by reducing P-gp efflux activity *in vitro* in MDR cell lines (HepG2-DR and K562-DR) (van Asperen et al., 2000). Citrus paradisi

(Grapefruit juice) has been reported to inhibit P-gp rhodamine-123 efflux in vivo in healthy volunteers. It was also found to increase the bioavailability of nifedipine in vivo in rats and talinolol *in vitro* in Caco-2 cells (Mohri & Uesawa, 2001; Di Marco, 2002). Other efflux transporters are the Multi-drug Resistance-associated Protein-2 (MRP2) or Breast Cancer Resistance Protein (BCRP). MRP2 is localized in the bile canalicular membrane of hepatocytes, and exports relatively large hydrophilic compounds like the glutathione, glucuronide and sulfate conjugates of endogenous and exogenous compounds from liver cells into the bile (Takano et al., 2006). MRP2 is also responsible for the biliary secretion of glucuronide, acetaminophen and camptothecin. Therefore, possible interactions of these with herbs or drugs affect the functioning of MRP2, i.e. there may be an increased effect of drugs which are effeluxed by this system (Nabekura et al., 2005). It is believed that herbs that show an ability to modulate P-gp activity which may also affect related efflux transporters. Cooray et al. report that some plant-derived polyphenols that interact with P-gp can also modulate BCRP activity *in vitro* (2004). Flavonoids like apigenin, genistein, biochanin A, and kaempferol from *Silybum marianum*, inhibits BCRP thereby enhancing the accumulation of the BCRP substrate mitoxantrone (Zhang et al., 2004). Naringin, a phytochemical in *Citrus paradisi* juice, inhibits the influx or uptake of active transporter organic anion transporting polypeptide (OATP) 1A2 consequently lowering the bioavailability of certain drugs (Dresser et al., 2002; Bailey et al., 2007). Inhibition of OATP1 and OATP3 by components of *Citrus sinensis* and *Malus domestica* juices may decrease drug uptake and lead to sub-therapeutic drug concentrations whilst over-induction of OATP may increase drug uptake and lead to toxic blood drug concentrations (Takano et al., 2006).

Herb-Drug Interactions at Metabolism Level

Pharmacokinetic herb-drug interactions occur when drug metabolic enzymes are induced or inhibited by concomitant herbal medicines. For example, induction of CYP enzymes often results in therapeutic failure because of lower plasma concentrations of the drugs. One of the well-studied herbal medicines, St. John's Wort (*Hypericium perforatum*), induces CYP3A4 and CYP2B6, resulting in a decrease in plasma levels of irinotecan and imatinib, which are two chemotherapeutic drugs. In general, inhibition of CYP enzymes would lead to an increase in plasma concentrations of the concomitant drug, and increased toxicity. Furano coumarins (e.g., naringenin and bergamottin) in paradisi juice, and *C. sinensis* increase the plasma concentration of a number of drugs, including cyclosporine, terfenadine, midazolam and felodipine, through mechanism-based inhibition of the CYP3A4 enzyme as 'suicide substrate' *in vitro* and *in vivo*. Some herbs such as meadowsweet and black willow, which contain pain-reducing salicylates, may displace highly protein bound drugs such as warfarin and carbamazepine, thus increasing the adverse effects of these drugs (Isnard et al., 2004).

Herb-Drug Interactions at Elimination Level

The major routes for the elimination of drugs remain via the kidney and bile, but there are no significant herb-drug interactions through bile elimination. Drugs that are chiefly excreted by the kidneys are involved in herb-drug interactions by different mechanisms such as competition at active transport sites, or alterations in glomerular filtration, passive renal tubular reabsorption or active secretion and urinary pH (Isnard et al., 2004). The mechanism of herbal diuresis is complex and non-uniform. Certain herbs increase the glomerular filtration rate but do not stimulate electrolyte secretion, while others act as direct tubular irritant (Crosby et al., 2001). For example, Impila (*Callilepis laureola*) causes damage to the proximal convoluted tubules and the loop of henle (Isnard et al., 2004). Whilst uvaursi (*Arctostaphylos uva ursi*), dandelion (*Taraxacum officinale*), goldenrod (*Solidago virgaurea*), juniper berry (*Juniperus communis*), parsley (*Petroselinum crispum*), horsetail (*Equisetum arvense*), asparagus root (*Asparagus officinalis*), and alfalfa (*Medicago sativa*) have been found to have diuretic properties and may increase the renal elimination of other drugs (Wojcikowski, 2009).

Pharmacodynamic Interactions

Pharmacodynamic interactions are herb-drug interactions that cause changes in pharmacological responses. Herb-drug pharmacodynamic interactions involve changes in the pharmacological effects of the drug through additive, synergistic or antagonistic actions (Izzo, 2005). Any single herbal preparation contains several components, many of them having unknown biological activities; therefore, a herbal medicine can potentially mimic, increase, or reduce the effects of co-administered drugs through simultaneous effects on the same drug targets. Toxicity may occur if the effect of the drug in combination with the herbal medicine is enhanced synergistically or by additive effects.

For example, ginger, garlic, ginseng, alfalfa, ginkgo, chamomile (*Matricaria recutita*), and danshen may enhance the anticoagulant activity of warfarin by targeting the same vitamin K epoxide reductase target (Greenblatt & von Moltke, 2005). Aspilia Africana, when used along with artemisinin, or chloroquine for malaria, has been reported to antagonize their effects (Abii & Onuoha, 2011). Ephedra is known to have risk for myocardial ischemia, tachycardia, hypertension and it may also produce ventricular arrhythmias when combined with anesthetics (White et al., 1997).

CAUSES OF HERBAL TOXICITY

Herbal toxicity can develop through incorrect identification leading to substitution of an innocuous herb with a toxic one; consumption of a herb with unknown toxicity; or deliberate or inadvertent contamination with nephrotoxic non-herbal drugs (e.g. non-steroidal anti-inflammatory agents), pesticides or chemicals (e.g. heavy metal contamination from soil or water); or potentiation of the toxic effect of a conventional drug due to interaction with a compound present in the herb; or consumption of meat from an animal that has grazed on toxic plants (e.g. hemlock). The kidney is the route of excretion of most of the substances present in the herbs. The high blood flow and large endothelial surface area of the kidneys ensures delivery of large amounts of toxin to the renal parenchyma. High concentrations may be reached in the medulla because of active tubular transport, especially during a state of fluid deprivation. Renal involvement associated with the use of traditional medicinal products can take several forms including acute kidney injury, tubular function defects, dyselectrolytaemias, systemic hypertension, chronic kidney disease (CKD), renal papillary necrosis, urolithiasis and urothelial cancer (Powell et al, 1998; Elvin-Lewis, 2001; Isnard et al., 2004; Luyckx & Naicker, 2008).

Herbal Remedies Used For Treatment of Kidney Diseases

Urolithiasis

Phyllanthus niruri (Freitas et al., 2002), *Dolichos biflorus* and *Orthosiphon grandiflorus* have been used in the prevention of urolithiasis, whilst fish stone is used as a method of stone expulsion. Although this treatment has also been evaluated in preliminary clinical trials, results are inconclusive (Barros et al., 2006; Kieley et al, 2008).

Glomerulonephritis and Urinary Tract Diseases

Native American tribes have been using Goldenrod extensively for treatment of urinary tract diseases (Melzig, 2004), and hydrangea root for promoting kidney and bladder health, for many years. Hydrangea root is also used as an anti-inflammatory agent in Chinese traditional medicine. There is evidence for *H. paniculata* for the treatment of glomerulonephritis (Zhang et al., 2013), and Gravel Root (*Eupatorium purpureum*), a well-known herb in the Eastern half of the United States, is used for promoting kidney and urinary health, although no scientific support is available yet for this. Arctostaphylos uva ursi (Bearberry) (*Taraxacum officinalis*) is reported as a prevention of urinary tract infections (Head, 2008). Dandelion (*Taraxacum officinale*) native to Europe, has been explored for use in kidney related disorders because of its antioxidant and anti-inflammatory activities, but more clinical evidence is needed (Gonzalez-Castejon, et al., 2012).

Diuretics

A number of plants species like *Spergularia purpurea*, *Hibiscus sabdariffa*, *Petroselinum sativum* and *Foeniculum vulgare*, *Lepidium latifolium* (Navarro et al., 1994), and *Lepidium sativum* (Maghrani et al., 2005); *Phyllanthus amarus*, and Sambucus (*Sambucus mexicana* and *Sambucus nigra*) have been reported to be beneficial in kidney related disorders as diuretics. Horsetail (*Equisetum arvense* L.) has been commonly known for its antioxidant properties (Mimica-Dukic et al., 2008). It has also been explored for diuretic properties (Gutierrez, 1985, Wright et al., 2007). *Vaccinium Macrocarpon* (Cranberry), Cranberry-Lingonberry, Berberine sulfate, and Arctostaphylos uva ursi have been used as botanical interventions for lower urinary tract infections. Use of herbs like *Agrimonia eupatoria* (agrimony), *Althea officinalis* (marshmallow), *Apium graveolens* (celery seed), *Arctium lappa* (burdock), *Elymus repens* (couchgrass), *Hydrangea aborescens* (hydrangea), *Juniperus communis* (juniper), dandelion, *Ulmus fulva* (slippery elm), and Zea mays (corn silk) have also been documented as diuretic (Yarnell, 2002).

Chronic Kidney Disease (CKD)

Astragalus is traditionally used either alone or in conjunction with *Angelica Sinensis* in China for CKD (Ma et al., 2002, Li & Wang, 2005). Successful use of astragalus has also been reported in the treatment of patients with nephrotic syndrome (Ahmed et al., 2007). Rhubarb (*Rheum palmatum*) is believed to increase the excretion of waste products in patients with CKD (Li, 1996; Wang et al., 2012) and renal failure through inhibition of lipopolysaccharide-induced expression of Toll-like receptor 4. *R. bupleuri* is used in China and Japan for the treatment of kidney diseases (Yoshikawa et al., 1997; Awazu et al., 2002). Triptolide, a diterpene triepoxide, major active components in T*ripterygium wilfordii* Hook F, have been extensively studied. Detailed discussions of this can be found in Zhou et al. (2012) and Sun et al. (2011). Studies have proven the potential of Curcumin in inhibiting renal cyst development (Gao et al., 2011). Curcumin is reported to slow down cyst formation in both a MDCK cyst model and an embryonic kidney cyst model with a dose-dependent response.

In India, a large number of herbal formulations (single or mixture) have been used to help in renal diseases. Herbs like punarnava, varuna, tribulus, shigru, apamarg etc. are described in ancient Ayurveda texts - 5000 B.C. for use in kidney diseases. These herbs reduce swelling and volume of accumulated fluid, thereby increasing the chances of reviving the kidneys. Some of the formulations are discussed here:

1. **Mutrakrichantak Churna:** The composition contains 8 medicinal plants/herbs namely *Crateva nurvala, Boerhavia diffusa, Tribulus terrestris, Chicorium intybus, Phyllanthus niruri, Albezzia lebbok, Moringa oleifera*. It is useful for kidney stones, urinary tract infections, high uric acid, or high urea and creatinine levels.
2. **Rencure Formula:** (Punarnava, gokshur, varun, palaash, and kaasni) is widely used to cure renal disorders and is believed to work on the ancient principle of Ayurveda.
3. **Varunadi vati:** Reduces pain caused by renal stones and maintains creatinine levels and clears the urinary passage.

Although no pre-clinical or clinical data about the efficacy and safety of these formulas could be found, there is enough literature available in support of these herbs for use in kidney diseases (Dash, 1991; Jouad et al., 2001; National Institutes of Health, 2005; Joshi et al., 2005; Prashanth et al., 2010; Kamboj et al., 2011; Parvin et al., 2011; Patel et al., 2011; Bhattacharjee et al., 2012; Khattar & Wal, 2012; Kulkarni et al., 2012).

HERBAL DRUG INTERACTIONS

Herbal Drug Interactions and Possible Effects

A book published by WHO listed some of the well-established interactions between herbs and conventional drugs (1999). Numerous examples are available in the literature, such as cranberries, known for their vitamin C content, increasing the effect of blood thinners (anticoagulants) like warfarin, leading to bruising or bleeding. If an herb inhibits or induces cytochrome P450 enzyme, it will show effects on other drugs which are metabolized by that enzyme. For example, warfarin is affected by herbs e.g. *Carica papaya, Harpago-phytum* that inhibit cytochrome P450. Herb-herb interactions are also reported such as the incompatibility of licorice with sargassum, veratrum with scrophularia, and raw aconite with raw pinellia. Aconite has hypotensive, diuretic, cardiac, depressant activities (Singh, 1986; Murayama, 1991) and raw aconite or pinellia products are extremely toxic. The aconite alkaloids have a narrow therapeutic index. *Pinellia ternata* was banned in 2004 in the US because of the presence of ephedrine alkaloids. These chemicals might cause serious side effects, such as heart attacks, stroke, or seizures. The combination of sargassum and glycyrrhizae has some toxic effects on rats' white blood cell and cardiac muscle and there is a correlation between toxicity and dose (Yan et al., 2007).

Herbs which reduce the effect of each other are also known such as *raphanus* which inhibits the action of ginseng; whilst ginseng inhibits that of pteropus. Similarly, clove affects the action of curcuma. Table 1 summarises the drug interaction of herbal drugs used in treatment of kidney disorders. Meanwhile, Table 2 discusses the herbs that produce various undesirable/unwanted effects if used with other modern medicines.

Table 1. Drugs used in kidney diseases and their possible drug interaction and effects

Plant/Herb	Pharmacological Effects	Possible Interaction With Other Drugs or Herbs	Possible Outcomes	Types of Study	References
Agrimony (*Agrimonia eupatoria*)	uricolytic effect, diuretic effect, hypotensive effect, hypoglycemic effect	May increase the risk of bleeding when taken with aspirin, anticoagulants (e.g. warfarin, heparin), anti-platelet drugs (e.g. clopidogrel) and non-steroidal anti-inflammatory drugs (NSAIDS) (e.g. ibuprofen). May lower blood sugar levels and blood pressure. Possible additive effect with hypotensive drugs contains up to 21% tannins, chronic ingestion may result in nephrotoxicity	Experimental studies in mice show limited evidence of a possible blood glucose lowering effect. There are no reported cases of decreases in clotting time.	Preclinical and experimental studies	Petkov, 1979; Giachetti, 1986; Gray & Flatt, 1998; Swanston-Flatt et. al., 1990, 2000
Astragalus, *Huangqi*, (*Astragalus membranaceus*)	CKD	Cyclosporine, azathioprine, methotrexate. inhibits CYP3A4	May affect the metabolism of certain drugs metabolized by CYP3A4 enzyme impairs intended immuno-suppressive effects of immunosuppressant, e.g. cyclophosphamide.	Pre-clinical studies	Wojcikowski et. al., 2000, 2010, Pao et al., 2012
Cordyceps sinensis	Known to increase immunity Hypoglycemic effect bronchitis, asthma, COPD	All Immunosuppressant drugs Antidiabetic drugs May affect drugs used in lung diseases	Impairs intended immuno-suppressive effects Potential for hypoglycemia, or diabetic shock	Clinical study	Guo & Zhang, 1995
Equisetum arvense L. (Horsetail)	Urinary antiseptic, diuretic, urolithiasis, cholelithiasis, hemostatic, stops bleeding, Anxiolytic, hypoglycemic, hepatoprotective and free radical scavenging activities.	Digitalis, Furosemide, CNS stimulants (e.g. caffeine), diabetic, gout, and hypertensive agents	Anxiolytic effect of cardiac stimulants (e.g. digitalis) as may potentiate their effect. Concurrently with diuretics can cause potassium loss (hypokalemia). Combining with CNS stimulants may cause over stimulation of the central nervous system May lead to diabetic shock increases production of uric acid and diuresis	Pre-clinical, Clinical studies	Lemus et al., 1996; Andrade Cetto, 2000; Baracho et. al., 2000, 2009, Duke, 2002; Gurbuz et. al., 2002; Oh, 2004; Soleimani, et al., 2007; Singh, 2011

continued on following page

Table 1. Continued

Plant/Herb	Pharmacological Effects	Possible Interaction With Other Drugs or Herbs	Possible Outcomes	Types of Study	References
Foeniculum vulgare	Diuretic and hypotensive effects	Inhibition of CYP3A4, significant interaction between ciprofloxacin Antihypertensive drugs	Affects all substrates of CYP3A4. Drugs mainly metabolized by this isozyme may be affected Decreases bioavailability and efficacy of ciprofloxacin Risk of hypotension	Pre-clinical studies	Zhu, 1999; Subehan et. al., 2006, 2007; Rahimi & Ardekani, 2013
Hibiscus sabdariffa L.	Diuretic effect and antihypertensive potential	Antihypertensive Agents, Hydrochlorothiazide (HCTZ)	Plasma clearance and elimination of HCTZ decrease. Therefore, possible increased diuresis, harmful as the body will lose water and minerals	Pre-clinical studies	Ndu et. al., 2000, 2011
Licorice root, *Glycyrrhiza glabra*	Urolithiasis, diuresis anti-diabetic effect, and hepatoprotective anti-inflammatory activities	anti-diabetic, and diuretic agents	Synergistic effects with antidiabetic agents. Hypokalemia	Preclinical and Clinical studies	Conn et al., 1968; Farese et. al., 1991; Elinav & Chajek-Shaul, 2003; Ferrari, 2009; Akila, 2011; Aksoy et al., 2012; Ming & Yin, 2013
Mulberry, Morus	Diuresis, Antidiabetic activity	Diuretic agents used in antihypertensive therapy, Antidiabetic agents, Anxiolytics	Hypoglycemia due to a synergistic effect Depression due to interaction with anxiolytics	Pre-clinical and human studies	Oku et. al., 2006; Lee et al., 2002; Yadav, 2008, Wang et al., 2011.
Petroselinum sativum	Diuretic and hypotensive activities Antidiabetic effect	Warfarin Chlorothiazide Lithium Antidiabetic agents	might increase blood clotting might cause the body to lose too much water lithium toxicity possible synergistic effect with antidiabetic agents	Pre-clinical studies	Campos, 2009; Shalaby, 2014; Yanardag, et. al., 2000, 2003; Ozoy-Sacan, 2006
Phyllanthus amarus	Midazolam through inhibition of CYP3A	Increased activity of midazolam substrates of CYP3A	May lead to oral bioavailability and metabolism of CYP3A substrates	Clinical and Pre-clinical studies	Thummel et al., 1996; Wilkinson, 1996; Wongnawa, 2014
R. bupleuri	CKD	Drugs which are primarily metabolized in the liver	Drug-induced pneumonitis and drug-induced acute hepatitis, e.g. ibuprofen, diclofenac, isoniazid Potentiation of other hepatotoxic agents, e.g. antitubercular drugs	Pre-clinical study, Case report	Aiba et al., 2007; Miyagawa et al., 2009

continued on following page

Table 1. Continued

Plant/Herb	Pharmacological Effects	Possible Interaction With Other Drugs or Herbs	Possible Outcomes	Types of Study	References
Rhubarb (*Rheum officinale*)	CKD	cardiac glycosides and antiarrhythmic agents	potentiating by reducing potassium via a laxative effect	Clinical study	Khan et al., 2014
Spergularia purpurea	Hypotensive effect Diuretic effect Hypoglycemic effect	Antidiabetic agents, antihypertensive agents	Synergetic effects on patient already on antidiabetic therapy or antihypertensive therapy	Pre-clinical study and surveys	Jouad et. al., 2000, 2001; Eddouks et. al., 2003
St. John's wort, *Hypericum perforatum* L	Urolithiasis Anti-inflammatory activity Antidepressant effect	acetaminophen / hydrocodone, amitriptyline / chlordiazepoxide; Induction of cytochrome P450 3A4 (CYP3A4) Anticonvulsants agents, e.g. carbamazepine, phenobarbitone, phenytoin	Hepatotoxicity Affects all substrates of CYP3A4 Reduced blood concentrations of other drugs like amitriptyline, cyclosporine, digoxin, fexofenadine, warfarin etc.	Pre-clinical and Clinical studies	Muller et al., 1997; Valentão, 2004; Chen et al., 2011; Neshat et al., 2011; Khalili et al., 2012
Uva ursi (*Arctostaphylosuvaursi*), dandelion (*Taraxacum officinale*), juniper berry (*Juniperuscommunis*), alfalfa (*Medicago sativa*)	Antioxidant and Antimicrobial activities Diuretic effect	May precipitate calcium May interact with antihypertensive agents and diuretics	Oxalate nephropathy, may increase the renal elimination of other drugs	Clinical and pre-clinical studies	Chen et al., 2001; Dearing, 2001; Wojcikowski, et al., 2009; Wu et al., 2011

Table 2. Herb drug interaction of herbs/natural compounds other than those used in kidney disorders with other medicines/drugs

Herb	Drug	Adverse Effects	Type of Study	References
Aloe vera gel and juice	Insulin or oral hypo-glycaemic agents	Potentiation in hypoglycemic effect	Clinical studies and case report	Aslam & Stockley, 1979; Yongchaiyuda, 1996
Bitter melon (Momardica Charantia)	Insulin or oral hypo-glycaemic agents	Potentiation in hypoglycemic effect	Clinical studies	Baskaran et al., 1990; "ESCOP," 1997, 1999; Blumenthal, 1998a
Chasteberry fruit (Vitex agnus-castus)	Metoclopramide	Might potentiate the actions of dopaminergic agonists (e.g. bromocriptine, levodopa), therefore counteracts dopaminergic agents like metoclopramide.	Pre-clinical studies	Blumenthal, 2000; Blumenthal et al., 1998a
Cinchona bark Procumbens Cinchona Pubescens	Warfarin	Possibly additive, potentiate warfarin's anticoagulant action.	Pre-clinical and clinical studies	Harris, 1995; Blumenthal et al., 1998a

continued on following page

Table 2. Continued

Herb	Drug	Adverse Effects	Type of Study	References
Devils claw (Harpago-phytum)	Warfarin	additive effects to warfarin; i.e. blood thinning increases	Pre-clinical and clinical studies	Harris, 1995; 'The world health report,' 1999; Blumenthal et al., 1998a
Ephedra (Ephedra sinica)	Guanethidine, ephedrine	Enhances a sympathomimetic effect of ephedra, Fatal Cardiac stimulation.	Clinical and pre-clinical studies	ESCOP, 1997, 1999; Blumenthal et al., 1998a; Blumenthal, 2000; Litt 2005
Feverfew (Tanacetum parthenium)	Warfarin	Retards absorption.	Clinical and Pre-clinical studies	Klepser & Klepser, 1999; Murphy, 1999
Flaxseed oil (Linum Usitatissimum)	Insulin or oral hypo-glycaemic agents	Delays absorption of drugs taken simultaneously in diabetics delays glucose absorption	Pre-clinical and clinical studies	ESCOP, 1997; Blumenthal, 1998; Ang, 1999
Garlic (Allium Sativum)	Warfarin	Additive effects (blood thinning increases) Potentiates warfarin's anticoagulant action.	Pre-clinical and clinical studies	Sunter, 1991; Harris, 1995; 'The world health report,' 1999
Ginger (Zingiber Officinale)	Warfarin	Additive effect; causes Immune Reconstitution Inflammatory Syndrome (iris), bleeding	Pre-clinical study and Case report	World Health Organization, 1999; Blumenthal, 2000
Ginkgo (Ginkgo biloba)	Aspirin	Increases the bleed clotting time, resulted in hyphema (pooling of blood inside the anterior chamber of the eye)	Clinical study	Rosenblatt & Mindel, 1997
Ginseng (Panax Ginseng)	Phenelzine, triazolam, lorazepam	Headaches, tremors, insomnia, irritability, visual hallucinations	Clinical study and case report	Gonzalez-Seijo et al., 1995; Harris, 1995.
Herbal sedatives Valerian (Valeriana officinalis)	Alcohol, antihistamines Phenytoin	Drowsiness, ability to use machinery; potentiates effects of antidepressants, anti-histaminic, antispasmodics	Clinical study	D'Arcy, 1993
Ma-huang, *Mahuang (Ephedra sinica)*	MAO inhibitors cardiac glycosides or halothane, caffeine, procainamide, quinidine	causes arrhythmia i.e. irregular heartbeat therefore might cause serious side effects including heart attack	Pre-clinical study	White et al., 1997
Papaya extract (Carica papaya)	Warfarin	Papain increased INR, damages mucous membranes of GI tract. Additive effect to warfarin	Pre-clinical and clinical studies	Harris, 1995; Blumenthal et al., 1998a; 'The world health report,' 1999
Pineapple enzyme (Ananas comosus)	Bromelian	Diarrhea, increased tendency for bleeding if used simultaneously with anticoagulants and inhibitors of thrombocytic aggregation due to modulation of the arachidonate cascade	Pre-clinical and clinical studies	Taussig & Batkin, 1988; Blumenthal, 2000
Psyllium seed (Plantago spp)	Coumarin derivatives, e.g. warfarin	Potentiates the effect of coumarin may cause bleeding	Pre-clinical studies	Harris, 1995; Blumenthal et al., 1998; 'The world health report,' 1999
Salicin containing herbals and oils (Salix spp.; Gaulthria procumbens Eucalyptu globulus)	Aspirin	Salicylism; hypersensitivity	Clinical studies	Malik et al., 1994; Ernst, 1998

continued on following page

Table 2. Continued

Herb	Drug	Adverse Effects	Type of Study	References
Shankha-phuspi (Centella asiatica, Convolvulus pluricaulis, Nardostachys jaatamansi, Nepteta elliptica, Nepeta hindostana and Onsosma bracteatum)	Alcohol, antihistamines. Phenytoin	Reduces plasma levels of phenytoin; seizure control lost	Clinical studies	(D'Arcy, 1991, 1993)

Reporting of Drug interactions

In 1968, the World Health Organization (WHO) promoted the "Programme for International Drug Monitoring", a pilot project aimed to centralize world data on adverse drug reactions (ADRs). Any medicine can cause adverse reactions/side effects, but sometimes rare adverse reactions aren't known. By collecting reports of adverse events, this helps to generate a signal regarding any new adverse events associated with a drug, and also enables judgement regarding the health risk associated with it according to the severity and prevalence of the adverse event. WHO adverse event monitoring program based in Uppsala, Sweden is a worldwide program to monitor adverse drug reactions. It has a number of offices in different countries. Any adverse drug reaction is reported to them where they take note of the information and forward for further processing. There are different methods for reporting, for example, the FDA provides options for online or offline reporting, whilst in the UK, there is a yellow card scheme which is completed with details of the adverse reaction and submitted. In India, the Pharmacovigilance program was started in collaboration with WHO's program.

CONCLUSION

The large increase in use of herbal medicine has led to increased concerns. Herbal medicines are comparatively safe when ingredients are pure and prescribed appropriately. Life-threatening events reported from them are rare, compared to pharmaceutical products. However, there are always risks when appropriate regulations do not mandate the appropriate formulation of the remedies, or when self-medication fosters abuse. Elvin-Lewis (2001) has given some basic rules for herb use guidelines:

- Be informed, seek out unbiased, scientific sources.
- Do not depend upon product claims alone.
- Inform your physician of self-medication regimens.
- Read labels carefully, know the benefits and risks and potential side effects.
- Know potential drug interactions.
- Never use if pregnant or nursing.
- Take care when giving to children or the elderly.
- Do not use for serious illnesses or for prolonged periods.

REFERENCES

Abii, T. A., & Onuoha, E. N. (n.d.). The chemical constituents of the leaf of *Aspilia africana* as a scientific backing to its tradomedical potentials. *Agric. J., 6*, 28–30.

Ahmed, M. S., Hou, S. H., Battaglia, M. C., Picken, M. M., & Leehey, D. J. (2007). Treatment of idiopathic membranous nephropathy with the herb Astragalus membranaceus. *American Journal of Kidney Diseases*, *50*(6), 1028–1032. doi:10.1053/j.ajkd.2007.07.032 PMID:18037104

Aiba, T., Takahashi, T., Suzuki, K., Okoshi, S., Nomoto, M., Uno, K., & Aoyagi, Y. (2007). Liver injury induced by a Japanese herbal medicine, sairei-to (TJ-114, Bupleurum and Hoelen Combination, Chai-Ling-Tang) R1. *Journal of Gastroenterology and Hepatology*, *22*(5), 762–763. doi:10.1111/j.1440-1746.2006.03373.x PMID:17444872

Akila, L. Kumar, P. A., Nirmala, P. (2011). Effect of a polyherbal formulation on ethylene glycol induced urolithiasis. *Internat. J. Pharma and Bio Sci., 4.*

Aksoy, N., Dogan, Y., Iriadam, M., Bitiren, M., Uzer, E., Ozgonul, A., & Aksoy, S. (2012). Protective and therapeutic effects of licorice in rats with acute tubular necrosis. *Journal of Renal Nutrition*, *22*(3), 336–343. doi:10.1053/j.jrn.2011.07.002 PMID:22047711

Andrade Cetto, A., Wiedenfeld, H., Revilla, M. C., & Sergio, I. A. (2000). Hypoglycemic effect of Equisetum myriochaetum aerial parts on streptozotocin diabetic rats. *Journal of Ethnopharmacology*, *72*(1-2), 129–133. doi:10.1016/S0378-8741(00)00218-X PMID:10967463

Aslam, M., & Stockley, I. H. (1979). Interaction between curry ingredient (karela) and drug (chlorpropamide). *Lancet*, *1*(8116), 607. doi:10.1016/S0140-6736(79)91028-6 PMID:85186

Awazu, M., Fujita, H., Omori, S., & Hida, M. (2002). The herbal medicine Sairei-to inhibits proliferation of rat mesangial cells. *Nephron*, *92*(3), 652–659. doi:10.1159/000064112 PMID:12372950

Bailey, D. G., Dresser, G. K., Leake, B. F., & Kim, R. B. (2007). Naringin is a major and selective clinical inhibitor of organic anion-transporting polypeptide 1A2 (OATP1A2) in grapefruit juice. *Clinical Pharmacology and Therapeutics*, *81*(4), 495–502. doi:10.1038/sj.clpt.6100104 PMID:17301733

Baracho, N. C., Vicente, B. B., Arruda, G. D., Sanches, B. C., & Brito, J. (2009). Study of acute hepatotoxicity of Equisetum arvense L. in rats. *Acta Cirurgica Brasileira*, *24*(6), 449–453. doi:10.1590/S0102-86502009000600005 PMID:20011829

Barros, M. E., Lima, R., Mercuri, L. P., Matos, J. R., Schor, N., & Boim, M. A. (2006). Effect of extract of Phyllanthus niruri on crystal deposition in experimental urolithiasis. *Urological Research*, *34*(6), 351–357. doi:10.1007/s00240-006-0065-1 PMID:16896689

Baskaran, K., Kizar Ahamath, B., Radha Shanmugasundaram, K., & Shanmugasundaram, E. R. (1990). Antidiabetic effect of a leaf extract from Gymnema sylvestre in non-insulin-dependent diabetes mellitus patients. *Journal of Ethnopharmacology*, *30*(3), 295–300. doi:10.1016/0378-8741(90)90108-6 PMID:2259217

Bhattacharjee, A., Chakrakodi, S. S. & Aswathanarayana (2012) Phytochemical and ethno-pharmacological profile of *Crataeva nurvala*, buch-hum (varuna): a review, *Asian Pacific J.Trop. Biomed.*, 1162-1168.

Blumenthal, M. (2000). Interactions between herbs and conventional drugs. *Introductory considerations. Herbalgram*, *49*, 52–63.

Blumenthal, M., Busse, W. R., Goldberg, A., Gruenwald, J., Hall, T., Riggins, C. W., & Rister, R. S. (Eds.). (1998). The Complete German Commission E Monographs, Therapeutic Guide to Herbal Medicines. Integrative Medicine Communications.

Blumenthal, M. N., Casale, T. B., Fink, J. N., Uryniak, T., & Casty, F. E. (1998). Evaluation of a non-chlorofluorocarbon formulation of cromolyn sodium (Intal) metered-dose inhaler versus the chlorofluorocarbon formulation in the treatment of adult patients with asthma: A controlled trial. *The Journal of Allergy and Clinical Immunology*, *101*(1), 7–13. doi:10.1016/S0091-6749(98)70186-1 PMID:9449494

Brandt, H., & Muller, G. J. (1995). Traditional medicines and acute poisoning. *CME*, *13*, 1053–1060.

Campos, K. E., Balbi, A. P. C., & Alves, J. Q. F. (2009). Diuretic and hypotensive activity of aqueous extract of parsley seeds (Petroselinum sativum Hoffm.) in rats. *J. Pharmacognosy*, *19*, 41–45.

Chan, L. M., Lowes, S., & Hirst, B. H. (2004). The ABCs of drug transport in intestine and liver: Efflux proteins limiting drug absorption and bioavailability. *European Journal of Pharmaceutical Sciences*, *21*(1), 25–51. doi:10.1016/j.ejps.2003.07.003 PMID:14706810

Chen, C. L., Fang, H. C., Chou, K. J., Wang, J. S., & Chung, H. M. (2001). Acute oxalate nephropathy after ingestion of star fruit. *American Journal of Kidney Diseases*, *37*(2), 418–422. doi:10.1053/ajkd.2001.21333 PMID:11157385

Chen, F. P., Chen, T. J., Kung, Y. Y., Chen, Y.-C., Chou, L.-F., Chen, F.-J., & Hwang, S.-J. (2007). Use frequency of traditional Chinese medicine in Taiwan. *BMC Health Services Research*, *7*(1), 26. doi:10.1186/1472-6963-7-26 PMID:17319950

Chen, X. W., Serag, E. S., Sneed, K. B., Liang, J., Chew, H., Pan, S. Y., & Zhou, S. F. (2011). Clinical herbal interactions with conventional drugs: From molecules to maladies. *Current Medicinal Chemistry*, *18*(31), 4836–4850. doi:10.2174/092986711797535317 PMID:21919844

Conn, J. W., Rovner, D. R., & Cohen, E. L. (1968). Licorice-induced pseudoaldosteronism. Hypertension, hypokalemia, aldosteronopenia, and suppressed plasma renin activity. *Journal of the American Medical Association*, *205*(7), 492–496. doi:10.1001/jama.1968.03140330034006 PMID:5695305

Cooray, H. C., Janvilisri, T., van Veen, H. W., Hladky, S. B., & Barrand, M. A. (2004). Interaction of the breast cancer resistance protein with plant polyphenols. *Biochemical and Biophysical Research Communications*, *317*(1), 269–275. doi:10.1016/j.bbrc.2004.03.040 PMID:15047179

Crosby, E. C., Dolan, R. L., Benson, J. E., Luetkemeier, M. J., Barton, R. G., & Askew, E. W. (2001). Herbal diuretic induced dehydration and resting metabolic rate. *Medicine and Science in Sports and Exercise*, *33*(5), S163. doi:10.1097/00005768-200105001-00920

D'Arcy, P. F. (1991). Adverse reactions and interactions with herbal medicines. Part 1. Adverse reactions. *Adverse Drug Reactions and Toxicological Reviews*, *10*(4), 189–208. PMID:1793770

D'Arcy, P. F. (1993). Adverse reactions and interactions with herbal medicines. Part 2--Drug interactions. *Adverse Drug Reactions and Toxicological Reviews*, *12*(3), 147–162. PMID:8218717

Dandekar, U. P., Chandra, R. S., Dalvi, S. S., Joshi, M. V., Gokhale, P. C., Sharma, A. V., & Kshirsagar, N. A. (1992). Analysis of a clinically important interaction between phenytoin and Shankhapushpi, an Ayurvedic preparation. *Journal of Ethnopharmacology*, *35*(3), 285–288. doi:10.1016/0378-8741(92)90026-N PMID:1548901

Dash, B. (1991). *Materia Medica of Ayurveda B*. New Delhi: Jain Publishers.

Dearing, D. M., Mangione, A. M., & Karasov, W. H. (2001). Plant secondary compounds as diuretics: An overlooked consequence. *American Zoologist*, *41*, 890–890.

Desmet, V. J. (1996). What more can we ask from the pathologist? *Journal of Hepatology*, *25*(Suppl 1), 25–29. PMID:8954188

Di Marco, M. P., Edwards, D. J., Wainer, I. W., & Ducharme, M. P. (2002). The effect of grapefruit juice and seville orange juice on the pharmacokinetics of dextromethorphan: The role of gut CYP3A and P-glycoprotein. *Life Sciences*, *71*(10), 1149–1160. doi:10.1016/S0024-3205(02)01799-X PMID:12095536

Dresser, G. K., Bailey, D. G., Leake, B. F., Schwarz, U. I., Dawson, P. A., Freeman, D. J., & Kim, R. B. (2002). Fruit juices inhibit organic anion transporting polypeptide-mediated drug uptake to decrease the oral availability of fexofenadine. *Clinical Pharmacology and Therapeutics*, *71*(1), 11–20. doi:10.1067/mcp.2002.121152 PMID:11823753

Duke, J. B. J., du Cellier, J., & Duke, P. (2002). Handbook of Medicinal Herbs. Boca Raton, FL: CRC Press.

Eddouks, M., Jouad, H., Maghrani, M., Lemhadri, A., & Burcelin, R. (2003). Inhibition of endogenous glucose production accounts for hypoglycemic effect of Spergularia purpurea in streptozotocin mice. *Phytomed.*, *10*(6-7), 594–599. doi:10.1078/094471103322331890 PMID:13678249

Elinav, E., & Chajek-Shaul, T. (2003). Licorice consumption causing severe hypokalemic paralysis. *Mayo Clinic Proceedings*, *78*(6), 767–768. doi:10.4065/78.6.767 PMID:12934789

Elvin-Lewis, M. (2001). Should we be concerned about herbal remedies. *Journal of Ethnopharmacology*, *75*(2-3), 141–164. doi:10.1016/S0378-8741(00)00394-9 PMID:11297844

Ernst, E. (1998). Harmless herbs? A review of the recent literature. *The American Journal of Medicine*, *104*(2), 170–178. doi:10.1016/S0002-9343(97)00397-5 PMID:9528737

ESCOP, European Scientific Cooperative on Phytotherapy. (1997). *ESCOP monographs on the medicinal uses of plant drugs*. Exeter, UK: ESCOP.

ESCOP, European Scientific Cooperative on Phytotherapy. (1999). *ESCOP monographs on the medicinal uses of plant drugs*. Exeter, UK: ESCOP.

Farese, R. V. Jr, Biglieri, E. G., Shackleton, C. H., Irony, I., & Gomez-Fontes, R. (1991). Licorice-induced hypermineralocorticoidism. *The New England Journal of Medicine*, *325*(17), 1223–1227. doi:10.1056/NEJM199110243251706 PMID:1922210

Freitas, A. M., Schor, N., & Boim, M. A. (2002). The effect of Phyllanthus niruri on urinary inhibitors of calcium oxalate crystallization and other factors associated with renal stone formation. *BJU International*, *89*(9), 829–834. doi:10.1046/j.1464-410X.2002.02794.x PMID:12010223

Gao, J., Zhou, H., Lei, T., Zhou, L., Li, W., Li, X., & Yang, B. (2011). Curcumin inhibits renal cyst formation and enlargement *in vitro* by regulating intracellular signaling pathways. *European Journal of Pharmacology*, *654*(1), 92–99. doi:10.1016/j.ejphar.2010.12.008 PMID:21187084

Giachetti, D., Taddei, E., & Taddei, I. (1986). Ricerche sull'attivita diuretica ed uricosurica di Agrimonia eupatoria. *Bollettino della Società Italiana di Biologia Sperimentale*, *62*, 705–711. PMID:3790308

Gonzalez-Castejon, M., Visioli, F., & Rodriguez-Casado, A. (2012). Diverse biological activities of dandelion. *Nutrition Reviews*, *70*(9), 534–547. doi:10.1111/j.1753-4887.2012.00509.x PMID:22946853

Gonzalez-Seijo, J. C., Ramos, Y. M., & Lastra, I. (1995). Manic episode and ginseng: Report of a possible case. *Journal of Clinical Psychopharmacology*, *15*(6), 447–448. doi:10.1097/00004714-199512000-00014 PMID:8748439

Gray, A. M., & Flatt, P. R. (1998). Actions of the traditional anti-diabetic plant, Agrimony eupatoria (agrimony): Effects on hyperglycaemia, cellular glucose metabolism and insulin secretion. *The British Journal of Nutrition*, *80*(1), 109–114. doi:10.1017/S0007114598001834 PMID:9797650

Greenblatt, D. J., & von Moltke, L. L. (2005). Interaction of warfarin with drugs, natural substances, and foods. *Journal of Clinical Pharmacology*, *45*(2), 127–132. doi:10.1177/0091270004271404 PMID:15647404

Gunjan, M., Naing, T. W., Saini, R. S., Ahmad, A. B., Naidu, J. R., & Kumar, I. (2015). Marketing trends & future prospects of herbal medicine in the treatment of various disease. *World J. Pharmaceut. Res.*, *4*, 132–155.

Guo, Q. C., & Zhang, C. (1995). Clinical observations ofadjunctive treatment of 20 diabetic patients with JinShuiBao capsule. *J. Admin. Tradit. Chin. Med.*, *5*, 22.

Gurbuz, I., Ustun, O., Yesilada, E., Sezik, E., & Akyurek, N. (2002). In vivo gastroprotective effects of five Turkish folk remedies against ethanol-induced lesions. *Journal of Ethnopharmacology*, *83*(3), 241–244. doi:10.1016/S0378-8741(02)00248-9 PMID:12426092

Head, K. A. (2008). Natural approaches to prevention and treatment of infections of the lower urinary tract. *Alternative Medicine Review*, *13*(3), 227–244. PMID:18950249

Isnard Bagnis, C., Deray, G., Baumelou, A., Le Quintrec, M., & Vanherweghem, J. L. (2004). Herbs and the kidney. *American Journal of Kidney Diseases*, *44*(1), 1–11. doi:10.1053/j.ajkd.2004.02.009 PMID:15211432

Izzo, A. A., & Ernst, E. (2009). Interactions between herbal medicines and prescribed drugs: An updated systematic review. *Drugs*, *69*(13), 1777–1798. doi:10.2165/11317010-000000000-00000 PMID:19719333

Joshi, V. S., Parekh, B. B., Joshi, M. J., & Vaidya, A. D. (2005). Herbal extracts of *Tribulus terrestris* and *Bergenia ligulata* inhibit growth of calcium oxalate monohydrate crystals *in vitro*. *Journal of Crystal Growth*, *275*(1-2), 1403–1408. doi:10.1016/j.jcrysgro.2004.11.240

Jouad, H., Eddouks, M., Lacaille-Dubois, M. A., & Lyoussi, B. (2000). Hypoglycaemic effect of spergularia purpurea in normal and streptozotocin-induced diabetic rats. *Journal of Ethnopharmacology*, *71*(1-2), 169–177. doi:10.1016/S0378-8741(99)00199-3 PMID:10904160

Jouad, H., Haloui, M., Rhiouani, H., El Hilaly, J., & Eddouks, M. (2001). Ethnobotanical survey of medicinal plants used for the treatment of diabetes, cardiac and renal diseases in the North centre region of Morocco (Fez-Boulemane). *Journal of Ethnopharmacology*, *77*(2-3), 175–182. doi:10.1016/S0378-8741(01)00289-6 PMID:11535361

Jouad, H., Lacaille-Dubois, M. A., Lyoussi, B., & Eddouks, M. (2001). Effects of the flavonoids extracted from *Spergularia purpurea* Pers. on arterial blood pressure and renal function in normal and hypertensive rats. *Journal of Ethnopharmacology*, *76*(2), 159–163. doi:10.1016/S0378-8741(01)00209-4 PMID:11390130

Kamboj, P., Aggarwal, P. M., Puri, S., & Singla, S. K. (2011). Effect of aqueous extract of *Tribulus terrestris* on oxalate-induced oxidative stress in rats. *Indian J. Nephrol.*, *21*(3), 154–159. doi:10.4103/0971-4065.83727 PMID:21886973

Khalili, M., Jalali, M. R., & Mirzaei-Azandaryani, M. (2012). Effect of hydroalcoholic extract of Hypericum perforatum L. leaves on ethylene glycol-induced kidney calculi in rats. *Urology Journal*, *9*(2), 472–479. PMID:22641490

Khan, I. A., Nasiruddin, M., Haque, S. F., & Khan, R. A. (2014). Evaluation of Rhubarb Supplementation in Stages 3 and 4 of Chronic Kidney Disease: A Randomized Clinical Trial. *Internat. J. Chronic Dis.*, *2014*, 1–6. doi:10.1155/2014/789340 PMID:26464863

Khattar, V., & Wal, A. (2012). Utilities of *Crataeva nurvala*. *Internat. J. Pharm. and Pharmaceut. Sci.*, *4*, 21–26.

Kieley, S., Dwivedi, R., & Monga, M. (2008). Ayurvedic medicine and renal calculi. *Journal of Endourology*, *22*(8), 1613–1616. doi:10.1089/end.2008.0020 PMID:18620498

Kulkarni, Y. R., Apte, B. K., Kulkarni, P. H., & Patil, R. R. (2012). Evaluation of nephroprotective and anti-nephrotoxic properties of rakta punarnava roots (*Boerhaavia diffusa*, l.) gokshur fruits (*Tribulus terrestris*, l.) in drug induced nephrotoxicity. *Internat. Res. J. Pharm.*, *3*, 329–334.

Kupiec, T., & Raj, V. (2005, October). Fatal seizures due to potential herb-drug interactions with Ginkgo biloba. *Journal of Analytical Toxicology*, *29*(7), 755–758. doi:10.1093/jat/29.7.755 PMID:16419414

Lee, S. H., Choi, S. Y., Kim, H., Hwang, J. S., Lee, B. G., Gao, J. J., & Kim, S. Y. (2002). Mulberroside F isolated from the leaves of Morus alba inhibits melanin biosynthesis. *Biological & Pharmaceutical Bulletin*, *25*(8), 1045–1048. doi:10.1248/bpb.25.1045 PMID:12186407

Lemus, I., Garcia, R., Erazo, S., Pena, R., Parada, M., & Fuenzalida, M. (1996). Diuretic activity of an Equisetum bogotense tea (Platero herb): Evaluation in healthy volunteers. *Journal of Ethnopharmacology*, *54*(1), 55–58. doi:10.1016/0378-8741(96)01444-4 PMID:8941869

Li, L. (1996). Rheum officinale: A new lead in preventing progression of chronic renal failure. *Chinese Medical Journal*, *109*(1), 35–37. PMID:8758359

Li, X., & Wang, H. (2005). Chinese herbal medicine in the treatment of chronic kidney disease. *Advances in Chronic Kidney Disease*, *12*(3), 276–281. doi:10.1016/j.ackd.2005.03.007 PMID:16010642

Luyckx, V. A., & Naicker, S. (2008). Acute kidney injury associated with the use of traditional medicines. *Nature Clinical Practice. Nephrology*, *4*(12), 664–671. doi:10.1038/ncpneph0970 PMID:18838981

Ma, X. Q., Shi, Q., Duan, J. A., Dong, T. T., & Tsim, K. W. (2002). Chemical analysis of R*adix Astragali* (Huangqi) in China: A comparison with its adulterants and seasonal variations. *Journal of Agricultural and Food Chemistry*, *50*(17), 4861–4866. doi:10.1021/jf0202279 PMID:12166972

Maghrani, M., Zeggwagh, N. A., Michel, J. B., & Eddouks, M. (2005). Antihypertensive effect of *Lepidium sativum* L. in spontaneously hypertensive rats. *Journal of Ethnopharmacology*, *100*(1-2), 193–197. doi:10.1016/j.jep.2005.02.024 PMID:15955648

Malik, A. S., Zabidi, M. H., & Noor, A. R. (1994). Acute salicylism due to accidental ingestion of a traditional medicine. *Singapore Medical Journal*, *35*(2), 215–216. PMID:7939826

Melzig, M. F. (2004). Goldenrod-a classical exponent in the urological phytotherapy. *Wiener Medizinische Wochenschrift, 154*(21-22), 523–527. doi:10.1007/s10354-004-0118-4 PMID:15638071

Mimica-Dukic, N., Simin, N., Cvejic, J., Jovin, E., Orcic, D., & Bozin, B. (2008). Phenolic compounds in field horsetail (*Equisetum arvense* L.) as natural antioxidants. *Molecules (Basel, Switzerland), 13*(7), 1455–1464. doi:10.3390/molecules13071455 PMID:18719517

Ming, L. J., & Yin, A. C. (2013). Therapeutic effects of glycyrrhizic acid. *Nat Prod Commun, 8*(3), 415–418. PMID:23678825

Miyagawa, T., Mochizuki, Y., Nakahara, Y., Kawamura, T., Sasaki, S., & Tsukamoto, H. (2009). A case of drug-induced pneumonitis due to Sai-rei-to. *Nihon Kokyuki Gakkai Zasshi, 47*(1), 47–51. PMID:19198236

Mohri, K., & Uesawa, Y. (2001). Effects of furanocoumarin derivatives in grapefruit juice on nifedipine pharmacokinetics in rats. *Pharmaceutical Research, 18*(2), 177–182. doi:10.1023/A:1011028401189 PMID:11405288

Muller, W. E., Rolli, M., Schafer, C., & Hafner, U. (1997). Effects of hypericum extract (LI 160) in biochemical models of antidepressant activity. *Pharmacopsychiatry, 30*(Suppl 2), 102–107. doi:10.1055/s-2007-979528 PMID:9342769

Murayama, M., Mori, T., Bando, H., & Amiya, T. (1991). Studies on the constituents of Aconitum species. IX. The pharmacological properties of pyro-type aconitine alkaloids, components of processed aconite powder kako-bushi-matsu: Analgesic, anti-inflammatory, and acute toxic activities. *Journal of Ethnopharmacology, 35*(2), 159–164. doi:10.1016/0378-8741(91)90068-O PMID:1809822

Murphy, J. M. (1999). Preoperative considerations with herbal medicines. *AORN Journal, 69*(1), 173–175. doi:10.1016/S0001-2092(06)62767-1 PMID:9932176

Nabekura, T., Kamiyama, S., & Kitagawa, S. (2005). Effects of dietary chemopreventive phytochemicals on P-glycoprotein function. *Biochemical and Biophysical Research Communications, 327*(3), 866–870. doi:10.1016/j.bbrc.2004.12.081 PMID:15649425

Navarro, E., Alonso, J., Rodriguez, R., Trujillo, J., & Boada, J. (1994). Diuretic action of an aqueous extract of Lepidium latifolium L. *Journal of Ethnopharmacology*, *41*(1-2), 65–69. doi:10.1016/0378-8741(94)90059-0 PMID:8170161

Ndu, O. O., Nworu, C. S., Ehiemere, C. O., Ndukwe, N. C., & Ochiogu, I. S. (2011). Herb-drug interaction between the extract of Hibiscus sabdariffa L. and hydrochlorothiazide in experimental animals. *Journal of Medicinal Food*, *14*(6), 640–644. doi:10.1089/jmf.2010.0117 PMID:21480802

Neshat, M., Azarmi, Y., Mehdi, Z. S., Doustar, Y., & Mousavi, G. (2011). Effects of *Hypericum perforatum* (St. Johns wort) extract on renal function after unilateral ureteral obstruction in rat. *Afr. J. Pharm. Pharmacol.*, *5*(4), 457–461. doi:10.5897/AJPP10.241

Nortier, J. L., & Vanherweghem, J. L. (2007). For patients taking herbal therapylessons from aristolochic acid nephropathy. *Nephrology, Dialysis, Transplantation*, *22*(6), 1512–1517. doi:10.1093/ndt/gfm167 PMID:17405785

Oh, H., Kim, D. H., Cho, J. H., & Kim, Y. C. (2004). Hepatoprotective and free radical scavenging activities of phenolic petrosins and flavonoids isolated from *Equisetum arvense*. *Journal of Ethnopharmacology*, *95*(2-3), 421–424. doi:10.1016/j.jep.2004.08.015 PMID:15507369

Oku, T., Yamada, M., Nakamura, M., Sadamori, N., & Nakamura, S. (2006). Inhibitory effects of extractives from leaves of Morus alba on human and rat small intestinal disaccharidase activity. *The British Journal of Nutrition*, *95*(5), 933–938. doi:10.1079/BJN20061746 PMID:16611383

Ozoy-Sacan, O., Yanardag, R., Orak, H., Ozgey, Y., Yarat, A., & Tunali, T. (2006). Effects of parsley (*Petroselimum crispum)* extract versus glibornuride on the liver of streptozotocin induced diabetic rats. *Journal of Ethnopharmacology*, *104*(1-2), 175–179. doi:10.1016/j.jep.2005.08.069 PMID:16223573

Pao, L. H., Hu, O. Y., Fan, H. Y., Lin, C. C., Liu, L. C., & Huang, P. W. (2012). Herb-drug interaction of 50 Chinese herbal medicines on CYP3A4 activity *in vitro* and in vivo. *The American Journal of Chinese Medicine*, *40*(1), 57–73. doi:10.1142/S0192415X1250005X PMID:22298448

Parvin, S., & Kader, A., Muhit, M. A., Haque, M. E, Mosaddik, M. A., & Wahed, M. I. I. (2011). Triterpenoids and phytosteroids from stem bark of *Crataeva nurvala* buch ham. *J. App. Pharmaceut. Sci*, *1*, 47–50.

Patel, M. V., Gupta, S. N., & Patel, N. G. (2011). Effects of Ayurvedic Treatment on 100 Patients of Chronic Renal Failure Other than Diabetic Nephropathy. *Ayu*, *32*(4), 483–486. doi:10.4103/0974-8520.96120 PMID:22661841

Perez Gutierrez, R. M., Laguna, G. Y., & Walkowski, A. (1985). Diuretic activity of *Mexican equisetum*. *Journal of Ethnopharmacology*, *14*(2-3), 269–272. doi:10.1016/0378-8741(85)90093-5 PMID:4094471

Petkov, V. (1979). Plants and hypotensive, antiatheromatous and coronarodilatating action. *The American Journal of Chinese Medicine*, *7*(3), 197–236. doi:10.1142/S0192415X79000180 PMID:574353

Powell, T., Hsu, F. F., Turk, J., & Hruska, K. (1998). Ma-huang strikes again: Ephedrine nephrolithiasis. *American Journal of Kidney Diseases*, *32*(1), 153–159. doi:10.1053/ajkd.1998.v32.pm9669437 PMID:9669437

Prashanth, G. S., Baghel, M. S., Ravishankar, B., Gupta, S. N., & Mehta, M. P. (2010). A clinical comparative study of the management of chronic renal failure with punarnavadi compound. *Ayu*, *31*(2), 185–192. doi:10.4103/0974-8520.72388 PMID:22131708

Rahimi, R., & Ardekani, M. R. (2013). Medicinal properties of *Foeniculum vulgare Mill.* in traditional Iranian medicine and modern phytotherapy. *Chinese Journal of Integrative Medicine*, *19*(1), 73–79. doi:10.1007/s11655-013-1327-0 PMID:23275017

Rosenblatt, M., & Mindel, J. (1997). Spontaneous hyphema associated with ingestion of *Ginkgo biloba* extract. *The New England Journal of Medicine*, *336*(15), 1108. doi:10.1056/NEJM199704103361518 PMID:9091822

Roshni, P. R., & Jyothylekshmi, V. (2014). Remya reghu, Vijayan, M. Renal disease with the use of herbal remedies Internat. *J. Pharmaceut. Chem. Biolog Sci*, *4*(2), 367–371.

Shalaby, M. A., & Hammouda, A. A. E. (2014). Nephroprotective, diuretic and antioxidant effects of some medicinal herbs in gentamicin-nephrotoxic rats. *J. Intercultural Ethnopharmacol.*, *3*(1), 1–8. doi:10.5455/jice.20131130022009

Shulman, A. (1997). Toxicological problems of traditional remedies and food supplements. *International Journal of Alternative and Complementary Medicine*, *1*, 9–10.

Singh, N. K. S., & Kaur, D. (2011). Anxiolytic effects of *Equisetum arvense* Linn. extracts in mice. *Indian Journal of Experimental Biology*, *49*, 325–356. PMID:21615059

Singh, S., Fadnis, P. P., & Sharma, B. K. (1986). Aconite poisoning. *The Journal of the Association of Physicians of India*, *34*(11), 825–826. PMID:2435703

Soleimani, S., Azarbaizani, F. F., & Nejati, V. (2007). The effect of Equisetum arvense L. (Equisetaceae) in histological changes of pancreatic beta-cells in streptozotocin-induced diabetic in rats. *Pakistan Journal of Biological Sciences*, *10*(23), 4236–4240. doi:10.3923/pjbs.2007.4236.4240 PMID:19086577

Subehan, U. T., Iwata, H., Kadota, S., & Tezuka, Y. (2006). Mechanism based inhibition of CYP3A4 and CYP2D6 by Indonesian medicinal plants. *Journal of Ethnopharmacology*, *105*(3), 449–455. doi:10.1016/j.jep.2005.12.001 PMID:16414224

Subehan, Z., Zaidi, S. F. H., Kadota, S., & Tezuka, Y. (2007). Inhibition on human liver cytochrome P450 3A4 by constituents of fennel (Foeniculum vulgare): Identification and characterization of a mechanism-based inactivator. *Journal of Agricultural and Food Chemistry*, *11*(25), 10162–10167. doi:10.1021/jf0713253 PMID:17988092

Sun, Y., Zhou, H., & Yang, B. X. (2011). Drug discovery for polycystic kidney disease. *Acta Pharmacologica Sinica*, *32*(6), 805–816. doi:10.1038/aps.2011.29 PMID:21642949

Sunter, W. H. (1991). Warfarin and garlic. *Pharmacol. J.*, *246*, 722.

Swanston-Flatt, S. K., Day, C., Bailey, C. J., & Flatt, P. R. (1990). Traditional plant treatments for diabetes. Studies in normal and streptozotocin diabetic mice. *Diabetologia*, *33*(8), 462–464. doi:10.1007/BF00405106 PMID:2210118

Swinyard, E. A., & Woodhead, J. H. (1982). Experimental detection quantificiation and evaluation of anticonvulsants. In D. M. Woodbury, J. K. Penry, & C. E. Pippenger (Eds.), *Antiepileptic Drugs*. New York, NY: Raven Press.

Takano, M., Yumoto, R., & Murakami, T. (2006). Expression and function of efflux drug transporters in the intestine. *Pharmacology & Therapeutics*, *109*(1-2), 137–161. doi:10.1016/j.pharmthera.2005.06.005 PMID:16209890

Taussig, S. J., & Batkin, S. (1988). Bromelain, the enzyme complex of pineapple (Ananas comosus) and its clinical application. An update. *Journal of Ethnopharmacology*, *22*(2), 191–203. doi:10.1016/0378-8741(88)90127-4 PMID:3287010

The World Health Report. (1999). *Making a difference*. Retrieved from http://www.who.int/whr/1999/en/

Thummel, K. E., OShea, D., Paine, M. F., Shen, D. D., Kunze, K. L., Perkins, J. D., & Wilkinson, G. R. (1996). Oral first-pass elimination of midazolam involves both gastrointestinal and hepatic CYP3A-mediated metabolism. *Clinical Pharmacology and Therapeutics*, *59*(5), 491–502. doi:10.1016/S0009-9236(96)90177-0 PMID:8646820

van Asperen, J., van Tellingen, O., & Beijnen, J. H. (2000). The role of mdr1a P-glycoprotein in the biliary and intestinal secretion of doxorubicin and vinblastine in mice. *Drug Metabolism and Disposition: the Biological Fate of Chemicals*, *28*(3), 264–267. PMID:10681369

Wang, C. P., Wang, Y., Wang, X., Zhang, X., Ye, J. F., Hu, L. S., & Kong, L. D. (2011). Mulberroside a possesses potent uricosuric and nephroprotective effects in hyperuricemic mice. *Planta Medica*, *77*(8), 786–794. doi:10.1055/s-0030-1250599 PMID:21154198

White, L. M., Gardner, S. F., Gurley, B. J., Marx, M. A., Wang, P. L., & Estes, M. (1997). Pharmacokinetics and cardiovascular effects of ma-huang (*Ephedra sinica*) in normotensive adults. *Journal of Clinical Pharmacology*, *37*(2), 116–122. doi:10.1002/j.1552-4604.1997.tb04769.x PMID:9055137

Wilkinson, G. R. (1996). Cytochrome P4503A (CYP3A) metabolism: Prediction of *in vivo* activity in humans. *Journal of Pharmacokinetics and Biopharmaceutics*, *24*(5), 475–490. doi:10.1007/BF02353475 PMID:9131486

Wojcikowski, K., Wohlmuth, H., Johnson, D. W., & Gobe, G. (2010). Effect of Astragalus membranaceus and Angelica sinensis combined with Enalapril in rats with obstructive uropathy. *Phytotherapy Research*, *24*(6), 875–884. PMID:19960445

Wojcikowski, K., Wohlmuth, H., Johnson, D. W., Rolfe, M., & Gobe, G. (2009). An *in vitro* investigation of herbs traditionally used for kidney and urinary system disorders: Potential therapeutic and toxic effects. *Nephrol.*, *14*(1), 70–79. doi:10.1111/j.1440-1797.2008.01017.x PMID:18808387

Wongnawa, M., Kawemeesri, P., Sriwiriyajan, S., Mahatthanatrakul, W., & Ridtitid, W. (2014). Effect of Phyllanthus amarus extract on the pharmacokinetics of midazolam in rabbits Songklanakarin. *J. Sci. Technol.*, *36*, 547–553.

Wright, C. I., Van-Buren, L., Kroner, C. I., & Koning, M. M. (2007). Herbal medicines as diuretics: A review of the scientific evidence. *Journal of Ethnopharmacology*, *114*(1), 1–31. doi:10.1016/j.jep.2007.07.023 PMID:17804183

Wu, S., Wang, S., Gao, J., Wu, Y., Chen, G., & Zhu, Y. (2011). Interactions between mercury and dry FGD ash in simulated post combustion conditions. *Journal of Hazardous Materials*, *188*(1-3), 391–398. doi:10.1016/j.jhazmat.2011.01.119 PMID:21334138

Yadav, A. K. L., & Nade, V. (2008). Effect of Morus alba L. (mulberry) leaves on anxiety in mice. *Indian Journal of Pharmacology*, *42*, 132–137. PMID:21264159

Yan, H., Wang, G. J., & Chen, J. (2007). Study of toxicity effect of different rate of Sargassum and Radix Glycyrrhizae on rats. *Zhongguo Zhong Yao Za Zhi*, *32*(16), 1700–1703. PMID:18027672

Yanardag, R., Bolkent, S., Tabakoglu-Oguz, A., & Ozsoy-Sacan, O. (2003). Effects of Petroselinum crispum extract on pancreatic B cells and blood glucose of streptozotocin-induced diabetic rats. *Biological & Pharmaceutical Bulletin*, *26*(8), 1206–1210. doi:10.1248/bpb.26.1206 PMID:12913280

Yarnell, E. (2002). Botanical medicines for the urinary tract. *World Journal of Urology*, *20*, 285–293. PMID:12522584

Yongchaiyuda, S., Rungpitarangi, V., Bunyapraphatsara, N., & Chokechaijaroenporn, O. (1996). Article. *Phytomedicine*, *3*, 241–243. doi:10.1016/S0944-7113(96)80060-2 PMID:23195077

Yoshikawa, N., Ito, H., Sakai, T., Takekoshi, Y., Honda, M., & Awazu, M. (1997). A prospective controlled study of sairei-to in childhood IgA nephropathy with focal/minimal mesangial proliferation. Japanese Pediatric IgA Nephropathy Treatment Study Group. *Nippon Jinzo Gakkai Shi*, *39*(5), 503–506. PMID:9283216

Zhang, S., Xin, H., Li, Y., Zhang, D., Shi, J., Yang, J., & Chen, X. (2013). Skimmin, a Coumarin from Hydrangea paniculata, Slows down the Progression of Membranous Glomerulonephritis by Anti-Inflammatory Effects and Inhibiting Immune Complex Deposition. *Evid.- Based Comp. Alternat Med*, *2013*, 1–10.

Zhou, Z. L., Yang, Y. X., Ding, J., Li, Y. C., & Miao, Z. H. (2012). Triptolide: Structural modifications, structure-activity relationships, bioactivities, clinical development and mechanisms. *Natural Product Reports*, *29*(4), 457–475. doi:10.1039/c2np00088a PMID:22270059

Zhu, M., Wong, P. Y., & Li, R. C. (1999). Effect of oral administration of fennel (Foeniculum vulgare) on ciprofloxacin absorption and disposition in the rat. *The Journal of Pharmacy and Pharmacology*, *51*(12), 1391–1396. doi:10.1211/0022357991777218 PMID:10678493

KEY TERMS AND DEFINITIONS

Additive Effect: An effect wherein two or more substances or actions used in combination produce a total effect. It is simple sum of two effects.

Anecdotal Interaction: Anecdotal interaction are based on anecdotal evidence i.e., evidence collected in a casual or informal manner and relying heavily or entirely on personal testimony.

CKD: Chronic Kidney Disease (CKD) is a condition characterized by a gradual loss of kidney function. That means loss of normal kidney function. The symptoms vary from mild to severe depending upon stage of the disease.

Compounding: Compounding is a practice in which a pharmacist or a physician or a person under the supervision of a licensed pharmacist, combines, mixes, or alters ingredients of a drug to create a medication tailored to the needs of an individual patient.

Cytochromes P450 Enzymes: Cytochromes P450 enzymes constitute a large superfamily of haem-thiolate proteins involved in the metabolism of a wide variety of both exogenous and endogenous compounds. The cytochrome P450 present throughout the body, but the highest concentrations are found in the liver (hepatocytes) and small intestine. These enzymes are responsible for the oxidative (Phase I) metabolism of a wide number of compounds, including many medications, biotransformation of lipophilic drugs to more polar compounds that can be excreted by the kidneys, etc. An individual enzyme of cytochrome P-450 may be able of metabolizing many different drugs, but a given drug may be primarily metabolized by a single enzyme.

Efflux Transport: Active efflux is a mechanism responsible for moving compounds, like neurotransmitters, toxic substances, and antibiotics, out of the cell; this is considered to be a vital part of xenobiotic metabolism, e.g. ABC transporters are a protein superfamily that all have an ATP binding site.

Nephropathy: Nephropathy means kidney disease or damage. Diabetic nephropathy is damage caused by diabetes to kidney.

Pharmacodynamics: The study of the biochemical and physiological effects of drugs and the mechanisms of their actions, including the correlation of their actions and effects with their chemical structure.

Pharmacokinetics: The study of action of drugs in the body over a period of time, including the processes of absorption, distribution, localization in tissues, biotransformation, and excretion.

Pharmacopoeia: It is an official book published usually under the jurisdiction of the government and containing a list of drugs, their formulas, and methods of identification, requirements and tests for their strength and purity, and other related information.

Synergistic Effect: An effect arising between two or more agents, entities, factors, or substances that produces an effect greater than the sum of their individual effects.

Traditional Chinese Materia Medica: The Materia Medica is regarded as the most complete and comprehensive medical book written in the history of traditional Chinese medicine. It lists all the plants, animals, minerals, and other items that were believed to have medicinal properties.

Chapter 9
Economic Evaluation of CAM Use

Li-Chia Chen
The University of Manchester, UK

Mayuree Tangkiatkumjai
Srinakharinwirot University, Thailand

ABSTRACT

Economic evaluation (EE) of health care interventions has been used to inform and affect policy decision-making by considering both costs and outcomes of the interventions. National guidelines in many countries consider cost-effectiveness evidence for making recommendations of healthcare interventions. In such case, EE of complementary and alternative medicine (CAM) is crucial to guide reimbursement decision-making. However, there is currently a lack of cost-effectiveness evidence of using CAM for kidney diseases. There are three types of full EEs, including a cost-benefit, cost-effectiveness, and cost-utility analysis, of which, results of cost-utility analysis is preferred and widely used by healthcare authorities in several developed countries. General approaches for EE of conventional medicine are likely to be applied to assess economic outcomes of CAM for kidney diseases. This chapter depicts the overall principles of EEs, interpretations of economic results and summaries the currently available EE for CAM.

DOI: 10.4018/978-1-5225-2882-1.ch009

INTRODUCTION

Increasing cost of health care expenditure is a global trend due to a variety of reasons such as changing population demographics, advances in medical technology, labour intensive nature of the health service and rising salaries, society's increasing expectations, defensive medicine, and impact of living habits on disease epidemiology (Elliott & Payne, 2005). Of which, the cost of pharmacological therapy is still the leading mainstay of the growing health care expenditure (Elliott & Payne, 2005). The increasingly expanding and expensive health service provision leads to scarcity of resources in health care systems, consequently the decisions to devise the maximum total benefit from finite resources, i.e. achieve efficiency of resource allocation, are being made every day. Allocating resources efficiently can be informed by economic evaluations (EEs). "The science which studies human behaviour as a relationship between ends and scarce means which have alternative uses" (Robbins, 1935, pg 16). Health economics is the application of economic principles to the production and consumption of health in the population.

The demand of applying EEs to inform health resource allocation was first raised by the United States (US) congress in 1967 (Tan-torres Edejert, et al., 2003), after which economic information started being used in health care decision making. In the late 1990s, the initiative of using health economic information was expended and consolidated into the Health Technology Assessment (HTA), which is a multidisciplinary field of policy analysis to study the medical, social, ethical and economic implications of the development, diffusion and use of health technology. It is used in the developed countries to provide input into decision making in policy and practice (Tan-torres Edejert, et al., 2003), and informs universal national health systems, such as in the UK, Canada, Australia, and Germany (Bridges et al., 2010; Canadian Agency for Drugs and Technologies in Health, 2006; National Institute for Health and Care Excellence, 2012).

EE is also relevant to the use of complementary and alternative medicine (CAM). The cost of CAM has been rapidly increasing over the last two decades (Davis & Weeks, 2012; Thomas et al., 2001; Xue et al., 2007), and the enquiry about whether it is rational to pay for integrative medicine instead of the conventional medicine has been raised by clinical practitioners (Spinks & Hollingsworth, 2009). Therefore the only valid expense maybe when CAM is an option for illnesses which fail to be treated by conventional medicine

(Singer & Adams, 2014). Many people believe that CAM is effective and cheaper than conventional medicine; however, there is lack of economic evidence to support that statement. In countries that employee HTA to inform decision making in choosing effective medicine with affordable costs, evidence from EEs are crucial to support the value claim of CAM. Given the increasing demand for CAM and the under-studied health economics of CAM, further research in this field is required. It is important to understand the methodology and challenges of conducting the economic evaluations, and carefully appraise the currently available economic evidence. Therefore, this chapter provides insights in the basic methodology, summarises existing evidence of EEs in CAM, and concludes by offering some suggestions for future economic evaluations of CAM in patients with kidney disease.

FOUNDATION OF ECONOMIC EVALUATION

Health EE is designed to assess two major components - the costs and outcomes of alternative healthcare strategies in order to provide a decision-making framework to ensure 'efficiency', i.e. to devise the maximum total outcome (benefit) from finite resources available (Donaldson & Gerard, 1993). In healthcare, allocative efficiency is to use resources across the whole economy, so that benefit is maximised (or the opportunity cost is minimized), i.e. moving resources from one programme to another. Technical efficiency means producing a given output for the least cost, or maximising output for a given cost, i.e. make best use of the resources you already have. For example, the cost-effectiveness comparing a pharmacist-led or physician-led smoking cessation programme. Methodology in EE is fast developing; numerous guidelines have been developed for conducting EEs, such as Cheers Guidelines (Husereau et al., 2013), and the principles of EE can also be applied to evaluate CAM. Similar to the previous chapter (Chapter 5), a clear research question and specific objectives are crucial to guide the development of an EE using a feasible study design. In assessing CAM modalities with inconclusive cost-effectiveness evidence, EE can be used to inform the evidence-based practice of healthcare professionals, price negotiation, or the development of clinical practice guidelines. It is important to present a clear and logical argument on the rationale of the need for an EE. An explicit objective of an EE should depict an evaluation of the costs and outcomes (or consequences) of interventions versus a comparator. A clear and justifiable study perspective, i.e. societal, provider, payer or patient viewpoint needs to be defined, as the perspective determines which cost to consider and whose values to use. In addition, target population and subgroups with their characteristics have to be identified and justified, as well as study setting and location, which will determine the methods of data collection, and values of all resources on which the decision needs to be made. Furthermore, target interventions, e.g. CAM programs, technologies, etc., and their comparators should also be identified and explained. A comparator might be an intervention currently practiced, normal or standard treatment as recommended in practice guidelines, no treatment or placebo. Finally, the time horizon, i.e. the length of time over which costs and outcomes are evaluated, should be described and justified, which should be long enough for researchers to assess the costs and consequences.

COSTS IN ECONOMIC EVALUATION

Type of Resource Use for Costing

True economic cost aims to evaluate all inputs in terms of 'opportunity cost', i.e., the value of resources in their best alternative use (Kobelt, 1996) and takes into account all the costs associated with an intervention or service. Therefore, all resources used to deliver the interventions must be identified, and valued by attaching the monetary value to the resource according to the specified perspective. From the viewpoint of society as a whole, three main categories of costs in health care including health service costs, costs borne by patients and their family, and external costs borne by the rest of society must be considered (Robinson, 1993c). Being valued in monetary terms, these costs are usually divided into direct, indirect, and intangible costs (Figure 1).

Direct costs are the most common costs included in economic evaluations. The direct costs of providing care (health service costs) comprises direct medical costs and direct non-medical costs. Direct medical costs are all costs occurring within the health sector, including costs associated with drug-related morbidity, and un-relieved conditions. Direct medical costs can be further categorised into fixed (incurred whatever the level of activity, e.g. heating and lighting), semi-fixed (e.g. staff), and variable (varied according to the level of activity, e.g. drugs and disposable equipment). The two major components of fixed costs are overheads (incurred by the running of the service, e.g. lighting, heating and cleaning), and capital costs (incurred by major capital

Figure 1. Categories of costs in economic evaluation

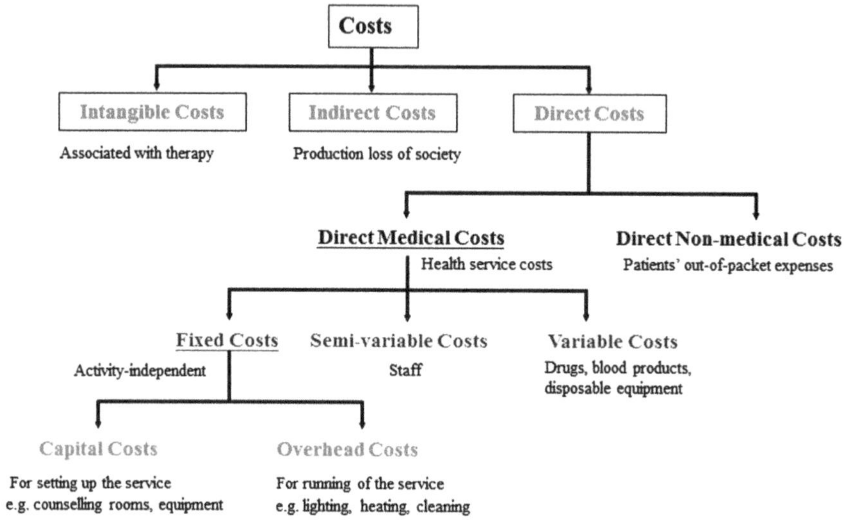

assets for the setting) (Robinson, 1993c). However, 'fixed costs' only exist in the short-term; in the long-term, all costs are variable. Direct non-medical costs are the costs not incurred by the health service but instead fall on other parts of the public sector or on patients and their families, such as patients' out-of-pocket expenses, 'informal' nursing care at home, or transportation costs of patients (Kobelt, 1996). Valuation of resources, in particular those related to direct medical costs, can be performed using a reference price, costs from a previous study, a standard cost list, retrospective or prospective data collection, interviews with patients or relatives (especially for informal care costs), and national databases for the ratio of 'hospital service' cost to charge (Shwartz et al., 1995).

Indirect costs are the costs to society, which relate to the lost productivity of an individual due to treatment, illness or death, or that of family members or friends if they attend to the patient. These costs include: time off work for the patients (sick leave, early retirement), time off work for family or friends, reduced productivity at work, or premature mortality. The methods of calculation of indirect costs such as human capital-cost (the lost gross income during the absence from work) (Weisbrod, 1961), or friction-cost (costs of replacing a sick worker) (Koopmanschap et al., 1995, 1996) raises an ethical issue, i.e. the inclusion of indirect costs favours interventions where most sufferers are those in work (Kobelt, 1996). Intangible costs are costs that cannot easily be measured, such as the pain and suffering experienced

Table 1. Example of costing health care resource use by different perspectives of economic evaluation

Cost	Example	Perspective Of Economic Evaluation			
		Societal	**Provider**	**3rd Party Payer Or Purchaser**	**Patient**
Direct medical costs of goods or services directly provided by the health care system	Medicine, laboratory, admission, home nursing	Cost	Cost	Reimbursement	Charge
	Value of side effects and future consequences linked to them				
Direct non-medical costs of goods or services not directly provided by the health care system	Transportation, meals, accommodation, facilities, equipment, services	Charge	-	-	Charge
	Informal care costs (e.g. family) who provide care without financial compensation	Productivity cost			Income loss
Indirect or productivity costs. Productivity losses relating to illness or death	Income loss from sick leave, permanent disability or premature death (morbidity and mortality)	Productivity cost	-	-	Income loss

by a patient as a consequence of treatment. These costs are particularly difficult to measure and value and as a result, are often left out of analyses. Current approaches used to assess intangible costs include the use of quality of life (QoL) instruments, or direct measurements within the framework of willingness-to-pay (WTP) assessments (Kobelt, 1996).

Speical Considerations in Cost Calculation

Interest and Depreciation

The costs of programs which will extend over several years will be affected by discounting and inflation. Investments in buildings, and equipment over a number of years give rise to capital costs. Generally, investment expenditure will be undertaken at the beginning of a project but the use of items of capital equipment will generate annual capital costs over the lifetime of the asset (Robinson, 1993c). These costs have two components, namely interest and depreciation. Interest costs should be included even if the asset was not acquired with borrowed money because tying up money in an item of capital equipment involves an opportunity cost that is interest foregone. Depreciation costs arise because of the wear and tear that an asset receives through use and the consequent reduction in the length of its useful life (Robinson, 1993c).

Discounting

Discounting is used in EE to reflect the fact that individuals prefer to have resources now rather than later. It is a method of calculation by which costs and benefits that occur at different times can be compared. Discounting converts the value of future costs and benefit into their present value, based on the assumption that generally people and society have a 'positive time preference' as they prefer to have something today rather than in the future (Kielhorn et al., 2000). EE 'weights' costs by a discount rate, according to the year in which they accrue, before adding them up and expressing total costs in current value terms (value in the current year) (Robinson, 1993c). The future monetary values must be adjusted to the present by the equation $PV = FV/(1+r)^t$, where PV is the present value, FV is the future value, r is the discounting rate, and t is the year from the beginning of the intervention or programme. Likewise, the past values must be adjusted to the present using the country's Consumer Price Index (CPI). The choice of discounting rate can have a significant effect on the result of EE. Many arguments exist regarding which discount rate to use and whether to discount costs and benefits at the same rate, or whether or not to discount benefits (Haycox & Walley, 1997). The governments of some countries have set discounting rates for the evaluation of public investment projects, e.g. 10% in USA and 5% in the Netherlands. In the various international guidelines on the EE of health services, the interest rates for discounting are usually 3-6%. In the UK, the discounting rate recommended by the Treasury for both costs and benefits is 3.5% (Haycox & Walley, 1997). In sensitivity analysis, the results are often compared with a calculation with no discounting (Kielhorn, et al., 2000).

Inflation

Most programs that extend over several years will be affected by inflation, and it is important to distinguish between changes in the general and relative price levels. In the case of general inflation, there will be no change in the relative cost of inputs (opportunity costs remain constant). However, some input prices are expected to increase more than others, such as the price for buying the same equipment may be £1000 this year and £1200 next year. The general rate of inflation may be used as a benchmark to adjust the future price of individual inputs, i.e. upwards or downwards by an amount that reflects the difference between their rate of inflation and the general rate. Thereafter, all costs should be discounted by a real (excluding inflationary effect) rate of interest (Robinson, 1993c).

OUTCOMES IN ECONOMIC EVALUATION

The outcome measure specified in an EE is related to whether the research is focused on technical or allocative efficiency. The commonly used outcomes measure includes effectiveness, QoL, utility, or WTP. As with the costs of interventions, outcomes also vary with time and future outcomes must be discounted (generally by 3%).

Effectiveness

Effectiveness is the outcome of an intervention or service measured in natural units, it is the most common type of outcome measure used in EEs. These natural units can be general outcome measures (such as cases successfully diagnosed, cases successfully treated, or life years gained) or clinical indicators (such as number of asthma attacks avoided, pain-free days, change in infection rate, percentage reduction in blood pressure, or nausea and vomiting frequency). Effectiveness measures are relatively simple to use and often reported in clinical trials of interventions. They are sometimes called intermediated or surrogate outcome measures (e.g. blood pressure or laboratory test results) because there is the implication that changes in them will extrapolate to an effect on the patient's ultimate health status.

Quality of Life

QoL is a multidimensional construct measuring at least four dimensions-mental state, social relations, functional competence and physical state, which are usually obtained through patient questionnaires. The instruments used to measure QoL can be divided into generic measures and disease-specific measures (see Chapter 4) (Kielhorn, et al., 2000).

Disease-specific QoL instruments are used for the quantitative determination of the subjective state of health or well-being in patients suffering from the same illness. These instruments usually have greater sensitivity to patients' symptoms within a disease because of the specific nature of the questions (Kielhorn, et al., 2000), such as the Kidney Disease Quality of Life 36 questionnaire, the Arthritis Impact Measurement Scale, Asthma Quality of Life Questionnaire or rhe Inflammatory Bowel Disease Questionnaire. The limitations of these measures are that since these questionnaires focus on individual aspects, not all aspects of QoL relevant to the illness or person are taken into account, and the results of these instruments cannot be used to compare different illnesses or health programmes (Kielhorn, et al., 2000). However, they may be more sensitive to detect the changes in different disease states.

Generic, i.e. general, QoL questionnaires are instruments for measuring health-related QoL and can be used for a wide range of illnesses of varying degrees of severity or for different types of treatment. They can be used for all types of ailments, as well as for healthy people, and can be used to compare outcomes in different patient groups. The questionnaires can generally be divided into two groups. In profile instruments, the results for the individual dimensions (physical pain, vitality, etc.) are usually given separately, such as the Short Form 36 (SF-36) (Medical Outcomes Trust, 2004), which includes eight values, one per dimension. In global index instruments, all of the dimensions are summed up in a single value, such as a 100 QoL value in the EuroQol (EuroQol Group, 2004) would mean that the patient is in sound health (Kielhorn, et al., 2000). The limitation with some generic QoL measures is that although they are informative, they are not presented on interval or ratio scales and cannot be analysed quantitatively, and so are not useful in economic evaluations (Elliott & Payne, 2005).

Utility

Health utility (or benefit) refers to the desirability of, or preference for, a particular state of health (Torrance, 1987), i.e. the unit of outcome relates to a person's pleasure or satisfaction with a programme and their level of wellbeing. Utility is a value attached by individuals, such as patients, health professionals or the general population, although the last is preferred (Jolicoeur et al., 1992). Different individuals may attach different values to a particular health state (Robinson, 1993b). It constructs a numerical representation of preferences for health states, and the value can be also used to "adjust" life expectancy. The utility values are often on a scale of 1.0 (normal health) to 0 (death). A health state considered worse than death is given a negative utility value (Jolicoeur, et al., 1992). A variety of approaches can be used to value health utility. It can be directly measured by visual analogue scales (VAS), time trade-off (TTO) or standard gamble (SG). Alternatively, indirect measures, such as EQ-5D (recommended by many countries), Health Utility Index (HUI), Quality of Well-being (QWB) or Short Form 6D (SF-6D) can be employed.

Direct utility measures are based on the value individuals place on not having a particular health-related scenario. Respondents (preferably a random sample of the general population) rate the desirability or undesirability of a health state relative to that of other health states. The VAS uses a linear scale with defined end-points and intervals that correspond to the differences in subjects' preferences for a health state (Drummond et al., 1998). In TTO, subjects are asked to trade off life years in a state of less than perfect health, with a shorter life span in a state of perfect health. The ratio of the number of years of perfect health that is equal to the longer life span in less than perfect health provides a measure of the preference for that state (Gold et al., 1996). In SG, subjects are offered two alternatives and asked to compare life in a particular given health state that is certain, to a gamble with a probability (p) that perfect health is the outcome, and probability (1-p) that immediate death is the outcome. The probability at which the expected utility of the two choices is equal is a measure of the preference for the health state (Gold, et al., 1996).

The most common and conventional way of using these utilities is to convert them into quality adjusted life years (QALYs). QALYs are calculated by multiplying the generic QoL measure by the years spent in that health state. For example, 10 years in a health state with a utility value of 0.5 would result in 5 QALYs, i.e. equivalent to 5 years of perfect health (Kielhorn, et al., 2000). However, when interpreting QALYs, it is important to consider the measurement property of the QALY states. For instance, the same QoL gain may not equal the same improvement in health status. Also, the same QALY gain may not equal the same health status, because QALY is the combination of QoL and time. Furthermore, a utility measure is limited in acute surgical patients with transient change of health status; it is more useful for measuring long-term health status.

Health utility methodologies and technologies are still being developed (Elliott & Payne, 2005). The health utility evaluation should be constructed from conceptualisation to measurement, i.e. measure something can be conceptualised, with considerations of study design, sample size, reliability (internal, test-retest, inter-rater), validity (criterion-related, content, construct, convergence), and responsiveness (Torrance, 1987). There are several drawbacks of health utility measurements: validity is still of concern; measurement is influenced by procesess; different methods do not yield identical results, and there is no consensus on the method (Drummond, et al., 1998).

Expressing Benefit as a Monetary Value

An alternative method for measuring outcomes is to convert these benefits to a monetary value, i.e. the monetary value attached to the health states produced by interventions. The value may be attached by patients, health professionals or by the general population, though the latter is preferred (Elliott & Payne, 2005). There are three main methods of doing this: the human capital approach (or per capital national income for productivity costs), revealed preference, and contingent valuation.

The human capital approach places monetary weights on time by using market wage rates, and the value of the programme is assessed in terms of the present value of future earnings. The valuation method had been criticised because it is not consistent with the principles of welfare economics. Revealed preference uses wage-risk studies, which examines the relationship between a particular health state associated with a hazardous job and wage rates that individuals require to accept the job. This approach is consistent with welfare economics, but established values have varied widely and estimation seems to be job-specific (Drummond, et al., 1998).

Contingent valuation uses survey methods to present subjects with hypothetical scenarios about the goods or service under evaluation and reveal the momentary value they will pay for benefits from the goods or services (Payne, 2000). Contingent valuation is gaining acceptance in the valuation of health care. There are two approaches to evaluate the monetary value of health services: stated preference, and discrete choice experiment.

The stated preference, i.e. WTP approach, is an evaluation method used to determine the maximum amount of money an individual is willing to pay to gain a particular benefit, e.g. receive a healthcare service (Robinson, 1993a). In the WTP approach, the outcome of a healthcare procedure and its alternative(s) are described and patients are asked how much they would be willing to pay (Torgerson & Raftery, 1999). Procedures with the highest values are preferred. Besides capturing non-health dimensions, this technique enables benefits to be expressed in monetary terms, allowing cost benefit analysis to take place (Palmer et al., 1999).

Discrete choice experiments present individuals with a list of pair-wise choices of a health intervention (Ryan & Shackley, 1995). For example, for inductive anaesthesia before surgery, would patients prefer inhalational anaesthetics with a cheaper price or injection anaesthetics with a higher price. The various attributes of the alternatives can be weighted to generate utilities. The option with the best cost utility ratio is the most efficient (Torgerson & Raftery, 1999). However, current empirical evidence and reviews, indicate that the ideal design for a contingent valuation study remains unresolved (Klose, 1999). The main issues include bias associated with value elicitation methods, the lack of consensus on payment vehicles, the influence of income on WTP, and the validity about the hypothetical nature of WTP (Elliott & Payne, 2005).

METHODS OF ECONOMIC EVALUATION

The framework of an EE involves comparison of the costs and benefits associated with alternative programmes or treatments. The characteristics of whether both cost and outcomes are examined, and whether two or more alternatives are compared, may be employed to distinguish and label several evaluation situations commonly encountered in health care evaluation literature (Drummond, et al., 1998) (Figure 2). There are four main forms of 'full economic evaluation', i.e. cost-minimisation analysis (CMA), cost-effectiveness analysis (CEA), cost-utility analysis (CUA), and cost-benefit analysis (CBA). Each method deals with costs but differs in the way that the consequences or outcomes of health care programmes are measured and valued (Reeder, 1995) (Table 2). Alternative methods of EE sometimes used are cost-of-illness or cost-consequence analysis. In general, CMA and CBA are not recommended for various reasons, such as difficulty in comparing or quantifying outcomes. CEA and CUA are the most commonly used and their results are computed in a ratio of incremental cost over incremental outcome (effectiveness or utility), i.e. the incremental cost-effectiveness ratio (ICER).

Figure 2. Differentiate different types of economic evaluations

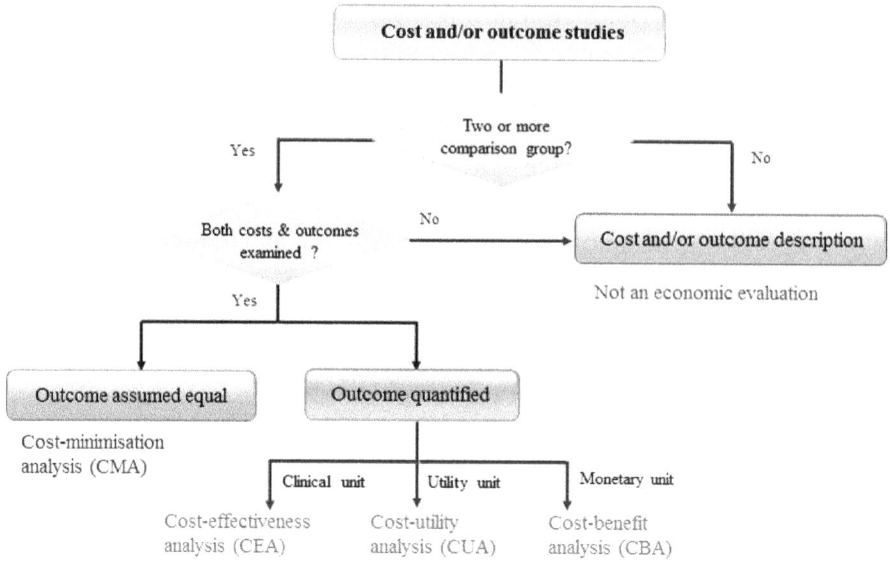

Table 2. The Major types of economic evaluation

Type of study	Measurement input / valuation of costs in both alternative	Identification of consequences	Measurement outcome / valuation of consequences	Use of result
Cost-minimization analysis (CMA)	(Direct medical) Cost / dollars	Identical in all relevant respects	None	Cost comparison (lowest cost to achieve an identical result): cost per case
Cost-effectiveness analysis (CEA)	Costs / dollars	Single effect of interest, common to both alternative, but achieved to different degree	Natural units: general outcome measures or clinical indicators, e.g. life-years gained, disability-days saved, points of blood pressure reduction, etc.	Comparison of interventions with the same unit of benefit but at a different magnitude: cost per unit of effect, an incremental cost-effectiveness ratio
Cost-utility analysis (CUA)	Costs / dollars	Single or multiple effects, not necessarily common to both alternatives	Healthy years equivalents or quality-adjusted life years Quality of life: generic or disease specific measures. Utility: rating scale, time trade off, and standard gamble.	Summary of multiple dimensions into one scales; comparison of treatments which initial different outcome measures: cost per QALY, incremental cost per QALY gained
Cost-benefit analysis (CBA)	Costs / dollars	Single or multiple effects, not necessarily common to both alternatives	Monetary benefit (dollars) Willing to pay: human capital approach, individual observed or stated preferences.	Cost minus benefit: cost/ benefit ratio

Cost-Effectiveness Analysis (CEA)

CEA is the most common form of EE. It compares the cost and consequence of alternative approaches to a common objective or outcome by using non-monetary (natural or physical) units as outcome measures (Drummond, et al., 1998). Published studies were typically relied on in the past for 'effectiveness' data (Payne, 2000). Uni-dimensional measures of outcome are used to assess the incremental difference in outcome between at least two alternatives of differing effectiveness. CEA differs from CBA in that outcomes are measured in non-monetary units, such as 'years of life gained' or 'cases correctly diagnosed', which must be identical for each alternative (Reeder, 1995). CEA developed in healthcare because the classic economic approach of CBA was much more difficult to apply. This difficulty arose from the methodological, theoretical, and philosphical difficulties associated with attaching a monentary value to health outcomes.

The costs are compared with one or more measurement of a treatment's effectiveness, i.e. the measured outcomes are expressed in terms of the cost per unit of success or effect, such as the cost per year of life saved, cost per treatment success, or cost per pain intensity decreased in pain control. The lower the cost-effectiveness ratio, the more this treatment should be preferred to another if resources were in short supply (Jolicoeur, et al., 1992). However, when one alternative is more effective but requires more resources than standard treatment, incremental economic analysis (see below) should be used for identifying differences (increments) in costs and outcomes between healthcare interventions. For CEA and CUA, calculate the expected costs and outcomes of all interventions studied, and most importantly compute the ICERs. Incremental economic analysis calculates an ICER which is derived from the difference in cost and difference in outcomes between healthcare interventions. ICERs are calculated as:

$$ICER = \frac{\Delta C}{\Delta E}$$

Where 'Δ C' refers to the difference in costs between the two alternatives, and 'Δ E' is the difference in effectiveness between the two alternatives, e.g. the cost per bleeding averted. The point estimate of the ICER is the best single estimate to evaluate the cost-effectiveness of different interventions. CEA cannot be used to compare treatments for different diseases or different health programmes if the units of outcome vary. For example, CEA could not be used to compare a heart surgery programme where outcomes were measured in life-years gained with a migraine treatment where outcomes were measured in pain-free days. Even using the same outcome unit, the value of life extension may not represent the function of the patient's state of health during that period; for example, comparing a year of life saved in a severely debilitated cancer patient with a year of life saved in a young patient with relatively mild asthma.

Cost-Minimisation Analysis (CMA)

If the effectiveness of different interventions is equal in CEA, the EE will become a cost-minimisation analysis (CMA). CMA is a simplified CEA. This method compares the costs of two or more alternatives that have equivalent outcomes; the objective being to identify the least expensive alternative (Reeder, 1995). Since the outcomes of the alternatives are assumed to be identical, CMA allows one to evaluate only the inputs or costs of each alternative (Jolicoeur, et al., 1992). Although CMA is the simplest method of economic-efficiency testing, due to the strict requirements of therapeutic equality, cost-minimization analysis is not commonly used (Jolicoeur, et al., 1992). However, this method can be useful when one is assessing the cost difference among dosage forms of the same drug, or different drugs for which patient outcomes have been shown to be the same (Drummond, et al., 1998).

Cost-Utility Analysis (CUA)

CUA compares the cost and consequence of alternative approaches to a common objective or outcome by using patient preferences or utility as outcome measures (Reeder, 1995). CUA is actually a form of CEA but utility is used instead of natural units to measure outcomes (Robinson, 1993b). The specific methods used to derive utility are complex and are still under development (Elliott & Payne, 2005). Generic QoL measures, such as the QALY and Healthy Year Equivalents (HYEs) are also sometimes used as measures of utility. Therefore, in CUA, evaluation of the consequences of programmes are adjusted by a health state preference score or utility weights, such as the quality of life-year gained or healthy years equivalents (Drummond, et al., 1998). In CUA, the results of the incremental economic analysis, i.e. ICERs, are usually expressed as the cost per QALY (Reeder, 1995). The decision rules for CUA are the same as CEA, i.e. unless one treatment dominates, the final decision resolves around how much decision makers are willing to pay for extra benefits. In theory, CUA can be used when deciding which services are allocated resources within the health care sector (Payne, 2000). Although different diseases and their effects on patient's health are very different, the analyses have all generated a common ICER, a cost per QALY. Therefore, healthcare services can be compared by their costs per QALY and ranked by their respective cost per QALY gained. CUA assumes that the decision-maker wants to maximise the possible numbers of QALYs gained from an intervention. This is the principle behind the use of league tables, which rank a list of interventions in order of cost per QALY, and compare different interventions. However, published league tables of CUAs need to be interpreted and used with caution. It is difficult to compare different costs per QALY as there is no 'gold standard' in many aspects of CUA (Elliott & Payne, 2005). Often the same perspectives are not used, costing methods are not comparable, the same methods of generating QALYs have not been used, and the discounting methods used are not the same (Johannesson, 1995).

Cost-Benefit Analysis (CBA)

CBA compares the costs and consequences of two or more alternatives and all costs (inputs) and benefits (consequences) of the alternatives are measured in monetary terms, i.e., the monetary value attached to the health states produced by the interventions. The outcome may be expressed as a ratio (benefit to cost) or in terms of net cost or benefit (benefit minus cost), and can be directly compared to the alternative (Drummond, et al., 1998) instead of ICERs. CBA is different from CEA or CUA because the inputs and outputs of the process are measured in the same unit. In CBA, a health care programme is considered good value for money when the benefit exceeds the total costs. Costs are ideally measured as opportunity costs, i.e. the best alternative benefit. Benefits are valued in monetary terms using the valuation of people's observed or stated preferences. These are usually based on the WTP approach. CBA uses economic welfare theory to inform the evaluation of interventions. It can be used to compare healthcare interventions that do not have comparable outcome measures, and thus helps decide how to allocate resources to those interventions (Elliott & Payne, 2005). CBA is particularly useful when resources are limited and only one program can be implemented (Jolicoeur, et al., 1992). In fact, CBA is considered to be the most comprehensive method of EE because it allows the returns on investment in health to be compared with the returns obtained from investments in other areas of the economy (Robinson, 1993a). However, there remains debate about the ability of current methods to accurately, and reliably, value outcomes in monetary terms (Payne, 2000). The difficulty in converting some non-monetary units, such as the number of medication errors avoided or years of life saved, into monetary units, is the major disadvantage (Jolicoeur, et al., 1992). Hence, CBA as a method, is not widely used at present, but is increasingly being applied in health care.

In terms of selecting an economic method for assessing the cost-effectiveness of CAM, the quality of life or an holistic health outcome is appropriate as it is associated with a CAM approach. The nature of CAM tends to provide a minor specific benefit, compared with conventional medicine. Therefore, CUA is more likely to suit CAM EE and the outcome over a longer follow up should be investigated (Coulter et al., 2013). Poor quality clinical trials in CAM has led to lack of proven efficacy therefore CEA is less like to be conducted in CAM research.

Other Forms of Evaluation Used to Assess Health Care Technologies

Cost-of-Illness Studies

Cost-of-illness (COI) studies (also known as burden-of-illness studies) attempt to represent the burden of disease from a particular ailment or medical condition in monetary terms (Drummond, 1992). Most COI studies are limited to estimating direct and indirect costs, though intangible costs are sometimes calculated. Costs can be analysed either on a prevalence or an incidence basis. As previously noted, such studies should not be categorised as EE as they do not examine clinical outcomes. Instead, they act as points of reference for economic analyses and provide information for health care policy-makers (Kobelt, 1996). Although these studies usually produce a large number of illnesses in terms of the cost to society (e.g. diabetes, heart disease), they do not consider what can be done to reduce this burden. Pharmaceutical companies are increasingly undertaking such studies in order to support product marketing, but the value to a health care provider's decision makers is often limited. From their perspective, EEs that show the relative costs and benefits of competing treatments to reduce the burden of disease are more useful.

Cost-Consequences Analysis

Cost-consequences analysis is a form of CEA. It was defined by Russell *et al.* (1996) as an analysis in which costs and effects are calaulated but not aggregated into QALYs or cost-effectiveness. In some cases, often multiple outcomes are relevant and it is difficult to determine which is the most important. It would be useful to present the results in a disaggregated form in order that all of the outcomes can be carefully considered (Goodacre & McCabe, 2002). It has been suggested that one of the key advantages of listing all the resource use, costs, and health outcomes in a transparent manner is that it allows decision-makers to choose whatever resource, cost or health outcomes are of particular interest to them to include in their economic analysis (Goodacre & McCabe, 2002). Most EEs usually present an aggregate result without being reported in disaggregated form. Although the aggregation of cost and outcome results, such as an ICER or a net benefit, can be implemented to a given decision rule (e.g. the ICER must be below a given threshold), the decision-maker may find it difficult to decompose the overall result or assumptions (Goodacre & McCabe, 2002).

There are ongoing debates on the whether the ECR or the cost-consequence format is more appropriate to inform healthcare decision-making. Mauskopf *et al.* (1998) suggested that cost consequence analysis provides the most comprehensive presentation of information describing the values of drug therapy or other healthcare intervention, and is also conceptually the simplest. Coast (2004) proposed that cost-consequences analysis would suit the objectives of decision makers and be easier to understand. However, the weakness of cost consequence analysis is that not all of the data are of comparable quality. Extrapolation and imputation are often necessary (Mauskopf, et al., 1998), hence the uncertainty surrounding decisions is important. Failure to consider uncertainty surrounding cost and effect can lead to misleading decisions (Claxton, 1999; Claxton et al., 2002). Moreover, decision-makers may objectively select the partial cost or outcome information and hence the decision-making may mislead. Lots of economists and methodologists still prefer to report aggregated results of EEs instead of disaggregated forms, such as ICERs or net benefit. Given a decision rule, i.e. the ICER much be below a given threshold (i.e. ceiling ratio), aggregated results compose quantified information to inform decision-making. Methodological developments in recent years, such as the analysis of stochastic data from clinical trials (Claxton, 1999), the development of probabilistic model, and Bayesian interpretations of data including the use of cost-effectiveness acceptability curve (CEAC) (Briggs, 2001, Drummond & McGuire, 2001), have improved the analysis in EE (Drummond & Sculpher, 2005).

Some methodological literature has demonstrated CEAC is an appropriate way to represent the uncertainty surrounding a decision to adopt a technology (Fenwick et al., 2001, 2004), although when considering more than two alternatives, it is difficult to interpret the results presented with uncertainty (e.g., scatter plots on a Cost Effectiveness plane). Claxton *et al.* (2005) argued that the use of simpler and more easily understood approaches (i.e. one-way or multi-way sensitivity analysis) either fail to account for the combined effect of uncertainty in all the parameters taken together or become impossible to interpret correctly.

ANALYSIS APPROACHES OF ECONOMIC EVALUATION

There are two major approaches, i.e. trial-based or model-based, to conduct an EE. These approaches synthesizes data derived from different evidence sources. The NHS Centre for Review and Dissemination (CRD) (1999) proposed a hierarchy of evidence (McKinnell et al., 1999). It notes that validity depends not only on the type of study but how well it was designed, conducted, and analysed. The input (cost) and outcome (effectiveness or benefit) data in EE may be adopted from different evidence sources. To use input and outcome data in an EE, Drummond and Jefferson (1996) suggest that the details of the study design, data synthesis and results should be presented if the effectiveness data is extracted from RCTs or meta-analysis. The research subjects (e.g. patients, members of the general public, health care professionals) and methods (e.g. time trade off, standard gamble, contingent valuation) used to measure the benefit data should also be detailed on the data of health benefits (Drummond & Jefferson, 1996).

Trial-Based Economic Evaluation

An EE study can be carried out using a prospective design, i.e. EEs alongside clinical trials, or model-based design based on data from various sources, such as data from clinical trials, prospective or retrospective studies, national databases, expert opinions, etc.

Randomised Controlled Trials (RCTs)

RCTs are considered to be the best method for proving causation and efficacy because they minimise the impact of potential confounding factors, thereby achieving high levels of 'internal validity' (Rittenhouse, 1996). Primary data from RCTs are preferred in economic analysis because they are stochastic and controlled for bias (Elliott & Payne, 2005). However, conducting RCTs in CAM is a challenge due to difficulties in randomising or blinding, finding an equal control group, and measuring specific outcomes. RCT data give a mean estimate of efficacy with quantified uncertainty. Associated uncertainty can be handled by sampling from an appropriate population and applying standard statistical methods to obtain an estimate representative of that population, i.e. randomised sampling, to give stochastic data and quantify the amount of uncertainty around that mean estimate in the form of 95%CI (Elliott & Payne, 2005). The quantitative measure of uncertainty is very useful in testing the robustness of an EE through sensitivity analysis. However, there are problems with the direct use of RCT evidence for policy-making (Brennan & Akehurst, 2000). These problems have been reviewed by Rittenhouse (1996), such as choice of comparison therapy, protocol-driven costs and outcomes, artificial environment, intermediate versus final outcomes, inadequate patient follow-up, and selected patient and provider population. The main limitation is the relevance of the study to practice situations, i.e. the 'external validity' or 'generalisability'. Evidence taken alone from RCTs can be misleading if endpoints are not translated into measures that are valued by patients, providers, insurers, and the general public (Elliott & Payne, 2005). A growing body of recent work has identified several problems with EEs undertaken alongside RCTs that can have potentially serious impact on the ability of decision-makers to draw valid conclusions (McCabe & Dixon 2000). When healthcare authorities need to make decisions on the licensing or reimbursement of a new drug, it is highly unlikely that there will be head-to-head clinical trials of the therapies concerned. The reasons may be partly because it is often costly and time-consuming to undertake a trial with sufficient power to detect the difference between therapies, or it is not possible to undertake a trial comparing two investigational therapies, and hence the indirect comparison is adopted. Adopting indirect comparisons in economic analysis is potentially subject to bias, because of the difference in baseline risk of patients, endpoints measured, and resource use in different settings (Drummond & Sculpher, 2005). To solve the problem of indirect comparison, modelling methods can be used to simulate the data from indirect comparisons in RCTs (Drummond & Sculpher, 2005). However, the scarcity of resource use data is a particular problem for RCTs, because resource use data are often not collected and the follow-up periods of most RCTs tend to be short. Alternatively, data from observational studies, retrospective case analysis or expert opinions are often used in EEs to provide outcome and resource use data associated with an intervention in the longer term.

Observational Studies

Data from observational (epidemiological) studies can provide estimates of effectiveness, especially for rare adverse events. The non-experimental designs often offer advantages in terms of cost, time, research design, and ethics (Rittenhouse, 1996). The main advantage of outcome data extracted from observational studies is external validity (or generalisability) suggesting the outcome is more applicable to clinical practice, because longitudinal data will have a longer follow-up period (than RCTs) thus are good for resource use data collection. Observational studies seem to be practical for CAM research as CAM needs to be examined for their long-term effect. Nevertheless, non-randomised study designs may cause different sources of biases and confounding factors which may lead to misleading results (Sackett et al., 1991).

Model-Based EE

Mathematical modelling has been used widely in EEs of health care technologies (Weinstein et al., 2003). A model is any mathematical structure that simplifies reality to a level that describes the essential consequences and complications of different options for decision-making (Rittenhouse, 1996). Decision analysis is a form of modelling (Payne, 2000). It is a systematic approach to decision-making under conditions of uncertainty (Elliott & Payne,

2005). This explicit, quantitative method, which may be prescriptive, breaks complex decisions into manageable parts, analyses these parts in detail, and combines them to suggest the best course of action (Thornton et al., 1992). The purpose of modelling in health-care evaluation is to structure evidence on clinical and economic outcomes in a format that can help to inform decisions about clinical practice and health-care resource allocation (Weinstein, et al., 2003). Decision analysis enables research questions to be answered without recourse to primary research (Rittenhouse, 1996), or enables further questions to be asked of trial-based studies. Although primary cost and outcome data emerges from prospective RCTs and therefore can achieve a high level of internal validity, the data collecting process is time and cost consuming, and the outcome measures may not be relevant to actual practice. In addition, the data on outcomes and costs of interventions are never presented in a single RCT. Therefore, an analytic model is often used in cost-effectiveness analysis to synthesise data from different sources of evidence, and most trial studies involve some element of modelling or synthesis.

In modelling studies, data from a wide range of sources (e.g. existing clinical trials, epidemiological studies, best-guess estimates) are synthesized using an economic model (Drummond & Sculpher, 2005). The model-based EE makes use of a decision tree (decision analysis) or Markov model (state transition model). The former provides outcome events in one direction without recursion, whereas the latter is employed when (1) the events occur more than once, i.e. a sequential or repetitive nature, (2) the risk of an event is ongoing over time and the timing of the events is crucial, or (3) diseases, especially chronic illnesses, progress through different disease states. The model is to extrapolate beyond the trial results based on the time horizon and cycle length. It also helps calculate expected costs and expected final outcomes, i.e. life expectancy or QALYs. However, for the EE the choice of model with its structure and assumptions underpinning it should be validated by experts in the field.

The principles of decision analysis are used to define the research question and express the interventions as a decision-analytical pathway. Each uncertain event can be characterised by a single number and illustrate the decisions and uncertain events diagrammatically with a decision tree (decision-analytical model) that incorporates strategies, probabilities of subsequent events and final outcomes (Elliott & Payne, 2005). A decision tree model emanates from the 'decision node' (the square in the decision tree) where clinicians choose different interventions for patients. These decisions lead to different outcomes by chance, the branches of these outcomes emanate from 'chance nodes' (the circles in the decision tree) with the probabilities associated with them. The sum of the probabilities of all of the branches at each chance node must equal one, and there is no overlap between outcomes at chance nodes (Rittenhouse, 1996). However, a simple decision tree may not be capable of modelling chronic disease states. A model trying to represent a chronic disease must be capable of reflecting changes in and out of health states. These may be referred to as random processes that evolve over time (Elliott & Payne, 2005). State-transition models, such as Markov models, are particularly useful for representing the use of an intervention to manage chronic health states (Briggs & Sculpher, 1995).

To obtain economic and clinical evidence to apply to the decision-analytic model, the data may come from primary sources, such as an RCT, an observational study, or other published evidence. Systematic reviews of economic and clinical data are often used to find and assess information to combine with the decision-analytical model. The combination of clinical and economic parameters within the decision model framework is used to derive cost-outcome ratios. This involves the analysis of the incremental effect of an intervention on overall resource use and outcome, compared with alternatives. The robustness of the ratios is examined using sensitivity analysis to determine the variation in which parameters have most effect on the conclusions drawn (Elliott & Payne, 2005). A model integrates the resource use and cost data and links these data to outcomes that are of interest to health-care decision makers via its logical mathematical framework. The value of a model lies not only in the results it generates, but also in its ability to reveal the logical connection between input and output in the form of valued consequences and costs (Weinstein, et al., 2003). However, there are limitations associated with the use of modelling, particularly the model structure and the data used to populate that model. A model should be able to piece together the process of care such that the model is realistic in terms of the alternatives under investigation and the sequence of events. Misspecification of the model will produce erroneous and misleading results. Furthermore, data used to populate models come from diverse sources and there is an assumption that it is appropriate to combine these data and use them as though they come from a homogenous source.

Sensitivity Analysis

In an EE, as with a model, all parameters, i.e. direct or indirect costs, outcomes and ICERs, are subject to uncertainty. The uncertainty can be determined using a sensitivity analysis, which examines the degree of influence that each value of parameters has on the conclusions of an economic study (Gold, et al., 1996). The estimates of key parameters are varied individually or collectively in order to assess the sensitivity of the study result to the various assumptions. There are four main types of sensitivity analysis: (1) simple, where one or more parameters are varied across a range; (2) threshold, which identifies a critical value; (3) analysis of extremes; and (4) probabilistic sensitivity analysis. Weinstein *et al.* (2003) proposed that a modelling study should include extensive sensitivity analyses of key parameters by using either deterministic (one-way or multi-way) and/or probabilistic sensitivity analyses (Weinstein, et al., 2003). Univariate analysis (one-way, threshold and extreme analysis) changes only single parameters at one time of analysis. The one-way sensitivity analysis is performed by setting the maximum and minimum values or percentages. Then new ICERS are calculated and compared with the base case to get the proportion (%) change. The result can be presented in a table or tornado diagram. For the threshold analysis, ICERs are varied, such as 0 vs. $10,000, to get the threshold cost. If the duration of health outcomes (or time horizon) is less than 30 years, both costs and outcomes should be varied with the rate of 0-6%. If the duration is equal to or longer than 30 years, the costs should be varied with the rate of 4% and outcomes with 2%.

Probabilistic sensitivity analysis (PSA) is a method of decision analysis in which probabilistic distributions (i.e. normal, gamma or beta distribution) are specified for each uncertain parameter (e.g., probabilities, utilities, costs). Non-parametric bootstrap simulation is performed whereby values of each parameter are randomly drawn from the corresponding distribution; and the resulting probability distribution of expected utilities (and cost) is displayed (Gold, et al., 1996). The type of distribution is informed by the nature of each variable (probability, cost, effect, relative risk). Monte Carlo simulation with appropriate iterations is the commonly used method to obtain 'simulated trial' with probability of ICERs at different levels. Calculate the mean result and assess decision uncertainty by PSA. PSA is a preferred method to deal with the uncertainty. Although sensitivity analysis has been recommended to be included in EE (Briggs et al., 1994), several reviews have shown that the approaches used are often inadequate (Briggs & Sculpher, 1995). The choice of parameters and their ranges for variation in sensitivity analysis are often not adequately justified. Moreover, studies often fail to combine the effect of several parameters varying at the same time, i.e. the majority of analysts conduct only a series of one-way sensitivity analyses (Drummond & Sculpher, 2005). Some approaches to sensitivity analysis, such as multi-way sensitivity analysis, threshold analysis, and scenario analysis, partly deal with this problem. Methodological developments in recent years, such as the analysis of stochastic data from economic clinical trials (Claxton, 1999), the development of probabilistic models (Drummond & McGuire, 2001), and Bayesian interpretations of data including the use of CEAC (Briggs, 2001), have improved the analysis of uncertainty in EE (Drummond & Sculpher, 2005).

INTERPRETATION AND PRESENTATION OF RESULTS

For CEA and CUA, the EE results can be presented based in deterministic and stochastic (probabilistic) ways.

Deterministic Results

Deterministic result presents a fixed set of parameter inputs (or mean values) against a fixed set of outcomes, and the result of ICER with its range (such as 25th and 75th percentiles). For example, comparing the cost-effectiveness of two interventions, e.g. A vs. B (control), the expected costs and outcomes with the corresponding ICER can be tabulated. Intervention A will be chosen if the ICER is less than the cost-effectiveness threshold (Figure 3). In the case of three or more interventions, a cost-effectiveness plane or table is utilised by plotting the expected costs against the y axis and expected outcomes against the x axis. A cost-effectiveness (CE) plane (Krahn et al., 1997; Van Hout et al., 1994) is often employed to show how decisions can be related to both costs and effects (Figure 3) (Briggs et al., 1998). The CE plane is divided into four quadrants indicating four possible situations in relation to the additional cost and outcomes of a new therapy compared to currently available therapy. Where one intervention is simultaneously cheaper and more effective than the other, it is clearly the treatment of choice and is said to dominate (i.e. the northwest or southeast quadrant) (Karlsson & Johannesson, 1996). Where one intervention is both more effective and costly (i.e. the southwest or northeast

Figure 3. The cost-effectiveness plane comparing a new treatment to a currently provided control treatment

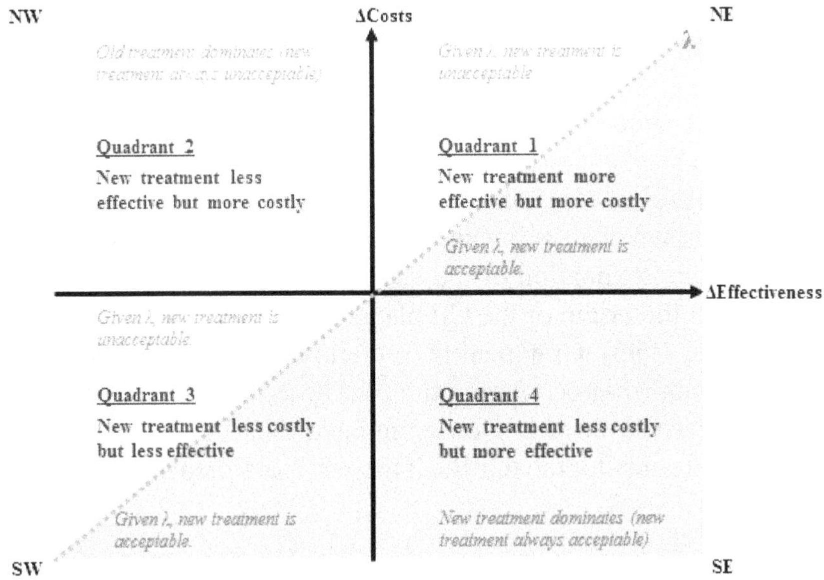

quadrant), a 'trade off' must be made between the additional outcomes and costs that must be committed to achieve those outcomes (Drummond & McGuire, 2001), and the final decision resolves around how much decision makers are willing to pay for extra benefits. The decision maker's willingness to pay, i.e. the cost-effectiveness threshold (also called the ceiling ratio, R_c or λ), depends on the interventions and country specific demographics, as well as the country's currency, inflation rate, etc. It has been suggested that $50,000 per QALY gained in the United States, £30,000 per QALY gained in the UK, and Bht 160,000 per QALY gained in Thailand are generally considered to be cost-effective.

(Note) NW = Northwest; NE = North-east; SW = Southwest; and SE = Southeast

Stochastic Results

Stochastic (probabilistic) results present a probability distribution or uncertainty of parameter inputs by simulation and produces the results from each distribution. It does not assume any known 'true' value of parameters. The simulated incremental costs and outcomes are plotted on the cost-effectiveness plane with lines showing the ceiling ratios (or thresholds).

Cost-Effectiveness Plane

The probabilistic simulation results of expected outcomes and costs of each intervention can be plotted on cost-effectiveness (CE) planes to visualize the variation within the bootstrapped samples of ICERs. The uncertainty of these ICERs can be shown by drawing an ellipse around 95% of the bootstrapped ICERs, and an approximation of the 95% confident intervals can be given by the rays from the origin of the CE plane that are tangential to the ellipse (Briggs & Fenn, 1998). Graphical presentations of ICER distributions are widely used in published economic studies. The 2.5% and 97.5% percentiles can also be extracted directly from simulated data to give a quantitative measure of uncertainty for the ICERs, if there are sufficient iterations (Elliott & Payne, 2005).

Cost-Effectiveness Acceptability Curve

The decision rules of cost-effectiveness for decision makers depend on two levels: uncertainty in the estimated values of cost effectiveness, and

Figure 4. A hypothetical example to demonstrate the cost-effectiveness plane

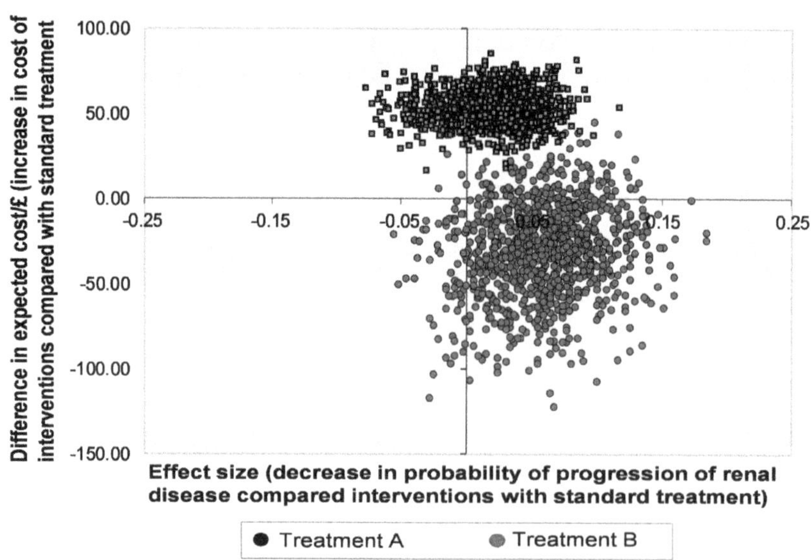

uncertainty about the maximum or ceiling cost effectiveness ratio that a decision maker would consider acceptable. CEACs can be defined in two equivalent ways, either in terms of the ICER estimator or the net-benefit (NB) estimator. The CEAC shows, for non-negative prices, the probability that a random realisation of the ICER estimator is below the price line on the CE plane or, equivalently, that a random realization of the NB estimator is above zero (Lothgren & Zethraeus, 2000). A 'net (monetary) benefit' is an alternative approach to ICER. It makes use of the cost-effectiveness threshold to value the health outcomes on the monetary scale. We usually accept the intervention if ICER is less than the ceiling ratio. A net benefit (or the optimal decision) depends on the cost-effectiveness threshold. It is feasible to calculate the probability of cost-effectiveness (or the proportion of iterations for which net benefit is greatest for that decision) at several thresholds. A cost-effectiveness acceptability curve (CEAC) is a plot of the probability of favouring each intervention being cost-effective against various ceiling ratios or WTP for a unit of outcomes. Multiple acceptability curves are used to present the results of three or more interventions. Although CEAC can present decision uncertainty, it ignores the magnitude of simulations and should not be used to determine the optimal intervention (Figure 4). A cost-effectiveness acceptability frontier demonstrates the decision uncertainty around the optimal choice (Figure 5). This can be augmented by the expected value of perfect information to render the potential gains for further research.

Figure 5. A hypothetical example to demonstrate the cost-effectiveness acceptability curve

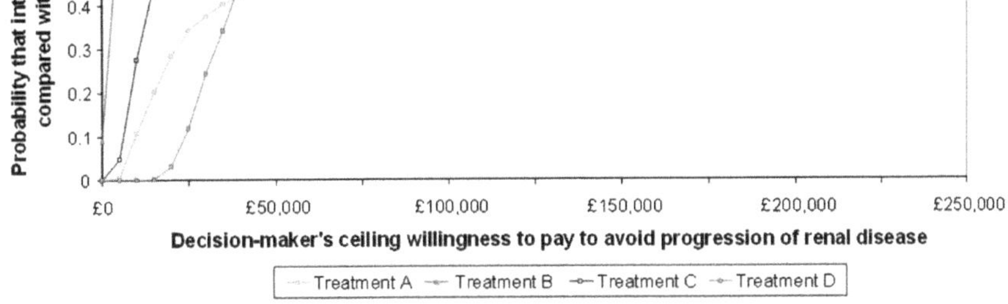

EXISTING EVIDENCE FOR EE IN COMPLEMENTARY AND ALTERNATIVE MEDICINE

There are more than 100 studies of EEs in various types of CAM, i.e. acupuncture, chiropractic, spinal manipulation, mind-body medicine, homeopathy, dietary supplements, and hypnosis (Pelletier et al., 2010). A CUA is the main form of EE required by national health guidelines (Canadian Agency for Drugs and Technologies in Health, 2006; National Institute for Health and Care Excellence, 2012). However, the evaluation of only cost and cost-effectiveness is frequently conducted in CAM (Ostermann et al., 2011). Despite the fact that the EE of CAM in patients with kidney disease is lacking, there are several systematic reviews recruited the EE of various CAM for different types of illnesses. A systematic review of studies (n = 204) published between 2001 and 2010 reported that manipulative and body-based practices, and acupuncture for back pain are the main CAMs, which were economically evaluated, followed by natural products for rheumatic disorders, cardiovascular disease, and diabetes (Herman et al., 2012). This review included CAM integrated with conventional medicine. Examples of manipulative and body-based practices are chiropractic, osteopathic manipulation, and massage. The authors found that 29% of 56 comparisons made in the high quality of studies of CUA reported that integrative medicine had better health outcomes and lower costs than usual therapy. Zhang et al. (2012) performed a systematic review of the EE of Traditional Chinese Medicine (TCM). Of the included RCTs (n = 31), acupuncture, and 'Tai Chi' were the main types of TCMs which had EE. They found inconsistent findings of TCM related to quality of life and concluded that TCM may contribute to better outcomes at a high cost (n = 10) (Zhang et al., 2012). Although herbal medicine is the most commonly used CAM and has a high number of RCTs, EE is still lacking. Baars and Kooreman (2014) compared healthcare costs and mortality rates in Dutch patients who received health care from either conventional general practitioners or CAM practitioners. They found no difference in the mortality rate between the two, although costs of the alternative care were lower than conventional care. Limitations of this study are that anthroposophic is the main CAM in this study, and the proportion of patients who received alternative care was very low (1.2%), compared with patients getting conventional care (98.8%).

Systematic Reviews and RCTs of Acupuncture for Various Illnesses

The most frequently reported EE of CAM is acupuncture. Several meta-analyses of acupuncture exist specific illness, e.g. headache and chronic pain (Ambrosio et al., 2012; Kim et al., 2012). Ambrosio et al. (2012) recruited eight EEs of acupuncture for chronic pain, dysmenorrhea, migraine, headache, or osteoarthritis. They found that the cost per QALY was below typical thresholds of WTP used by the UK National Institute for Health and Clinical Excellence. Seven cost-utility analyses showed the clinical effectiveness of acupuncture had a higher cost. Therefore, acupuncture for chronic pain may not be cost-effective and further studies are required. A systematic review reported that acupuncture for dysmenorrhea, allergic rhinitis, or headaches in Germany and UK is cost-effective (reported by CUA), compared with usual care (Kim, et al., 2012). Acupuncture was provided with or without conventional medicine. One included RCT of acupuncture for migraine in China, reported that acupuncture is likely to be cost-effective (Deng et al., 2012).

EEs of Other CAMs for Various Illnesses

A CUA recruited 60 people with constipation in Sweden (Lämås et al., 2010). The authors found that abdomen massage may be cost effective over a long term compared with laxatives. Furthermore, this intervention may be suitable for patients who do not respond to conventional medicine. Hollinghurst et al. (2008) performed a cost-effective analysis in 579 patients with chronic or recurrent low back pain. They reported that exercise with sessions in Alexander technique were cost-effective, compared with normal care (Hollinghurst et al., 2008). There is also a retrospective observational study of registered CHM integrated with conventional medicine for ischemic stroke in China between 2006 and 2010 (n=12,009) (Li et al., 2014). The authors reported that this integrative medicine is likely to be cost effective. However, further RCTs are needed to confirm this finding. Finally, Solomon et al. (2013) found that St. John's wort for mild to moderate depression may be cost effective in the long term, compared with venlafaxine and sertraline. This study was analysed using net monetary benefits and conducted in Australia. Thus, these studies provide the argument that CAM maybe cost-effective.

FUTURE RESEARCH DIRECTIONS

CHM is the main CAM for kidney diseases. There is a challenge of conducting EE of CHM due to their inconsistent outcomes in quality of life. A CUA is the preferred form of EEs in CAM (the same as in conventional medicine). Traditional herbal medicine (THM) is commonly used in Africa and Asia. Patients using THM believe that this medicine is cheaper than conventional medicine. However, studies of the cost-effectiveness of THM are rare and needed to investigate both patient's and policy maker's perspectives.

CONCLUSION

EEs provide evidence to inform healthcare decision making. There are a variety of methods that are available to investigate different research questions. The methodologies for assessing cost and outcome, controlling uncertainty and applying EE results are still developing. Although the principle approaches for EE of conventional medicine is likely to be applied to assess economic outcomes of CAM for kidney diseases. The currently available evidence showed that acupuncture for pain, headache, and rhinitis is the most common CAM supported by EE. Despite several meta-analyses of CHM for chronic kidney disease, there is a lack of evidence for EE. EEs have been found widely used at the central decision-making level, e.g. reimbursement policy or recommendations in national guidelines, however, they have not been adopted locally mainly due to the discrepancy in key decision-making considerations. A manual of national guidelines in many countries has recommended that treatment should be researched using CUA before their national health system decides whether this treatment will be used. However, EEs are not routinely conducted for registration purposes and decision makers often need to make a decision based on imperfect or insufficient information. In addition, the transferability of EE results across different countries is generally poor due to different perspectives of decision makers as well as different costs and outcome measures. Assessing the cost-effectiveness of CAM requires evidence for both benefits and costs of CAM, however, the main challenge to evaluate economic outcomes in CAM is the uncertain benefits of CAM. This chapter has provided healthcare practitioners and academic researchers an overview about the principles of health EEs that may be considered for either conducting or appraising further economic studies. However, as the methodology and application of EE are fast developing, it is necessary to keep updating the knowledge around this area.

REFERENCES

Ambrosio, E. M. M., Bloor, K., & MacPherson, H. (2012). Costs and consequences of acupuncture as a treatment for chronic pain: A systematic review of EEs conducted alongside randomised controlled trials. *Complementary Therapies in Medicine*, *20*(5), 364–374. doi:10.1016/j.ctim.2012.05.002 PMID:22863652

Baars, E. W., & Kooreman, P. (2014). A 6-year comparative EE of healthcare costs and mortality rates of Dutch patients from conventional and CAM GPs. *BMJ Open*, *4*, e005332. doi:10.1136/bmjopen-2014-005332 PMID:25164536

Brennan, A., & Akehurst, R. (2000). Modelling in health EE- what is its place? what is its value? *PharmacoEconomics*, *17*(5), 445–459. doi:10.2165/00019053-200017050-00004 PMID:10977387

Bridges, J. F., Cohen, J. P., Grist, P. G., & Mühlbacher, A. C. (2010). International experience with comparative effectiveness research: Case studies from England/Wales and Germany. *Advances in Health Economics and Health Services Research*, *22*, 29–50. doi:10.1108/S0731-2199(2010)0000022005 PMID:20575227

Briggs, A., & Fenn, P. (1998). Confidence intervals or surfaces? Uncertainty on the cost-effectiveness plane. *Health Economics*, *7*(8), 723–740. doi:10.1002/(SICI)1099-1050(199812)7:8<723::AID-HEC392>3.0.CO;2-O PMID:9890333

Briggs, A., & Sculpher, M. (1995). Sensitivity analysis in EE: A review of published studies. *Health Economics*, *4*, 355–371. doi:10.1002/hec.4730040502 PMID:8563834

Briggs, A., Sculpher, M., & Buxton, M. (1994). Uncertainty in the EE of health care technologies: The role of sensitivity analysis. *Health Economics*, *3*(2), 95–104. doi:10.1002/hec.4730030206 PMID:8044216

Briggs, A. H. (2001). A Bayesian approach to stochastic cost-effectiveness analysis. An illustration and application to blood pressure control in type 2 diabetes. *International Journal of Technology Assessment in Health Care*, *17*(1), 69–82. doi:10.1017/S0266462301104071 PMID:11329846

Canadian Agency for Drugs and Technologies in Health. (2006). *Guidelines for the EE of health technologies*. Author.

Claxton, K. (1999). The irrelevance of inference: A decision-making approach to the stochastic evaluation of health care technologies. *Journal of Health Economics*, *18*(3), 341–364. doi:10.1016/S0167-6296(98)00039-3 PMID:10537899

Claxton, K., Sculpher, M., & Drummond, M. (2002). A rational framework for decision making by the National Institute For Clinical Excellence (NICE). *Lancet*, *360*(9334), 711–715. doi:10.1016/S0140-6736(02)09832-X PMID:12241891

Claxton, K., Sculpher, M., McCabe, C., Briggs, A., Akehurst, R., Buxton, M., & OHagan, T. et al. (2005). Probabilistic sensitivity analysis for NICE technology assessment: Not an optional extra. *Health Economics*, *14*(4), 339–347. doi:10.1002/hec.985 PMID:15736142

Coast, J. (2004). Is EE in touch with societys health values? *British Medical Journal*, *329*(7476), 1233–1236. doi:10.1136/bmj.329.7476.1233 PMID:15550430

Coulter, D., Herman, P. M., & Nataraj, S. (2013). Economic analysis of complementary, alternative, and integrative medicine: Considerations raised by an expert panel. *BMC Complementary and Alternative Medicine*, *13*(1), 191. doi:10.1186/1472-6882-13-191 PMID:23885789

Davis, M. A., & Weeks, W. B. (2012). The concentration of out-of-pocket expenditures on complementary and alternative medicine in the United States. *Alternative Therapies in Health and Medicine*, *18*(5), 36–42. PMID:22894889

Deng, Z., Zheng, H., Zhao, L., Zhou, S. Y., Li, Y., & Liang, F. R. (2012). Health EE of acupuncture along meridians for treating migraine in China: Results from a randomized controlled trial. *BMC Complementary and Alternative Medicine*, *12*, 75. doi:10.1186/1472-6882-12-75 PMID:22697367

Donaldson, C., & Gerard, K. (1993). *Economics of healthcare financing: the visible hand*. London: Macmillan. doi:10.1007/978-1-349-22512-5

Drummond, M. (1992). Cost-illness studies: A major headache? *PharmacoEconomics*, *2*(1), 1–4. doi:10.2165/00019053-199202010-00001 PMID:10146974

Drummond, M., & Jefferson, T. (1996). Guidelines for authors and peer reviewers of economic submissions to the BMJ. The BMJ EE Working Party. *British Medical Journal*, *313*(7052), 275–283. doi:10.1136/bmj.313.7052.275 PMID:8704542

Drummond, M., & McGuire, A. (2001). *EE in health care: merging theory with practice*. Oxford, UK: Oxford University Press.

Drummond, M., O'Brien, B., & Stoddart, G. (1998). *Methods for the EE of health care programmes* (2nd ed.). New York: Oxford Medical Publications.

Drummond, M., & Sculpher, M. (2005). Common methodological flaws in EEs. *Medical Care*, *43*(7 Suppl.), 5–14. PMID:16056003

Elliott, R., & Payne, K. (2005). *Essentials of EE in healthcare*. London: Pharmaceutical Press.

EuroQol Group. (2004). *Website of the EuroQol Group*. Retrieved from http://www.euroqol.org/

Fenwick, E., Claxton, K., & Sculpher, M. (2001). Representing uncertainty: The role of cost-effectiveness acceptability curves. *Health Economics*, *10*(8), 779–787. doi:10.1002/hec.635 PMID:11747057

Fenwick, E., Claxton, K., Sculpher, M., & Briggs, A. (2000). *Improving the efficacy and relevance of health technology assessment: the role of iterative decision analytic modelling*. Academic Press.

Fenwick, E., OBrien, B. J., & Briggs, A. (2004). Cost-effectiveness acceptability curvesfacts, fallacies and frequently asked questions. *Health Economics*, *13*(5), 405–415. doi:10.1002/hec.903 PMID:15127421

Gold, M., Siegel, J., Russell, L., & Weinstein, M. (1996). *Cost-effectiveness in health and medicine*. New York: Oxford University Press.

Goodacre, S. W., & McCabe, C. (2002). An introduction to EE. *Emergency Medicine Journal*, *19*(3), 198–201. doi:10.1136/emj.19.3.198 PMID:11971826

Haycox, A., & Walley, T. (1997). Pharmacoeconomics: Evaluating the evaluators. *British Journal of Clinical Pharmacology*, *43*(5), 451–456. doi:10.1046/j.1365-2125.1997.00575.x PMID:9159558

Herman, P. M., Poindexter, B. L., Witt, C. M., & Eisenberg, D. M. (2012). Are complementary therapies and integrative care cost-effective? A systematic review of EEs. *BMJ Open*, *2*, e001046. doi:10.1136/bmjopen-2012-001046 PMID:22945962

Hollinghurst, S., Sharp, D., Ballard, K., Barnett, J., Beattie, A., Evans, M., & Little, P. et al. (2008). Randomised controlled trial of Alexander technique lessons, exercise, and massage (ATEAM) for chronic and recurrent back pain: Economic evauation. *BMJ (Clinical Research Ed.)*, *337*(dec11 2), a2656. doi:10.1136/bmj.a2656 PMID:19074232

Husereau, D., Drummond, M., Petrou, S., Carswell, C., Moher, D., & Greenberg, D. (2013). Consolidated Health EE Reporting Standards (CHEERS) statement. *Cost Effectiveness and Resource Allocation*, *11*(1), 6.

Johannesson, M. (1995). The relationship between cost-effectiveness analysis and cost-benefit analysis. *Social Science & Medicine*, *41*(4), 483–489.

Jolicoeur, L. M., Jones-Grizzle, A. J., & Boyer, J. G. (1992). Guidelines for performing a pharmacoeconomic analysis. *American Journal of Hospital Pharmacy*, *49*(7), 1741–1747. PMID:1621734

Karlsson, G., & Johannesson, M. (1996). The decision rules of cost-effectiveness analysis. *PharmacoEconomics*, *9*(2), 113–120. doi:10.2165/00019053-199609020-00003 PMID:10160090

Kielhorn, A., & Graf von der Schulenburg, J.-M. (2000). The health economics handbook (2nd ed.). Glaxo Wellcome Group of Companies.

Kim, S. Y., Lee, H., Chae, Y., Park, H. J., & Lee, H. (2012). A systematic review of cost-effectiveness analyses alongside randomised controlled trials of acupuncture. *Acupuncture in Medicine*, *30*(4), 273–285. doi:10.1136/acupmed-2012-010178 PMID:23099289

Klose, T. (1999). The contingent valuation method in health care. *Health Policy (Amsterdam)*, *47*(2), 97–123. doi:10.1016/S0168-8510(99)00010-X PMID:10538292

Kobelt, G. (1996). *Health Economics: An introduction to EE*. London: Office of Health Economics.

Koopmanschap, M. A., & Rutten, F. F. (1996). A practical guide for calculating indirect costs of disease. *PharmacoEconomics*, *10*(5), 460–466. doi:10.2165/00019053-199610050-00003 PMID:10172868

Koopmanschap, M. A., Rutten, F. F., van Ineveld, B. M., & van Roijen, L. (1995). The friction cost method for measuring indirect costs of disease. *Journal of Health Economics*, *14*(2), 171–189. doi:10.1016/0167-6296(94)00044-5 PMID:10154656

Krahn, M. D., Naglie, G., Naimark, D., Redelmeier, D. A., & Detsky, A. S. (1997). Primer on medical decision analysis: Part 4Analyzing the model and interpreting the results. *Medical Decision Making*, *17*(2), 142–151. doi:10.1177/0272989X9701700204 PMID:9107609

Lämås, K., Lindholm, L., Engstrom, B., & Jacobsson, C. (2010). Abdominal massage for people with constipation: A cost utility analysis. *Journal of Advanced Nursing*, *66*(8), 1719–1729. doi:10.1111/j.1365-2648.2010.05339.x PMID:20557387

Li, Y., Xi, H. X., Zhu, S., Yu, N., Wang, J., Li, Y., & Zhao, L. et al. (2014). Cost-effectiveness analysis of combined Chinese medicine and Western medicine for ischemic stroke patients. *Chinese Journal of Integrative Medicine*, *20*(8), 570–584. doi:10.1007/s11655-014-1759-9 PMID:25087603

Lothgren, M., & Zethraeus, N. (2000). Definition, interpretation and calculation of cost-effectiveness acceptability curves. *Health Economics*, *9*(7), 623–630. doi:10.1002/1099-1050(200010)9:7<623::AID-HEC539>3.0.CO;2-V PMID:11103928

Mauskopf, J. A., Paul, J. E., Grant, D. M., & Stergachis, A. (1998). The role of cost-consequence analysis in healthcare decision-making. *PharmacoEconomics*, *13*(3), 277–288. doi:10.2165/00019053-199813030-00002 PMID:10178653

McCabe, C., & Dixon, S. (2000). Testing the validity of cost-effectiveness models. *PharmacoEconomics*, *17*(5), 501–513. doi:10.2165/00019053-200017050-00007 PMID:10977390

McKinnell, I., Elliot, J., & Frankish, R. (1999). *The Cochrane Library self-training guide*. York: NHS Centre for Reviews and Dissemination.

Medical Outcomes Trust. (2004). *SF-36.org*. Retrieved from http://www.rand.org/health/surveys_tools/mos/36-item-short-form.html

National Institute for Health and Care Excellence. (2012). *Process and methods guides: The guidelines manual*. Retrieved from https://www.nice.org.uk/process/pmg6/chapter/introduction

Ostermann, T., Krummenauer, F., Heusser, P., & Boehm, K. (2011). Health EE in complementary medicine: Development within the last decades concerning local origin and quality. *Complementary Therapies in Medicine*, *19*(6), 289–302. doi:10.1016/j.ctim.2011.09.002 PMID:22036521

Palmer, S., Byford, S., & Raftery, J. (1999). Economics notes: Types of EE. *British Medical Journal*, *318*(7194), 1349. doi:10.1136/bmj.318.7194.1349 PMID:10323827

Payne, K. (2000). *The economic impact of decision-making in relation to the introduction of drug into practice*. Academic Press.

Pelletier, K. R., Herman, P. M., Metz, R. D., & Nelson, C. F. (2010). Health and medical economics applied to integrative medicine. *Explore (New York, N.Y.)*, *6*(2), 86–99. doi:10.1016/j.explore.2009.12.009 PMID:20362266

Reeder, C. E. (1995). Overview of pharmacoeconomics and pharmaceutical outcomes evaluations. *American Journal of Health-System Pharmacy*, *52*(19Suppl 4), S5–S8. PMID:8846244

Rittenhouse, B. (1996). *Uses of models in EEs of medicines and other health technologies*. London: Office of Health Economics.

Robbins, L. (1935). *An Essay on the Nature and Significance of Economic Science* (2nd ed.). London: Macmillan.

Robinson, R. (1993a). Cost-benefit analysis. *British Medical Journal*, *307*(6909), 924–926. doi:10.1136/bmj.307.6909.924 PMID:8241859

Robinson, R. (1993b). Cost-utility analysis. *British Medical Journal*, *307*(6908), 859–862. doi:10.1136/bmj.307.6908.859 PMID:8401133

Robinson, R. (1993c). Costs and cost-minimisation analysis. *British Medical Journal*, *307*(6906), 726–728. doi:10.1136/bmj.307.6906.726 PMID:8401098

Russell, L. B., Gold, M. R., Siegel, J. E., Daniels, N., & Weinstein, M. C. (1996). The role of cost-effectiveness analysis in health and medicine. Panel on Cost-Effectiveness in Health and Medicine. *Journal of the American Medical Association*, *276*(14), 1172–1177. doi:10.1001/jama.1996.03540140060028 PMID:8827972

Ryan, M., & Shackley, P. (1995). Assessing the benefits of health care: How far should we go? *Quality in Health Care*, *4*(3), 207–213. doi:10.1136/qshc.4.3.207 PMID:10153432

Sackett, D., Haynes, R., Guyatt, G., & Tugwell, P. (1991). Clinical epidemiology: a basic science for clinical medicine (2nd ed.). Boston: Little Brown.

Shwartz, M., Young, D. W., & Siegrist, R. (1995). The ratio of costs to charges: How good a basis for estimating costs? *Inquiry*, *32*(4), 476–481. PMID:8567084

Singer, J., & Adams, J. (2014). Integrating complementary and alternative medicine into mainstream healthcare services: The perspectives of health service managers. *BMC Complementary and Alternative Medicine*, *14*(1), 167. doi:10.1186/1472-6882-14-167 PMID:24885066

Solomon, D., Adams, J., & Graves, N. (2013). EE of St. Johns wort (*Hypericum perforatum*) for the treatment of mild to moderate depression. *Journal of Affective Disorders*, *148*(2-3), 228–234. doi:10.1016/j.jad.2012.11.064 PMID:23291009

Spinks, J., & Hollingsworth, B. (2009). Are the economics of complementary and alternative medicine different to conventional medicine?. *Expert Rev Pharmacoecon Outcomes Res*, *9*(1), 1–4. doi:10.1586/14737167.9.1.1 PMID:19371170

Tan-Torres Edejert, R. A., Baltussen, T., Hutubessy, R., Acharya, A., Evans, D. B., & Murray, C. J. L. (2003). Making choices in health: WHO guide to cost-effectiveness analysis. Geneva: World Health Organization.

Thomas, K. J., Nicholl, J. P., & Coleman, P. (2001). Use and expenditure on complementary medicine in England: A population based survey. *Complementary Therapies in Medicine*, *9*(1), 2–11. doi:10.1054/ctim.2000.0407 PMID:11264963

Thornton, J. G., Lilford, R. J., & Johnson, N. (1992). Decision analysis in medicine. *British Medical Journal*, *304*(6834), 1099–1103. doi:10.1136/bmj.304.6834.1099 PMID:1530694

Torgerson, D., & Raftery, J. (1999). Economics notes: Measuring outcomes in EEs. *British Medical Journal*, *318*(7195), 1413. doi:10.1136/bmj.318.7195.1413 PMID:10334758

Torrance, G. (1987). Utility approach to measuring health-related quality of life. *Journal of Chronic Diseases*, *40*(6), 593–603. doi:10.1016/0021-9681(87)90019-1 PMID:3298297

Van Hout, B. A., & Maiwenn, J. A. (1994). Costs, effects and C/E-ratios alongside a clinical trial. *Health Economics*, *3*(5), 309–319. doi:10.1002/hec.4730030505 PMID:7827647

Weinstein, M. C., OBrien, B., Hornberger, J., Jackson, J., Johannesson, M., McCabe, C., & Luce, B. R. (2003). Principles of good practice for decision analytic modeling in health-care evaluation: Report of the ISPOR Task Force on Good Research Practices Modeling Studies. *Value in Health*, *6*(1), 9–17. doi:10.1046/j.1524-4733.2003.00234.x PMID:12535234

Weisbrod, B. (1961). The valuation of human capital. *Journal of Political Economy*, *69*(5), 425–436. doi:10.1086/258535

Xue, C., Zhang, A., Lin, V., Da Costa, C., & Story, D. (2007). Complementary and alternative medicine use in Australia: A national population-based survey. *Journal of Alternative and Complementary Medicine (New York, N.Y.)*, *13*(6), 643–650. doi:10.1089/acm.2006.6355 PMID:17718647

Zhang, F., Kong, L., Zhang, Y. Y., & Li, S. C. (2012). Evaluation of impact on health-related quality of life and cost effectiveness of traditional Chinese medicine: A systematic review of randomized clinical trials. *Journal of Alternative and Complementary Medicine (New York, N.Y.)*, *18*(12), 1108–1120. doi:10.1089/acm.2011.0315 PMID:22924383

KEY TERMS AND DEFINITIONS

Cost-Effectiveness Analysis: A method of comparing the cost and effectiveness of two or more alternatives to allow the decision maker to determine whether the value of an intervention justifies its cost.

Cost-Utility Analysis: An alternative method of cost-effectiveness analysis to compare costs of different interventions with their outcomes measured in 'utility based' units, i.e. units that relate to a person's level of wellbeing, and the most commonly used unit is the quality adjusted life year (QALYs). It enables QALYs to be calculated and interventions ranked according to cost per QALY gained.

Cost-Benefit Analysis: A method estimating and summing up the equivalent money value of the benefits and costs of different interventions to enable the calculation of the net cost or benefit associated with the intervention.

Economic Evaluation: A study that compares the costs and benefits of two or more alternative interventions in order to inform decision-making for achieving efficiency in using finite resources.

Quality Adjusted Life Year: A utility measure that is calculated by estimating the total life years gained from an intervention and weighting each year to reflect the quality of life in that year.

Utility: A numerical value the individuals attached for a particular health state based on preference.

Willingness to Pay: The maximum sum an individual (or a government) is willing to pay to acquire some good or service, or the maximum sum an individual (or government) is willing to pay to avoid a prospective loss.

Chapter 10
Integrative Medicine and Prospective Research on CAM

Mayuree Tangkiatkumjai
Srinakharinwirot University, Thailand

Annalisa Casarin
The NIHR Research Design Service East of England, UK

ABSTRACT

There is a link between integrative medicine (IM) and prospective research on complementary and alternative medicine (CAM). IM is the future direction of CAM and research is needed to support clinical practice. Meaning of IM, proposed models of IM, and existing research on IM will be presented. Prospective research on CAM will cover methodologies presenting randomised controlled trials, harms studies of CAM in kidney disease, and a gap of CAM research. Study design and outcome measures are current challenges in CAM/IM research. Several networks of CAM research worldwide are still working on them and have proposed possible alternative approaches, such as pragmatic clinical trials and cohort multiple randomised controlled trials. These approaches would solve some limitations of randomised controlled trials in CAM research.

DOI: 10.4018/978-1-5225-2882-1.ch010

INTRODUCTION

The World Health Organization (WHO) Traditional Medicine Strategy 2014-2023 suggested promoting universal health coverage by integrating CAM into conventional medicine (World Health Organization, 2013). Three Asian countries provide full coverage of traditional medicine integrated into their national health system, i.e. China, South Korea and Vietnam. In Switzerland, partial integration of CAM is employed (World Health Organization, 2013). Integrative medicine (IM) is a new term in the CAM field, compared with the terms complementary or alternative medicine. There is no consensus on the definition of IM. One definition of this term focused on its meaning is 'IM is the use of CAM integrated into conventional medicine, which should be supported by evidence' (Walach, 2010). Hu et al. (2015) proposed five key elements of IM as described by an expert consensus: (1) presence of aspects of both CAM and conventional medicine; (2) goals of health and healing; (3) holistic approach; (4) optimum treatment; and (5) uses the body's innate healing response.

Patients with chronic diseases tend to use CAM with their conventional medicine as they hope that CAM could complement it, including patients with kidney disease (Tangkiatkumjai et al., 2014). Several chronic diseases are frequently treated by IM, such as asthma, rheumatic disease, chronic inflammatory bowel disorder, and chronic pain (Dobos & Tao, 2011). Patients need to know how to integrate CAM with their conventional medicine in order to obtain both higher efficacy and lower adverse effects of conventional medicine. Both CAM and conventional systems have their own advantages and disadvantages, so their integration would be an option for some illnesses that cannot be fully treated by one system. CAM users and conventional practitioners are also concerned about the interaction between them, which may be either synergistic or antagonistic. Research on IM is therefore required to support clinical decision-making. This chapter will describe existing IM models, research on IM and a checklist for reporting research on IM. The section of prospective research on CAM methodologies will: (1) discuss a research approach to building up evidence for CAM; (2) highlight major issues of methodologies of randomised controlled trials (RCTs) in CAM/IM research; (3) propose plausible solutions for those issues; and (4) provide prospective research on CAM/IM in kidney diseases.

Some models of an IM service have been proposed in primary care in many countries, which includes 1) the choice between systematic or individual IM; and 2) the need for collaboration between CAM and conventional practitioners (Templeman & Robinson, 2011). Such IM models would give an idea for practitioners who would like to develop an IM service in their setting. However, outcome studies of IM services are very limited. Khorsan et al. (2011) and Grant et al. (2015) systematically reviewed IM research and faced a challenge of inconsistently defined IM, which was an obstacle to analyzing the findings. To promote robust reporting evidence on IM, Hu et al. (2015) proposed a checklist for standard reporting clinical trials of IM. Regarding CAM research, Fønnebø et al. (2007) proposed 'Reverse research strategies' between conventional and alternative medicine, which seems to be suitable for CAM/IM research. CAM research should start with what people use in practice, followed by the safety and efficacy of CAM, and pre-clinical studies. This strategy reverses research on conventional medicine, which starts with *in vitro* and *in vivo*, followed by phase I clinical trials to test its safety, then RCTs to prove its efficacy. For example, in the case of herbal medicine, its safety should be investigated prior to its effectiveness and mechanism of action. If positive and negative effects of herbal medicine were examined in the same way as conventional medicine, it would be costly and time consuming. Further studies are required to provide robust evidence for the efficacy and safety of CAM. This chapter focuses on the methodology of RCTs. As the methodology of choice, RCTs have been criticised by CAM researchers because they are inappropriate for CAM. Fischer et al. (2012) systematically reviewed several RCTs of CAM methods and effectiveness, and found five key issues of methodological problems: (1) double-blinding; (2) randomisation; (3) standardised CAM modalities; (4) defined outcomes in CAM; and (5) a choice of a proper control group. They have also suggested pragmatic clinical trials (PCTs) for CAM research, rather than RCTs, as an appropriate methodology for CAM research, and solutions for such issues that will be described later. However, Relton (2013) disagreed that PCTs were suitable for CAM research as these trials may increase some biases, such as cognitive measurement and selection biases. She proposed a new approach for CAM research: 'cohort multiple randomised controlled trial' design (cmRCT). This method is promising to solving unsuccessful recruitment, randomisation and blinding in CAM research. In addition, a mixed methods study is another approach for CAM research. The qualitative method alongside a clinical trial will better understand the effects of interventions and how they are experienced by patients (Lewin et al., 2009).

INTEGRATIVE MEDICINE

This section describes and discusses models of IM, research on IM and a checklist for reporting research on IM.

Models of Integrative Medicine

Templeman and Robinson (2011) reviewed IM models and found two issues in IM models which are: (1) the choice between systematic or individual IM; and (2) the need for collaboration between CAM and conventional practitioners. The systematic IM is defined as the integration of the best effectiveness of both CAM and conventional medicine in order to provide an optimal health outcome for a patient. This model has been employed in the UK and Australia, although it is quite difficult to implement if there is a lack of rigorous scientific evidence regarding which CAM has the highest effectiveness for what illness. The individual IM adopts both holistic and patient-centred approaches and a practitioner needs to select the CAM and conventional medicine that is well suited to an individual patient, based on his/her need, which consists of mind, body, emotion and spirit. This concept is therefore quite abstract for a conventional health practitioner. Whereas, CAM practitioners instinctively adopt such concepts as they assess their patient's medical need by considering all of those elements. Limitations of this model are that some practitioners may not assess all elements and be skillful at providing integration of CAM and conventional medicine. This model is more likely to serve patient satisfaction, however, a patient treated by this model should be evaluated for his/her clinical outcomes as well. The major concern of both models is whether or not CAM and conventional medicine have an interaction regarding adverse events. Therefore, further research on IM is in great demand. Table 1 shows types of IM models in each country. It is important to keep in mind that the development of IM models in each country is ongoing, so such models may be changed in the future.

Regarding collaboration between CAM and conventional practitioners, three models are: (1) a multidisciplinary team of CAM and conventional practitioners; (2) a referral system; or (3) clinicians who have been trained in both conventional medicine and CAM. Firstly, CAM practitioners become a member of a multidisciplinary team of health professionals. Theoretically this model seems to provide more effective outcomes for a patient as all practitioners have a chance to discuss and solve their patient's problems

Table 1. Integrative medicine experience in primary care

Country	Model	Common Types of CAM Modality	Limitation
Australia	Referral system Conventional medicine practitioners with training CAM	Chiropractic Osteopathy Naturopathy	Inconsistency of the IM system Limited access to IM
China	GPs with training both conventional medicine and TCM	Acupuncture TCM	Time-consuming for the training programme
Germany	Multidisciplinary team of health professionals	Naturopathy Anthroposophic therapy TCM Homeopathy Acupuncture	Time-consuming for a multidisciplinary team meeting
Thailand	Direct-working within a hospital Prescribed herbal medicine by GPs	Massage Herbal medicine	Lack of knowledge about herbal medicine amongst GPs
UK	Referral system Direct-working within the same setting Biomedical practitioners with training in CAM, e.g. acupuncture	Acupuncture Homeopathy Chiropractic Aromatherapy Massage Reflexology Hypnotherapy	Inconsistency of the IM system Limited access to IM Little financial support in some settings Poor communication channel between CAM and conventional practitioners
USA[a]	Referral system Direct-working within the same setting	Acupuncture/TCM Chiropractic Mental health care Naturopathy Yoga Massage	Inconsistency of the IM system Limited access to IM

GPs = General Practitioners; TCM = Traditional Chinese Medicine

[a]IM has been most frequently used for five conditions in the US: chronic pain, gastrointestinal disorders, depression or anxiety, cancer and stress (Horrigan et al., 2012).

together. However, pragmatic clinical trials are required to confirm the benefits of this model. This model is more likely to be appropriate for patients with multiple co-morbidities as their illnesses are more complex and need several specialists for different aspects. Simple illnesses may not require this model if one system can cure it. In this case, IM may become a luxury asset and may be inappropriate for health care system in developing countries.

An example of the German model is a multidisciplinary team of an IM model in hospitalised patients. The German health care system has established the official German Operationen- und Prozedurenschlüssel or OPS (Operation and Procedure Code), which is a code for the diagnosis of complex illnesses requiring IM (Romeyke & Stummer, 2015). For instance, OPS 8-975 is Naturopathic and Anthroposophic medical complex therapy.

The OPS is linked to a hospital payment system in Germany and provide 'the flat-rate pay system diagnosis-related group', i.e. the government will reimburse a fixed cost for a list of diseases treated by IM. Advantages of the German model are that due to the firm structure of an IM service, there is a consistent system across the country.

The collaboration between CAM and conventional practitioners model was adopted in the US and UK, and to a lesser extent in Australia (Templeman & Robinson, 2011). Sundberg et al. (2007) reported a plausible model for IM services in Swedish primary care in which a general practitioner is a gatekeeper to discuss a care plan with their patients. If CAM is considered as necessary by way of a consensus of an IM team, it will be included in the care plan. Additionally, a collaborative system of both conventional and alternative medicine practitioners was developed in Denmark (Skovgaard et al., 2012). The concept of a multidisciplinary team was also applied in South Korea, Zambia and Uganda and showed successful collaboration between both (Park et al., 2014; Sundberg et al., 2014). A drawback of the collaborative model is that it is time-consuming for both CAM and conventional practitioners. Therefore, further research on cost-effectiveness of the IM model is required to evaluate whether or not an IM system outweighs a conventional medicine system or CAM alone. Secondly, a referral system is where a conventional medicine practitioner refers their patient to a CAM practitioner if necessary. They need to build their referral network in order to work together. This model requires a sufficient number of CAM practitioners. It is more practical to apply in any countries where they are relying primarily on a conventional medical service. A self-referral system is frequently used in Western countries where patients would like to use CAM. Limitations of this model may be lack of coordination between both systems, lack of CAM practitioners, and expense of patients to pay for their CAM. Many countries, e.g. Africa, depend on traditional medicine as a mainstream service and may be unsuitable for this model due to limited access to conventional medicine.

The final model is where clinicians who have been trained in both conventional medicine and CAM. For example, doctors in China must be trained in both, so they can diagnose and treat their patients using both approaches depending on which approach is most suited to their patient's condition. From the authors of this chapter's opinion, this model seems to provide the optimal outcome for a patient, compared with the first two models. However, the clinicians need to study and be trained for a long time. The Chinese model is an example of a successful model for IM services and could be applied to a country which relies on traditional medicine. For instance, the government of India aims to develop universal health coverage by integrating Indian traditional medicine into conventional medicine by 2020 and will learn from the Chinese experience (Patwardhan & Mutalik, 2014). Likewise, many biomedical doctors in Western countries have been trained acupuncture; therefore, they can suggest an alternative choice of treatment for their patient where appropriate. The UK has adopted all of the three models of IM.

The key components of achieving the establishment of an IM system are shared philosophy of care, interprofessional relationships and trust in referrals (Gray & Orrock, 2014). Both CAM and conventional medicine practitioners should share their philosophy in order to understand each other. This component would lead to building up their relationship and trust. However, these models may be inappropriate for all settings and some settings may want to design their own model. A mixed methods study has been suggested to investigate new models of IM (Sundberg, et al., 2014).

Some barriers to implement IM are that if conventional medicine practitioners do not accept CAM due to a lack of rigorous evidence of the effectiveness of IM modalities, and it is difficult to form collaborations between CAM and conventional medicine practitioners. Research on IM is needed to establish robust scientific evidence of the effectiveness, safety, and cost-effectiveness of IM. Rigorous evidence on IM would lead to IM being embedded in clinical practice guidelines, and then the costs of IM would be covered by the national health system or insurance. At the moment IM cannot be fully reimbursed in some countries, e.g. Sweden.

Research on Integrative Medicine

Integrative medicine needs research to design IM models and evaluate their efficacy and safety in order to provide what IM model suits each setting. There are only a small number of existing RCTs and PCTs aimed to evaluate outcomes of IM services. This is due to difficulties designing a study of IM, inconsistent definitions, and lack of defined appropriate outcomes of IM. Research on IM faces more challenges than CAM research. Discussion and recommendations for appropriate methodologies is presented below. Most of the current studies are in cancer or chronic pain. Unfortunately, clinical trials of IM services in kidney diseases were not found. The existing evidence for evaluating IM services is: (1) two systematic reviews assessing existing IM services in Sweden, the UK and US; (2) a meta-analysis of RCTs evaluating the effectiveness and safety of IM services in China; (3) a study evaluating a comparative economic outcome of an IM service in the Netherlands; and (4) a survey of existing healing services in the UK.

Firstly, Khorsan et al. (2011) systematically reviewed studies of IM modalities in order to assess the level of evidence for IM research and suggest further research on IM and found four RCTs and two clinical trials in patients with cardiovascular diseases or breast cancer. These studies indicated most research evaluated existing IM clinics and measured an outcome before and after implementing IM clinics. The authors suggest that observational studies are suitable for evaluating existing IM clinics as the intervention has been already implemented. In 2015, another systematic review of clinical trials of IM modalities in patients with low back pain was published (Grant et al., 2015). This systematic review included two RCTs, two PCTs and one case-control study. Humanistic outcomes, e.g. quality of life, symptom relief and patient self-assessment, were the main outcomes and one study reported the crude costs of IM services. The weaknesses of the included studies were lack of blinding of health care providers and participants, and outcome measurements. Both systematic reviews faced the challenge of defining IM modalities in order to recruit more relevant studies. Secondly, a meta-analysis determined the effectiveness and safety of IM modalities for treating low back pain, and included 56 RCTs (n = 6,616) (Hu, et al., 2015). The intervention was the integration of CAM and conventional medicine at the same setting in China. Examples of such interventions were: (1) acupuncture together with traction; (2) Chinese herbal medicine (CHM) integrated with acupuncture; (3) conventional medicine and traction; and (4) acupuncture with conventional medicine. The control groups received standard medicine, usual care or CAM. The primary outcome, pain symptoms, was measured using validated self-report questionnaires, such as the Roland Morris Disability Questionnaire or the Oswestry Disability Index. The authors reported that IM was significantly superior to conventional medicine alone (mean difference [MD] in pain scores: -12.8; 95%CI: -14.1,-11.5, I^2: 38%), or CAM (MD: -5.1; 95%CI: -7.6,-2.5, I^2: 85%) in the short-term ($\leq$3 months). The results had a high heterogeneity due to small sample sizes and poor quality of the included studies, e.g. lack of blinding and unclear allocation concealment. Therefore, this finding should be interpreted with caution. Additionally, 28% of RCTs reported adverse effects i.e. acupuncture caused soreness, pain, circulation problems, bruising and lightheadedness, and CHM induced dizziness, nausea and vomiting.

Thirdly, Baars and Kooreman (2014) aimed to compare total annual healthcare costs in the last year of life and mortality rates between patients with terminal illnesses who had a conventional general practitioner (GP), or had a GP who were trained CAM. Most IM practitioners were trained in anthroposophathy. They found that the healthcare costs of the patients who received IM, reduced costs by 10%, compared with those with conventional medicine, although there was no difference in mortality rate. This study showed that such IM models seems to save costs in patients with terminal illnesses. However, limitations of this study are lack of other clinical outcomes, and selection/intervention bias between the two groups. Participants with a CAM GP may be healthier than those with a GP also a CAM GP may give better care than a GP. Therefore, further studies are needed to confirm this finding and examine what elements of treatment with CAM GPs are related to decreased health cost. Finally, a survey recruited 67 patients with cancer (Lorenc et al., 2010). Healing techniques, i.e. Reiki, therapeutic touch and healing touch, integrated into conventional medicine was a common IM choice for patients with cancer in the UK. A self-referral system was used and the findings suggested that multidisciplinary health professionals in the UK seem to accept these treatments and perceived benefits.

Checklist for Reporting Research on Integrative Medicine

To promote robust reporting evidence of IM, Hu et al. (2015) proposed a checklist for standard reporting of clinical trials of integrative medicine as the Consolidated Standards of Reporting Trials (CONSORT) is not well suited for IM. This checklist guides how to conduct high quality IM research as well:

- **Title:** Identification of IM in the title
- **Background:**
    - Rationale of chosen interventions providing the potential optimum treatment for the target condition
    - Literature on both CAM and conventional medicine
        - Details of each intervention
        - Theoretical background in an IM regimen and/or each intervention
        - Existing evidence for the efficacy and safety of an IM regimen and/or each intervention
- **Study Design:**

- Explanation and justification of the appropriate study design and methodologies, e.g. pragmatic clinical trials
- Integrative methods of diagnosis
  - It may involve both conventional medicine tests and CAM theory
  - Use of any conventional medical or CAM diagnostic guidelines
- Details of all practitioners: licensing, education background, length of training
- Details of the IM model when a different intervention is provided by different practitioners
  - Interdisciplinary/multidisciplinary teamwork
  - Referral network
  - Methods of communication amongst practitioners
- Details of each intervention and the IM regimen
  - Regimen: number of treatment sessions, frequency and duration of treatment sessions, when and how each intervention was provided
  - When and how treatments were integrated
  - Any take home or self-care/lifestyle/family care or general advice
- Clinical setting
- Outcome measures addressing multiple dimensions, e.g. physical, mental, safety and economic conditions

- **Results:**
  - If used both quantitative and qualitative approaches, triangulation of the results
  - Any harm caused or interactions between/among interventions
  - Cost

However, this checklist does not detail how to report the discussion and the authors suggest that this checklist still requires further development. The authors of this chapter suggest that the CONSORT could be applied to reporting the discussion and research limitations, also how to generalise and interpretation of the findings.

PROSPECTIVE RESEARCH ON CAM METHODOLOGIES

Several biomedical researchers and practitioners criticise the poor quality of clinical trials in CAM, resulting in a scarcity of rigorous evidence of the effectiveness of CAM, and a lack of safety evidence (Choi et al., 2014; Li et al., 2014). As a result, conventional medicine practitioners suggest that their patients should not use CAM. Many CAM bodies and practitioners, particularly in Europe, established a novel approach to methodology in CAM research in order to build up scientific evidence on CAM. Fønnebø et al. (2007) proposed a new approach in CAM research called 'Reverse Research Strategies', which seems to be more relevant to the nature of CAM. It is a paradigm shift from conventional medicine to IM since no one can refuse patient preferences.

Research Strategies for CAM

In general, evaluating the efficacy and safety of conventional medicine is required by both pre-clinical studies, i.e. *in vitro* and *in vivo,* and in clinical trials before their use in clinical practice is approved. On the other hand, CAMs have been through a non-scientific process of trial and error before the scientific revolution, supported mainly by anecdotal evidence. The safety and efficacy of CAM now needs to be based on clinical practice evidence (Figure 1). In this reversed approach, traditional wisdom would inform which CAM is likely to work for which illness. Then, such CAM will be firstly tested for its safety, then its efficacy will be confirmed through clinical trials

Figure 1. Reverse research strategies adapted from Fønnebø et al. (2007)

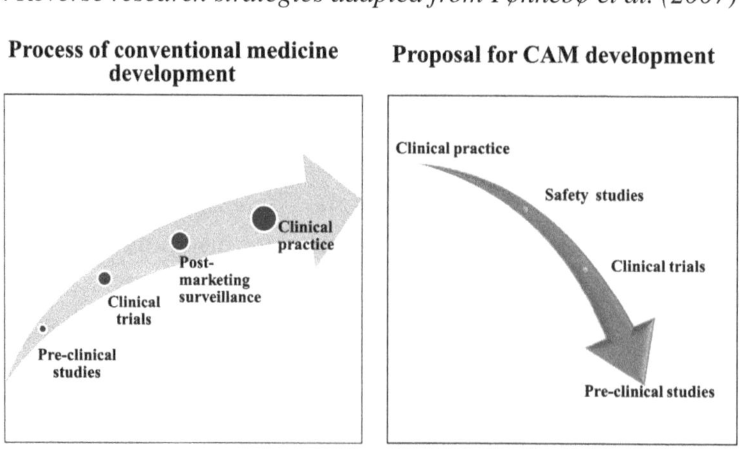

and pre-clinical studies, respectively (Fønnebø et al., 2007). If the process of CAM development, particularly herbal medicine, was similar to conventional medicine, it would be expensive and time consuming.

Randomised Controlled Trials in CAM

Known as randomised controlled trial (RCT), this methodology is a gold standard methodology to prove the efficacy and safety of both conventional and alternative medicines. Several systematic reviews report the poor quality of RCTs in CAM. As a result, the findings from these RCTs may lead to positive results bias and are less likely to convince conventional medicine practitioners to use CAM. The limitations of RCTs in CAM will be discussed and suggest guidelines of clinical trials of CAM that provide how to improve the quality of RCTs in CAM. Currently, we still need to improve both quality and quantity of RCTs in CAM.

Poor Quality of RCTs in CAM

Herbal medicine is the main CAM used for kidney diseases, so this section mainly focuses on studies of herbal medicine. The CONsolidated Standard of Reporting Trials (CONSORT) extension for herbal interventions was implemented in 2006 to improve the RCT methodology and scientific reports on herbal medicine. Since then, the quality of RCTs of herbal medicine has been slowly improving (Choi, et al., 2014). However, several systematic reviews report the poor quality of RCTs of herbal medicine when assessed using the CONSORT, particularly from Asian countries (Gagnier et al., 2006; Pratoomsoot et al., 2015). The major problems, as found by the reviews, were; (1) a lack of describing characteristics of herbal medicine treatment, e.g. amounts of active ingredients, the type or dosage of herbal preparation; (2) incomplete reporting of allocation concealment and type of analysis, e. g. an intention-to-treat analysis; and (3) poor accounting of adverse effects of herbal medicine. In addition, Li et al. (2014) assessed the quality of RCTs of traditional Chinese medicine published by China National Knowledge Infrastructure database from 2005 to 2012 and found the similar problems as Choi's study: limited reports on randomisation, blinding methods and adverse effects of traditional Chinese medicine (Li, et al., 2014). Therefore, further clinical trials of herbal medicine need to improve such issues and follow CONSORT and the Dalhousie Assessment Instrument for natural products, which standardise the description of the characteristics of herbal medicine (Jurgens et al., 2009). Details of these validated assessment tools have been described in Chapter 5.

As for RCTs on herbal medicine, reporting of RCTs of acupuncture has been slowly improving after implementing the STandards for Reporting Interventions in Clinical Trials of Acupuncture (STRICTA) (details of the STRICTA have been explained in Chapter 5) (Ma et al., 2016). This has mainly enhanced reports on randomisation (Kim et al., 2014). The missing items in the incomplete reporting of RCTs on acupuncture are similar to the ones in reporting RCTs on herbal medicine described above. Many of the studies lack an outcome definition, sample size calculation or the flow diagram of participants (Kim, et al., 2014). Further studies of acupuncture should address such issues.

In summary, testing the efficacy and safety of some types of herbal medicine and acupuncture may benefit from the use of RCT methodology, so researchers should follow recommendations from CONSORT and STRICTA in order to build up rigorous scientific evidence in this field. However, many CAM researchers have argued that RCTs are less likely to fit several CAM and IM modalities that are more complex. Several new approaches to study design of a complex interventions have been proposed, i.e. pragmatic clinical trials, cohort multiple randomised controlled trials, and mixed method studies.

Limitations of RCTs in CAMs and Guidelines for Clinical Trials of CAM

An explanatory RCT has intrinsic limitations such as generalisation or transferability, and may not suit some CAMs. For instance, findings from RCTs that focus on a specific study sample are likely to not be applicable to other populations, who differ from participants in the studies, and therefore have poor external validity. Moreover, the intervention in a RCTs needs to be explicit and standardised (Table 2). Meanwhile, CAM interventions are more complex, e.g. acupuncture, Ayurveda and meditation, and are likely to integrate usual practice. It is difficult to find an appropriate placebo. Clinical outcomes of RCTs of conventional medicine are mainly measured by biological markers or quantitative data, whilst health outcomes in a CAM therapy seem to be investigated via Patient Reported Outcome Measures (PROM), such as quality of life scales or patient satisfaction. Therefore, CAM or IM research that aims to prove their effectiveness in practice seems to suit pragmatic clinical trials (PCTs) rather than RCTs (Fischer et al., 2012). The PCTs can offer broader generalisation (or higher external validity) and are a more simple design than RCTs. However, PCTs require a larger sample size and have limited applications in different settings (Zwarenstein et al., 2008). For example, the effectiveness of an intervention in European countries may not translate to Asian countries on account of different health care systems and practitioner backgrounds.

Chinese herbal medicine (CHM) has its own characteristics, which differ from other CAMs. For example, after diagnosing, practitioners are likely to prescribe a specific remedy that may contain many mixed ingredients. Decoctions are the main dosage form of CHM and the process of preparing decoctions may produce new active ingredients which may provide synergistic effects. CHM has a distinctive smell and taste, so it is difficult to disguise the medicine or prepare a matching placebo. Another key issue of CHM is that even when patients are diagnosed with a same condition, they will not be prescribed exactly the same remedy with the same ingredients. Traditional Chinese Medicine (TCM) philosophy employs a concept of personalised medicine. Thus, physicians commonly adjust the ingredients and a dosage regimen, based on individual conditions. The unique characteristics of the intervention may result in a lack of standardisation due to each intervention being based on a particular condition in an individual patient. Due to these

Table 2. Key differences between explanatory and pragmatic trials adapted from the CONSORT extension for Pragmatic Trials (2009)

Key Feature	Explanatory Trial	Pragmatic Trial
1. Objective of a study	Investigate the efficacy of intervention	Ascertain effectiveness of intervention in normal practice
2. Participants	Highly selected Participants may not relevant to patients in the real world	Less likely to select Participants are quite similar to patients in clinical practice
3. Intervention	Standardised intervention	Treatment in normal practice A combination of interventions
4. Control group	Placebo	Best care Usual care No care
5. Biases	Minimised confounding factors	More likely to have confounding factors than RCTs
6. Outcomes	Biological/Specific effects	Patient and practitioners' perspective: Health outcomes, e. g. quality of life
7. Generalisation	Limited external validity	Improved external validity

issues, Flower et al. (2014) proposed guidelines for RCTs investigating CHM. The guidelines provide pragmatic options for the type of research on CHM, how to describe the details of the interventions, which include both standardised CHM and TCM, defining best practice of CHM, how to deal with a placebo, and outcomes.

Fischer et al. (2012) systematically reviewed RCTs of CAM and found some methodological problems in CAM research. They proposed recommendations on how to standardise CAM, assess specific and non-specific outcomes, choose a proper control group (s), report the randomisation procedure, and achieve double-blinding. Recommendations for CAM research shown in Table 3 have been also suggested by the CONSORT extension for Pragmatic trials (2008), Power and Hopayian (2011), Relton (2013) and the CAMbrella project (Fischer et al., 2014; Power & Hoyayian, 2011; Relton, 2013). Such recommendations could be applied to IM research as well. Regarding study populations choices, it is acknowledged that CAM research often focuses on a metropolitan population, even if rural area inhabitants are more likely

Table 3. Proposal for pragmatic clinical trials in CAM

Methodological Problem	Proposal for CAM research	Potential Bias	Recommendation
1. Double-blinding	Open-labelled trials	Cognitive measurement biases	▪ Blinding an assessor if blinding of participants and practitioners may be impossible ▪ Measure objective data ▪ New approach of trials: Cohort multiple randomised controlled trial
2. Randomisation	Preference trial	Selection bias	▪ Control similar baseline characteristics between an intervention and control groups ▪ New approach of trials: Cohort multiple randomised controlled trial
3. Standardised intervention	Semi-standardised intervention	Performance bias	▪ Semi-standardised intervention ▪ Develop a protocol of CAM/IM intervention
4. Outcomes	Measure overall outcomes	Cognitive measurement biases	▪ Clarify primary and secondary outcomes ▪ Using validated tools to measure subjective data ▪ Measure objective data if applicable ▪ Distinguish between true placebo effects and cognitive measurement biases
5. A control group	Active control		Clarify non-specific outcomes (a control effect) and true placebo effects (may be a CAM effect)

to use CAM. A research group from Australia, explored rural communities' attitudes towards CAM. The researchers identified gaps to be addressed: the use, practice and decision making processes around CAM among rural patients and practitioners; the environmental and social transformation impact on CAM use; the professional role of rural CAM professionals in terms of privacy and boundaries; the interaction between conventional and CAM practitioners, since the former healthcare dimension is highly regarded and powerful; and the evaluation and comparison with experiences and behaviour in other countries (Wardle et al., 2012).

Double-Blinding and Randomisation

On the blinding issue, some CAM researchers suggest designing an open-labelled pragmatic clinical trial (PCT) as participants in CAM research prefer to receive treatment rather than a placebo. When they are informed that they may receive a placebo, they may withdraw from the study. This leads to attrition bias and failure to complete recruitment. Additionally, they may be disappointed with the control treatment that may influence participants to report negative effects. Meanwhile, participants who know that they will receive a CAM therapy, may report positive effects of CAM. Therefore, open-labelled PCTs may cause cognitive measurement biases, which are 'errors of attribution, recollection or reporting that leads to systematic errors in outcome measurements.' (Power & Hoyayian, 2011). The use of objective outcome measures may reduce this bias. It is important to keep in mind that objective data on health outcomes in some CAMs may not be possible, such as with mood disorders where the outcomes are mostly always self-report.

Relton (2013) proposed a new approach that is 'cohort multiple randomised controlled trial' design (cmRCT), which could avoid the disadvantages of PCTs. Key points of cmRCTs are: (1) recruiting a large observational cohort of patients with the condition of interest; (2) regularly measuring health outcomes over a long period; (3) conducting multiple RCTs over a period of time; and (4) identifying all eligible patients for all RCTs; (5) participants being randomly selected from all eligible patients in the cohort, and then given the intervention of the study. Regarding the comparison of the outcomes of a study, (6) the results of the intervention group are compared to those receiving the control in the same cohort. The final key point is (7) 'patient centred' informed consent. Informed consent will be collected from each group of participants separately. Patients receiving the control will not be told about the treatment intervention and vice versa. This could prevent the control group feeling disappointment. The first feature of cmRCTs allows a high number of eligible patients to be recruited. In addition, eligible patients who prefer intervention will enter the treatment group. Likewise, all eligible patients who prefer usual care will be randomly selected as a control group. This design could diminish the failure of recruitment in CAM.

Standardised Intervention

An intervention in RCTs needs to be standardised in order to provide a similar effect for each participant. Most CAM interventions are more complex than conventional medicine. Professionals also have their own specific technique, so is less feasible to be standardised. In the case of having to standardise CAM, it may be difficult to generalise to other populations due to the effectiveness of some interventions based on the experience of practitioners. This is because most CAMs are considered individualised therapy. Fischer et al. (2012) suggest using semi-standardised treatment regimens. Further studies are still required to develop and validate a protocol of the semi-standardised intervention of CAM or IM. The authors suggest that the validation process should be performed only on key features of CAM practice, which mainly influence the effectiveness of the intervention. For example, aromatherapy combined with massage seems to have an effect on relieving itching in patients with end-stage renal disease. The key feature of such intervention is massage, so researchers should standardise massage technique, rather than the standardising of the aromatic oil.

Assessment of Specific and Overall Outcomes

Some CAM interventions are integrated with more than one therapy. Expected outcomes are likely to result from a mixture of features of CAM interventions, such as the presence of an experienced practitioner, specific settings, particular diagnostic systems of CAM and the patient-practitioner relationship. CAM/IM interventions are, therefore, appropriate for evaluating a humanistic outcome as a whole rather than a specific outcome. CAM/IM research also should measure an overall outcome as described below (Fischer, et al., 2012). However, researchers should be concerned about measuring non-specific outcomes as a placebo sometimes may contribute to such outcomes, which may be called a true placebo effect. Therefore, Power and Hopayian (2011) suggest that CAM research should be able to differentiate between a true placebo effect and a non-specific outcome where appropriate. They also criticised that such suggestions are likely to increase cognitive measurement bias in the case of measuring subjective data as an outcome. It is a challenge in CAM research to distinguish between true placebo effects and cognitive measurement biases. To minimise the cognitive bias, an overall outcome for CAM/IM modalities needs to be well defined and should be measured by validated tools. For example, using the short form 36 health survey (SF-36) to measure the quality of life (Ware et al., 1992). Symptom relief after using CAM can be evaluated by the Measure Yourself Medical Outcome Profile (MYMOP) (Paterson, 1996). Other examples of validated questionnaires to measure the quality of life and symptoms in patients with kidney disease are shown in Chapter 4.

A systematic review evaluating patients' questionnaires for use in IM reported that available questionnaires, e.g. the MYMOP-2 (Polus et al., 2011), the Arizona Integrative Outcomes (Bell et al., 2004), the Complementary and Integrative Medicine Outcome Scale (CIMOS) (Eton et al., 2005) and SF-36, need to be tested for their validity and reliability of measuring IM outcomes (Hunter et al., 2013). If the available questionnaires cannot detect an overall health outcome of CAM or IM appropriately, there are greater demands on defining a new overall outcome and a mixed-methods study has been recommended for defining and validating the new outcome (Fischer, et al., 2012).

A Choice of Proper Control Group (s)

CAM researchers find it difficult to provide and allocate a placebo when evaluating complex intervention. It is also less easy to blind in CAM/IM studies, when compared to conventional medicine, so participants may know that they are receiving a placebo. This would influence the study outcome, particularly if measuring subjective data as the outcome. Active control groups or usual care could be an optimal choice in CAM/IM research. For instance, an RCT of acupuncture could use a different technique of acupuncture in a control group that is less likely to affect an overall outcome. This would be more appropriate than a real placebo, i.e. needling a sham point because needling may cause false negative results (Paterson & Dieppe, 2005).

Mixed Methods in CAM

Mixed methods is a combination of quantitative and qualitative methods. A qualitative component could complement a clinical trial for example. The qualitative study alongside a trial aims to better understand the effects of interventions and how they are experienced by patients (Lewin, et al., 2009). Bishop and Holmes (2013) systematically reviewed mixed methods studies in CAM research and frequently found limited reporting of the qualitative section, i.e. unclear sampling methods and participation rates, and low methodological quality when compared with the quantitative component. To improve the value of a mixed methods study, further mixed methods studies should be better performed and described. It is also necessary to explain why the researchers chose a mixed method design and provide the limitations of the study. The qualitative study needs to clearly discuss the researchers' impact on the outcomes and the broader context of the findings and transparently report data analysis methods (Bishop & Holmes, 2013). Interpretation of the findings from the qualitative component should explain how they add to the results from the quantitative component. Wishing to reach a deeper understanding of the patients' experiences, the CAM researcher can adopt social science methodologies such as interview analysis, diary analysis or focus groups (Broom & Adams, 2007). In-depth interviews, diaries and focus group analysis examine patients' lived experience, but, while interviews and focus groups provide a snapshot of the situation, diary analysis gives insight on the whole process. Since diseases and treatments evolve overtime, a diary is a powerful tool to follow the patients' experience embedded in their social context.

Two other social science methods, i.e. Action research and the Delphi process, can be useful in IM and CAM research. Action research is used with the aim of problem solving. The study is carried out in the course of action in order to improve the intervention. According to the process, the results are directly fed back to the researcher in order for him/her to take action and change the intervention. This type of research is therefore participatory, democratic and contributes to change (Broom & Adams, 2007). The Delphi process is a consensus technique involving experts and patients in the field. The collective judgment of specialists provide better understanding of the researched topic, and their final decision is used to create guidelines (Broom & Adams, 2007).The process goes through rounds of enquiries and feedback until a consensus has been made.

Example of Study Design for Research on IM

Designing a study for IM research is more difficulty than for CAM research because of issues like semi-standardised IM modalities and difficulties in double-blinding. Herman et al. (2014) designed a protocol for evaluating clinical and cost outcomes of an IM model in primary care in the US. A mixed methods design was used and outcomes were measured before and after the implementation of the IM service. The first phase of this study designed the IM model. Afterwards, a comparative effectiveness of the model was conducted. An intervention group received the IM, which was a collaboration between conventional physicians and CAM practitioners. This was compared with two matched control groups who received usual care. The qualitative component explored the effect of the IM model. Several outcomes were measured with validated self-assessment questionnaires of symptom relief (pain, fatigue, depression and anxiety), quality of life and well-being, e.g. the Perceived Stress Scale and the 9-item Pittsburgh Sleep Quality Index (Buysse et al., 1989), the 12-Item Short Form Medical Outcomes Survey (SF-12) (Ware et al., 1996) and the 5-item World Health Organization Well-Being Index (WHO-5) (Bech et al., 2003).

This protocol reflects the nature of research on IM. The authors designed the study to minimise as much bias as possible, despite the lack of a standardised protocol for the intervention, double-blinding or randomisation. Several outcomes were measured in order to assess patients as a whole, which is related to the concept of IM. Unfortunately, an example of IM research on kidney disease was not found.

Guidelines for Safety Studies of CAM

There are often poorly reported adverse effects of CAM in RCTs as assessed by the CONSORT extension for harms (Turner et al., 2011). The CAM methods which have poor reporting of these are; herbal medicine, dietary supplements, acupuncture or chiropractic. To improve recording of safety issues of CAM, the CAMbrella project suggests that researchers should routinely report common adverse effects of CAM and clarify the definition of safety in CAM where appropriate. They also should be encouraged to report serious adverse effects even if only a single case was found (Fischer, et al., 2014). Observational studies, clinical studies, and case studies have been recommended in order to identify the adverse effects of CAM. Moreover, the CONSORT extension for harms should be used when reporting CAM adverse effects in RCTs (Loannidis et al., 2004) (Table 4).

Table 4. The quality of reporting adverse effects of CAM in RCTs based on the CONSORT extension for harms (2004)

Item	Description
Title and abstract	1. Title and abstract should state both harms and benefits if the study collects data on both.
Introduction	2. The introduction should state harms as well as benefits if the study aims to investigate both.
Method	3. Expected and unexpected adverse effects should be defined.
	4. Method of collecting data on harms should be clarified, e.g. passive, active, mode of data collection, and timing.
	5. Describe plans for presenting and analysing information on harms.
Results	6. Describe for each arm the participant withdrawals that are due to harms and the experience with the allocated treatment.
	7. Provide the denominators for analyses in harms.
	8. Present the absolute risk of each adverse event.
	9. Describe any subgroup analyses and exploratory analyses for harms.
Discussion	10. Provide a balanced discussion of benefits and harms with emphasis on study limitations, generalisation, and other sources of information on harms.

Harm Research in Kidney Diseases

Conventional practitioners are concerned about the safety of CAM in patients with renal insufficiency due to limited evidence, particularly with herbal medicine. The first research priority in this field is the safe use of CAM, e.g. herbal medicine, followed by efficacy. Some CAMs may not have a major benefit compared to conventional medicine, but may improve the quality of life in these patients. If such a CAM is safe and patients prefer to use it, it is possible to allow the patient to do so. Regarding nephropathy due to CAM, single case reports and observational studies, i.e. case-control and cohort studies, and post-marketing surveillance, are required to provide evidence. Such research should focus on acute kidney injury related to herbal and dietary supplements (HDS) as there is a major risk of this (Tangkiatkumjai et al., 2015). Kidney stones caused by HDS should be also explored. Several HDS may cause hyperphosphatemia and hyperkalemia in patients with advanced chronic kidney disease, so herbal products should be further investigated for these issues as well. There is underreporting of nephropathy from HDS due to several barriers among practitioners, i.e. lack of knowledge regarding where to report, how to report, and limited time. These issues should also be addressed.

International, Regional and National Organisations of CAM Research

CAM researchers in several regions have collaborated and built up an international or regional organisation of CAM research. These networks aim to promote CAM research, foster researchers in CAM, build up robust evidence for CAM, and provide archives of CAM information. The International Society for Complementary Medicine Research (ISCMR) was launched in 2008. It collaborates with researchers and practitioners in Asia, Canada and Europe. This organisation holds a conference every year in order to disseminate CAM knowledge, train new researchers and communicate with researchers worldwide (www.iscmr.org [last accessed 29/03/17]).

CAMbrella is a CAM research network in Europe which was launched in 2010. It aimed to assess the situation of CAM in Europe between 2010-2012 and found that the overall aim of EU CAM researchers was to strengthen the CAM research infrastructure such as improving the sources of independent funding, and supporting European research coordination (Fischer, et al., 2014). The research group of CAMbrella identified 6 clinical and epidemiological key areas for CAM research (www.cambrella.eu [last accessed 29/03/17]):

- CAM prevalence in the EU.
- Needs and attitudes of citizens and professionals.
- Information about safety and the risk benefit ratio of CAM.
- Comparative effectiveness research and pragmatic clinical trials including health economic evaluations.
- Understanding to what extent the clinical effects of CAM (and conventional medicine) are due to meaning value and context.
- Different CAM integration models such as "opposition", "integration" and "pluralism".

National organisations of CAM research in Australia, the US and Canada were established prior to these international networks. The Australasian Integrative Medicine Association was established in 1992 www.aima.net.au [last accessed 28/08/16]). In 1998, the National Center for Complementary and Integrative Health in the US was set up (www.nccih.nih.gov [last accessed 28/08/16]), and in 2004 the Interdisciplinary Network of Complementary and Alternative Medicine was launched (www.incamresearch.ca [last accessed 28/08/16]). These three networks have collaborate with each other.

CONCLUSION

Integrative medicine is likely to be suitable for illnesses failed by either conventional or alternative medicine therapies, e.g. cancer, kidney disease, etc., and patients who suffer from serious adverse effects from conventional medicine. This approach aims to provide the advantages of both systems and diminish disadvantages. The possibly successful model of IM in many countries is due to the collaboration between conventional and CAM practitioners. However, if this model is inappropriate, qualitative methods have been suggested in order to design new IM models. There is a scarcity of IM research. Although the RCT design is a gold standard for inference of causality between treatments and effects, it does not suit IM research due to a lack of suitable placebos, difficulties in double blinding, randomization, standardising interventions, and suitable objective outcomes. Alternatively, a PCT seems to be more suitable for assessing the treatment outcomes of CAM, as it simulates the actual practice in terms of patient's characteristics and CAM modalities. Additionally, cohort multiple randomised controlled trials have been suggested as a choice of CAM research. Mixed-methods design may also be appropriate.

REFERENCES

Baars, E. W., & Kooreman, P. (2014). A 6-year comparative economic evaluation of healthcare costs and mortality rates of Dutch patients from conventional and CAM GPs. *BMJ Open*, *4*(8), e005332. doi:10.1136/bmjopen-2014-005332 PMID:25164536

Bech, P., Olsen, L. R., Kjoller, M., & Rasmussen, N. K. (2003). Measuring well-being rather than the absence of distress symptoms: A comparison of the SF-36 Mental Health subscale and the WHO-Five well-being scale. *International Journal of Methods in Psychiatric Research*, *12*(2), 85–91. doi:10.1002/mpr.145 PMID:12830302

Bell, I. R., Cunningham, V., Caspi, O., Meek, P., & Ferro, L. (2004). Development and validation of a new global well-being outcomes rating scale for integrative medicine research. *BMC Complementary and Alternative Medicine*, *4*(1), 1. doi:10.1186/1472-6882-4-1 PMID:14725717

Bishop, F. L., & Holmes, M. M. (2013). Mixed methods in CAM research: a systematic review of studies published in 2012. *Evid Based Complement Alternat Med, 2013*, ID 187365.

Broom, A., & Adams, J. (2007). Current issues and future directions in complementary and alternative medicine (CAM) research. *Complementary Therapies in Medicine*, *15*(3), 217–220. doi:10.1016/j.ctim.2006.08.001 PMID:17709067

Buysse, D. J., Reynolds, C. F. III, Monk, T. H., Berman, S. R., & Kupfer, D. J. (1989). The Pittsburgh Sleep Quality Index: A new instrument for psychiatric practice and research. *Psychiatry Research*, *28*(2), 193–213. doi:10.1016/0165-1781(89)90047-4 PMID:2748771

Choi, J., Jun, J. H., Kang, B. K., Kim, K. H., & Lee, M. S. (2014). Endorsement for improving the quality of reports on randomized controlled trials of traditional medicine journals in Korea: A systematic review. *Trials*, *15*(1), 429. doi:10.1186/1745-6215-15-429 PMID:25373427

Dobos, G., & Tao, I. (2011). The model of Western integrative medicine: The role of Chinese medicine. *Chinese Journal of Integrative Medicine*, *17*(1), 11–20. doi:10.1007/s11655-011-0601-x PMID:21258891

Eton, D. T., Koffler, K., Cella, D., Eisenstein, A., Astin, J. A., Pelletier, K. R., & Riley, D. (2005). Developing a self-report outcome measure for complementary and alternative medicine. *Explore (New York, N.Y.)*, *1*(3), 177–185. doi:10.1016/j.explore.2005.02.007 PMID:16781527

Fischer, F. H., Lewith, G., Witt, C. M., Linde, K., von Ammon, K., Cardini, F., & Brinkhaus, B. et al. (2014). High prevalence but limited evidence in complementary and alternative medicine: Guidelines for future research. *BMC Complementary and Alternative Medicine*, *14*(1), 46. doi:10.1186/1472-6882-14-46 PMID:24499316

Fischer, H. F., Junne, F., Witt, C., von Ammon, K., Cardini, F., Fønnebø, V., & Brinkhaus, B. et al. (2012). Key issues in clinical and epidemiological research in complementary and alternative medicine - a systematic literature review. *Forschende Komplementarmedizin*, *19*(s2), 51–60. doi:10.1159/000343126 PMID:23883945

Flower, A., Witt, C., Liu, J., Ulrich-Merzenich, G., Muir, K., & Yu, H. (2014). GP-TCM unabridged guidelines for randomised controlled trials investigating Chinese herbal medicine (CHM). *European Journal of Internal Medicine*, *6*(2), 186–210.

Fønnebø, V., Grimsgaard, S., Walach, H., Ritenbaugh, C., Norheim, A. J., & MacPherson, H. et al.. (2007). Researching complementary and alternative treatments-the gatekeepers are not at home. *BMC Complementary and Alternative Medicine*, *7*(7).

Gagnier, J. J., DeMelo, J., Boon, H., Rochon, P., & Bombardier, C. (2006). Quality of reporting of randomized controlled trials of herbal medicine interventions. *The American Journal of Medicine*, *119*(9), 800.e801–800.e811. doi:10.1016/j.amjmed.2006.02.006 PMID:16945616

Grant, S. J., Frawley, J., & Bensoussan, A. (2015). Process of care in outpatient integrative healthcare facilities: A systematic review of clinical trials. *BMC Health Services Research*, *15*(1), 322. doi:10.1186/s12913-015-0976-z PMID:26264852

Gray, B., & Orrock, P. (2014). Investigation into factors influencing roles, relationships, and referrals in integrative medicine. *Journal of Alternative and Complementary Medicine (New York, N.Y.)*, *20*(5), 342–346. doi:10.1089/acm.2013.0167 PMID:24437357

Herman, P. M., Dodds, S. E., Logue, M. D., Abraham, I., Rehfeld, R. A., Grizzle, A. J., & Maizes, V. H. et al. (2014). IMPACT - Integrative Medicine PrimAry Care Trial: Protocol for a comparative effectiveness study of the clinical and cost outcomes of an integrative primary care clinic model. *BMC Complementary and Alternative Medicine*, *14*(1), 132. doi:10.1186/1472-6882-14-132 PMID:24708726

Horrigan, B., Lewis, S., Abrams, D., & Pechura, C. (2012). Integrative medicine in America: How integrative medicine is being practiced in Clinical centers across the United States. *Glob Adv Health Med*, *1*(3), 18–94. doi:10.7453/gahmj.2012.1.3.006

Hu, X. Y., Chen, N. N., Chai, Q. Y., Yang, G. Y., Trevelyan, E., Lorenc, A., & Robinson, N. et al. (2015). Integrative treatment for low back pain: An exploratory systematic review and meta-analysis of randomized controlled trials. *Chinese Journal of Integrative Medicine*. doi:10.1007/s11655-015-2125-2 PMID:26501693

Hu, X. Y., Lorenc, A., Kemper, K., Liu, J. P., Adams, J., & Robinson, N. (2015). Defining integrative medicine in narrative and systematic reviews: A suggested checklist for reporting. *European Journal of Internal Medicine*, *7*, 76–84.

Hunter, J., & Leeder, S. (2013). Patient questionnaires for use in the integrative medicine primary care setting - a systematic literature review. *European Journal of Internal Medicine*, *5*(3), 194–216.

Jurgens, T., Whelan, A. M., MacDonald, M., & Lord, L. (2009). Development and evaluation of an instrument for the critical appraisal of randomized controlled trials of natural products. *BMC Complementary and Alternative Medicine*, *9*(11). PMID:19389240

Khorsan, R., Coulter, I. D., Crawford, C., & Hsiao, A. F. (2011). Systematic review of integrative health care research: randomized control trials, clinical controlled trials, and meta-analysis. *Evid Based Complement Alternat Med, 2011*, ID 636134.

Kim, K. H., Won, K. J., Lee, M. S., & Lee, J. D. (2014). Assessment of the quality of reporting in randomised controlled trials of acupuncture in the Korean literature using the CONSORT statement and STRICTA guidelines. *BMJ Open*, *4*(7), e005068. doi:10.1136/bmjopen-2014-005068 PMID:25079926

Lewin, S., Glenton, C., & Oxman, A. D. (2009). Use of qualitative methods alongside randomised controlled trials of complex healthcare interventions: Methodological study. *BMJ (Clinical Research Ed.)*, *339*(sep10 1), b3496. doi:10.1136/bmj.b3496 PMID:19744976

Li, J., Liu, Z., Chen, R., Hu, D., Li, W., Li, X., & Liao, L. et al. (2014). The quality of reports of randomized clinical trials on traditional Chinese medicine treatments: A systematic review of artices indexed in the China National Knowledge Infrastructure database from 2005 to 2012. *BMC Complementary and Alternative Medicine*, *14*(1), 362. doi:10.1186/1472-6882-14-362 PMID:25256890

Loannidis, J. P., Evans, S. J., Gotzsche, P. C., ONeill, R. T., Altman, D. G., & Schulz, K. et al.. (2004). Better reporting of harms in randomized trials: An extension of the CONSORT statement. *Annals of Internal Medicine*, *141*(10), 781–788. doi:10.7326/0003-4819-141-10-200411160-00009 PMID:15545678

Lorenc, A., Peace, B., Vaghela, C., & Robinson, N. (2010). The integration of healing into conventional cancer care in the UK. *Complementary Therapies in Clinical Practice, 16*(4), 222–228. doi:10.1016/j.ctcp.2010.03.001 PMID:20920808

Ma, B., Chen, Z. M., Xu, J. K., Wang, Y. N., Chen, K. Y., Ke, F. Y., & Wang, Y. et al. (2016). Do the CONSORT and STRICTA checklists improve the reporting quality of acupuncture and moxibustion randomized controlled trials published in Chinese journals? a systematic review and analysis of trends. *PLoS ONE, 11*(1), e0147244. doi:10.1371/journal.pone.0147244 PMID:26808550

Park, S. U., Cho, S. Y., Park, J. M., Ko, C. N., Park, H. J., & Walls, B. L. et al.. (2014). Integrative treatment modalities for stroke victims in Korea. *Complementary Therapies in Clinical Practice, 20*(1), 37–41. doi:10.1016/j.ctcp.2013.10.007 PMID:24439643

Paterson, C. (1996). Measuring outcomes in primary care: A patient generated measure, MYMOP, compared with the SF-36 health survey. *BMJ (Clinical Research Ed.), 312*(7037), 1016–1020. doi:10.1136/bmj.312.7037.1016 PMID:8616351

Paterson, C., & Dieppe, P. (2005). Characteristic and incidental (placebo) effects in complex interventions such as acupuncture. *BMJ (Clinical Research Ed.), 330*(7501), 1202–1205. doi:10.1136/bmj.330.7501.1202 PMID:15905259

Patwardhan, B., & Mutalik, G. (2014). Search of novel model for integrative medicine. *Chinese Journal of Integrative Medicine, 20*(3), 170–178. doi:10.1007/s11655-014-1745-2 PMID:24615209

Polus, B. I., Kimpton, A. J., & Walsh, M. J. (2011). Use of the measure your medical outcome profile (MYMOP2) and W-BQ12 (Well-Being) outcomes measures to evaluate chiropractic treatment: An observational study. *Chiropr Man Therap, 19*(1), 7. doi:10.1186/2045-709X-19-7 PMID:21418608

Power, M., & Hopayian, K. (2011). Exposing the evidence gap for complementary and alternative medicine to be integrated into science-based medicine. *Journal of the Royal Society of Medicine, 104*(4), 155–161. doi:10.1258/jrsm.2011.100271 PMID:21502214

Pratoomsoot, C., Sruamsiri, R., Dilokthornsakul, P., & Chaiyakunapruk, N. (2015). Quality of reporting of randomised controlled trials of herbal interventions in ASEAN plus six countries: A systematic review. *PLoS ONE*, *10*(1), e108681. doi:10.1371/journal.pone.0108681 PMID:25633206

Relton, C. (2013). Implications of the placebo effect for CAM research. *Complementary Therapies in Medicine*, *21*(2), 121–124. doi:10.1016/j.ctim.2012.12.011 PMID:23497816

Relton, C., Torgerson, D., OCathain, A., & Nicholl, J. (2010). Rethinking pragmatic randomised controlled trials: Introducing the cohort multiple randomised controlled trial design. *BMJ (Clinical Research Ed.)*, *340*(mar19 1), c1066. doi:10.1136/bmj.c1066 PMID:20304934

Romeyke, T., & Stummer, H. (2015). Evidence-based complementary and alternative medicine in inpatient care: Take a look at Europe. *J Evid Based Complementary Altern Med*, *20*(2), 87–93. doi:10.1177/2156587214555714 PMID:25404750

Skovgaard, L., Bjerre, L., Haahr, N., Paterson, C., Launsø, L., Boesen, F., & Søndermark, K. et al. (2012). An investigation of multidisciplinary complex health care interventions - steps towards an integrative treatment model in the rehabilitation of people with multiple sclerosis. *BMC Complementary and Alternative Medicine*, *12*(1), 50. doi:10.1186/1472-6882-12-50 PMID:22524586

Sundberg, T., Halpin, J., Warenmark, A., & Falkenberg, T. (2007). Towards a model for integrative medicine in Swedish primary care. *BMC Health Services Research*, *7*(1), 107. doi:10.1186/1472-6963-7-107 PMID:17623105

Sundberg, T., Hok, J., Finer, D., Arman, M., Swartz, J., & Falkenberg, T. (2014). Evidence-informed integrative care systems - The way forward. *European Journal of Internal Medicine*, *6*, 12–20.

Tangkiatkumjai, M., Boardman, H., Praditpornsilpa, K., & Walker, D.-M. (2014). Reasons why Thai patients with chronic kidney disease use or do not use herbal and dietary supplements. *BMC Complementary and Alternative Medicine*, *14*(1), 473. doi:10.1186/1472-6882-14-473 PMID:25481733

Tangkiatkumjai, M., Boardman, H., Praditpornsilpa, K., & Walker, D.-M. (2015). Association of herbal and dietary supplements with progression and complications of chronic kidney disease: A prospective cohort study. *Nephrology (Carlton, Vic.)*, *20*(10), 679–687. doi:10.1111/nep.12531 PMID:26040915

Templeman, K., & Robinson, A. (2011). Integrative medicine models in contemporary primary health care. *Complementary Therapies in Medicine*, *19*(2), 84–92. doi:10.1016/j.ctim.2011.02.003 PMID:21549259

Turner, L. A., Singh, K., Garritty, C., Tsertsvadze, A., Manheimer, E., Wieland, L. S., & Moher, D. et al. (2011). An Evaluation of the completeness of safety reporting in reports of complementary and alternative medicine trials. *BMC Complementary and Alternative Medicine*, *11*(1), 67. doi:10.1186/1472-6882-11-67 PMID:21859470

Walach, H. (2010). Complementary or integrative - ideas and notions. *Forschende Komplementarmedizin*, *17*(4), 215–220. doi:10.1159/000317639 PMID:20848756

Wardle, J., Lui, C. W., & Adams, J. (2012). Complementary and alternative medicine in rural communities: Current research and future directions. *The Journal of Rural Health*, *28*(1), 101–112. doi:10.1111/j.1748-0361.2010.00348.x PMID:22236320

Ware, J. E. Jr, Kosinski, M., & Keller, S. D. (1996). A 12-Item short-form health survey: Construction of scales and preliminary tests of reliabity and validity. *Medical Care*, *34*(3), 220–233. doi:10.1097/00005650-199603000-00003 PMID:8628042

Ware, J. E. Jr, & Sherbourne, C. D. (1992). The MOS 36-item short-form helth survey (SF-36). I. Conceptual framework and item selection. *Medical Care*, *30*(6), 473–483. doi:10.1097/00005650-199206000-00002 PMID:1593914

World Health Organization. (2013). WHO traditional medicine strategy: 2014-2023. Geneva: WHO.

Zwarenstein, M., Treweek, S., Gagnier, J. J., Altman, D. G., Tunis, S., Haynes, B., & Moher, D. et al. (2008). Improving the reporting of pragmatic trials: An extension of the CONSORT statement. *BMJ (Clinical Research Ed.)*, *11*(337), a2390. doi:10.1136/bmj.a2390 PMID:19001484

KEY TERMS AND DEFINITIONS

Intervention: The treatment is given by practitioners. It includes one type of complementary and alternative medicine or integration of both conventional and alternative medicine.

Integrative Medicine: The treatment comprises of both conventional and alternative medicine.

Mixed-Methods: A research method consists of both quantitative and qualitative methods.

Model of Integrative Medicine: A pattern of the treatment provides a combination of both conventional and alternative medicine.

Outcome of Integrative Medicine: A result of the treatment consists of multiple results, e.g., physical health, mental health, spiritual outcome, and quality of life.

Patient-Centred Care: A care is focused on patient's needs.

Randomised Controlled Trial: A study in human is that participants are randomised in order to receive either an intervention or control groups.

About the Authors

Mayuree Tangkiatkumjai registered as a pharmacist in 2000 having graduated the previous year with a BSc in pharmacy from Chulalongkorn University in Thailand. She obtained MSc in clinical pharmacy from the same University and have worked as a lecturer in Faculty of Pharmacy, Srinakharinwirot University, Thailand since 2002. She has taught about clinical skills, pharmaceutical care in chronic kidney disease, herbal and drug safety. With the sponsorship from the Royal Thai Government, she pursued my PhD studies in University of Nottingham, the UK and obtained a PhD in 2014. Her research interests are the use of herbal and dietary supplements in patients with chronic illnesses, pharmacovigilance, adverse events of medicines and herbal medicines, particularly nephrotoxicity, and pharmaceutical care in chronic kidney disease.

Annalisa Casarin is a medical doctor, specialised in Anaesthesia, Critical Care and Pain Management with an interest in Complementary Medicine (Traditional Chinese Medicine and Acupuncture). She trained in Italy then worked as a Critical Care Clinical Fellow in Toronto (Canada), Cambridge (UK) and London (UK). After repatriating, she spent two and half years as a Pain Management Consultant in Italy using integrative medicine. In 2013 she returned to the UK as Research Fellow, she has been involved in the MoDUS RCT, the AWARE2 Trial, and a number of audits and observational trials. She appears in several peer reviewed publications. She is currently undertaking a part-time Masters in Public Health – Health Services Research at the University of Sheffield, UK, and works part-time for the NIHR Research Design Service, East of England, as a Research Adviser. Her main areas of interest are quantitative studies in Critical Care, Complementary Medicine and Health Services Research methodology.

Li-Chia Chen is a pharmacist trained in pharmacy practice research, specialising in evidence-based medicine, drug utilisation, pharmacoepidemiology, and health economics. She has a progressing and balanced professional and academic profile and an insightful scope of international teaching and research of pharmacy in higher education institutes. Dr Chen received foundation pharmacy qualification in Taiwan and trained in a prestigious Master Programme for clinical pharmacy, and soon escalated her career from a clinical pharmacist to Director of Pharmacy in hospitals. Sponsored by Taiwan Ministry of Education, she completed a PhD programme at the University of Manchester and then a post-doctoral research in the U.K., when she acquired expertise in the systematic review, meta-analysis, economic modelling and qualitative research. Thereafter, Dr Chen taught at a postgraduate programme in Taiwan as an Assistant Professor for all subjects of her expertise, and she also established skills in secondary healthcare database analysis. She took a lectureship at the University of Nottingham in 2010 and worked as a Senior Lecturer at the University of Manchester since 2017.

Dawn-Marie Walker is an Associate Professor at the University of Southampton where she teaches statistics. As a psychologist by background, she is particularly interested in placebo for healing, which is where her interest in complementary medicines stemmed from. She is an extremely well published academic writer with numerous journal papers, chapters, and has edited a book previously. Her research method of choice is mixed methods, but also has conducted and published a number of systematic reviews and meta-analyses.

* * *

Mymoona Akhter holds Ph.D. Pharmaceutical Sciences, M. Pharma in Pharmaceutical Chemistry from Jamia Hamdard (Hamdard University) New Delhi. Akhter is working as an Associate Professor of Medicinal Chemistry in School of Pharmaceutical Education and Research and is Deputy Co-ordinator of the Bioinformatics Facility Jamia Hamdard. Akhter has been bestowed with several honors like the SERB- fast track research project award for young scientists by Department of Science and Technology, Govt. of India (2012), the Career award for young Teachers by All India Council of Technical Education (2010), SERC Visiting Fellowship by DST (2005). She is supervising scientific research of the post-graduation and the doctoral level.

She has guided/under guidance about 18 theses of M. Pharm. and M.Tech Bioinformatics and 5 theses of Ph. D. She has presented his research work in 43 conferences held in India and abroad. She has a list of more than 50 manuscripts in journals and has co-authored a book on Practical Pharmaceutical Analytical Chemistry.

Chatchai Kreepala completed his MD degree (Doctor of Medicine) at Srinakharinwirot University in 2000, Diploma of Nephrology Mahidol University, Bangkok, Thailand in 2007, and obtained the Certification of Clinical/research fellow in renal transplantation from the University of Alberta, Edmonton, Alberta, Canada in 2013. He worked as a clinical instructor and lecturer at the Division of Nephrology, Department of Internal Medicine, Srinakharinwirot University in Thailand during 2008. He attended Dr. Halloran's laboratory training program during 2011. One of his studies focused on molecular expression acute kidney injury patients who received renal allografts. After the completion of his certification in transplantation, he moved back to the Srinakharinwirot University where he started working as the Head of Organ Donation and Transplantation Unit of HRH Princess MahaChakriSirindhorn Medical Center (MSMC). At MSMC, he has become a nephrology and transplantation specialist.

Win Winit-Watjana obtained his first degree in pharmacy from Chulalongkorn University in Bangkok, MSc in Clinical Pharmacy from Mahidol University and PhD in Pharmacy Practice from King's College London. After his graduation, he worked as a hospital pharmacist in Saraburi Province, Thailand. After that, he became a pharmacy academic with various positions in Thailand and abroad, i.e. Rangsit University (1991 – 1993), Chulalongkorn University (1993 – 2006), University of Sunderland in the UK (2006 – 2013), University of Dammam in Saudi Arabia (2013 – 2014) and University of Bahrain (2014 – 2015). He is currently an Associate Professor in Pharmacy Practice at International Medical University in Malaysia. His teaching and research interests are in the areas of international pharmacy practice, older people and medication use (gerontology and geriatric pharmacotherapy), and pharmacy education. Additionally, he is also interested in complementary and alternative medicine (CAM) that is a crucial part of health care nowadays. He has published some papers in international journals regarding the disclosure of CAM use by patients, perceived CAM efficacy and safety, and attitudes and perceptions of pharmacy students about CAM modalities.

Index

D

E

F

H

I

www.ingramcontent.com/pod-product-compliance
Lightning Source LLC
LaVergne TN
LVHW081334300926
849161LV00008B/1968
* 9 7 8 1 5 2 2 5 2 8 8 2 1 *